T0331078

Clinical Case Studies in Long-Term Care Psychiatry

Clinical Case Studies in Long-Term Care Psychiatry

Navigating Common Mental Health Challenges in Geriatric Care

Matthew Gibfried
Saint Louis University School of Medicine, Missouri

George T. Grossberg
Saint Louis University School of Medicine, Missouri

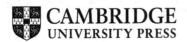

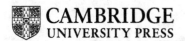

Shaftesbury Road, Cambridge CB2 8EA, United Kingdom

One Liberty Plaza, 20th Floor, New York, NY 10006, USA

477 Williamstown Road, Port Melbourne, VIC 3207, Australia

314–321, 3rd Floor, Plot 3, Splendor Forum, Jasola District Centre, New Delhi – 110025, India

103 Penang Road, #05–06/07, Visioncrest Commercial, Singapore 238467

Cambridge University Press is part of Cambridge University Press & Assessment,
a department of the University of Cambridge.

We share the University's mission to contribute to society through the pursuit of
education, learning and research at the highest international levels of excellence.

www.cambridge.org
Information on this title: www.cambridge.org/9781108722322

DOI: 10.1017/9781108630344

When citing this work, please include a reference to the
DOI 10.1017/9781108630344

First published 2025

A catalogue record for this publication is available from the British Library

Library of Congress Cataloging-in-Publication Data
Names: Gibfried, Matthew, author. | Grossberg, George T., author.
Title: Case studies in long-term care psychiatry : navigating common mental health challenges in geriatric care / Matthew
    Gibfried, George T. Grossberg.
Description: Cambridge ; New York, NY : Cambridge University Press, 2025. | Includes bibliographical references and index. |
    Summary: "A compilation of compelling real-life cases on the psychiatric care of older adults in the long-term care setting.
    Cases cover the various common psychiatric disorders alongside more complex cases on psychiatric multimorbidity and
    psychotropic polypharmacy. Essential reading for healthcare practitioners who work regularly with older adults"– Provided
    by publisher.
Identifiers: LCCN 2024020601 (print) | LCCN 2024020602 (ebook) | ISBN 9781108722322 (paperback) | ISBN 9781108630344
    (epub)
Subjects: MESH: Mental Disorders | Aged | Long-Term Care–methods | Geriatric Psychiatry–methods | Case Reports
Classification: LCC RC451.4.A5 (print) | LCC RC451.4.A5 (ebook) | NLM WT 150 | DDC 618.97/689–dc23/eng/20240627
LC record available at https://lccn.loc.gov/2024020601
LC ebook record available at https://lccn.loc.gov/2024020602

ISBN 978-1-108-72232-2 Paperback

....

Contents

v

Preface

When I tell friends, family, and even medical colleagues about my clinical and academic interest in geriatric psychiatry, I am usually greeted with a look somewhere between quizzical and sympathetic. Statements that follow have become somewhat predictable and tend to reflect the general misunderstanding of the lay public and medical community about the field. "That must be *really* hard," "I'm sure there is such a need for *that*," "That must be sad a lot of the time . . . what you see," and "Oh good! . . . now I know who to call about my older patients that need antipsychotics!" Questions usually follow such as, "How in the world did you become interested in that?!" "Is that its own specialty?" and "How does an internist end up in geriatric psychiatry?"

I love telling friends and colleagues about the field for as long as they will listen. I usually start by telling them how often I would encounter patients in my geriatric-focused internal medicine practice suffering from a wide variety of psychiatric conditions and often feeling that I had just enough knowledge to recognize pathology but not enough to truly understand and help these patients and their families as much as they deserved. The shortage of geriatric mental health providers is acute and I experienced it nearly every day in my internal medicine practice. Wait times for referrals to geriatric psychiatrists can be months, if they are taking new patients at all. General adult psychiatrists are nearly always as busy as their geriatric counterparts and can be potentially less comfortable with the medical frailty, polypharmacy, and comorbidities often seen with my older adult patients. Those older adults in acute psychiatric crisis will often be admitted for several days for "psychiatric stabilization" and then discharged back to their long-term care facility into an environment that contributed to their pathology without necessary psychiatric follow-up. The need for more geriatric psychiatrists or those well versed in its principles is real.

Few things give me the rush and satisfaction of seeing a long-term care resident in my care in the depths of a deep and anxious depression improve and once again achieve a sense of meaning and purpose in their life. Guiding a family past the stages of shock and sadness and into feelings of hope and understanding when discovering a new diagnosis of a major neurocognitive disorder in their loved one is also a deeply fulfilling experience as a clinician.

The pursuit of excellence in the field of geriatric psychiatry also fosters those skills I most value and want to improve in myself. Active listening, empathy, compassion, and connection are skills that set apart those clinicians perceived as exceptional by their patients, families, and colleagues alike.

Why a case-based format for a text on geriatric psychiatry? Many hours of reading journals and textbooks, listening to lectures, and attending professional meetings have added to my knowledge base for sure. But the best lessons I have learned have been from the patients themselves. Their pain inspires me to listen better, learn more, be more empathic, and try harder to foster that ever-important therapeutic connection. I will always remember the most challenging cases because they have often taught me the most. Lessons learned from them will continue to influence my clinical practice for the rest of my career.

The cases in this book are based on real-life situations. The stories, of course, are edited for content and details that could jeopardize the anonymity of the subjects. I purposely tried to include a wide variety of cases to touch on topics in all areas of geriatric psychiatric pathology, including mood disorders, anxiety disorders, psychotic disorders, major neurocognitive disorders, substance use disorders, and personality disorders. Hopefully, the reader will find value and will be able to apply the principles taught in these cases to their own clinical practice in the long-term care setting.

This book is written for the benefit of any provider who cares for those in long-term care, but is also likely to provide insights into geriatric psychiatric disorders for those who practice in the office setting as well. After finishing this book, I realized that the experience and learning involved in writing it provided more benefit to me than anyone. Revisiting and analyzing the cases and researching the topics were a capstone to my fellowship experience and humbled me with knowing how much more there is still to learn about these topics.

As mentioned earlier, I came to the field of geriatric psychiatry through a different path than most. My training in internal medicine provided me with a wonderful foundation for the understanding of pathophysiology and treatment of multiple organ systems. My pull toward geriatric medicine developed over time and, eventually, I spent the majority of my time caring for older adults in long-term care settings. It was in this practice setting that my lack of a better understanding of major neurocognitive disorders and other neuropsychiatric disorders felt more acute. A friend, geriatric psychiatrist, and mentor of mine, Dr. Buntee Co, inspired me to further my career by pursuing a fellowship in geriatric psychiatry and encouraged me to reach out to one of the pillars of the field, Dr. George T. Grossberg, at St. Louis University School of Medicine. I am very thankful for the support of both of these outstanding clinicians and teachers.

Dr. Grossberg pulled me into his world without hesitation and has been a consistent source of inspiration since the day of our introduction and even before, as I tried to read as many of his publications as possible prior to my first day of fellowship. It took me only several hours of reading to realize that Dr. Grossberg has been more instrumental in furthering the field of geriatric psychiatry than anyone I will likely have the pleasure to know. His trainees are now scattered throughout the world and are training and inspiring learners themselves just as he did. His skills as a teacher, clinician, writer, and researcher are unmatched by anyone I have had the privilege to work with.

I would like to thank Dr. Grossberg for gently pushing me toward this opportunity to research, write, and publish this book. He has acted as my editor, cowriter, and motivator throughout the project. He assists me still in clinical practice as I often ask myself "What would Dr. Grossberg do?" when confronted with difficult clinical situations.

As a side note, I would like to encourage any mid-career medical provider to consider pursuing advanced clinical training in a subspecialty that interests them. I feel that a mid-career fellowship has reenergized my practice and provided me with some much-needed professional development that will benefit me throughout the rest of my career.

My family has been stoically supportive of me throughout the months of mornings and evenings researching and writing this book. My partner, Doug, will probably be happy to no longer have to patiently ask, "How's the book coming?" as he has done countless times over the past year. Our now eight- and nine-year-old kids will someday hopefully understand why their dad was sometimes not much fun on the weekends and seemed "super grouchy!" after spending hours typing and staring at his computer screen.

To those who have chosen to read this book, I hope it helps you on your journey to become better mental health providers. Hopefully it will inspire a few to pursue even further learning in geriatric psychiatry and pass along their knowledge to the next generation of clinicians who will be caring for us in the future.

Matthew Gibfried, MD

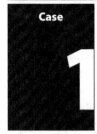

"I've Fallen ... and I Can't Get Up"
Sundowner Syndrome

Mr. S is an 80-year-old gentleman with a significant medical history of a kidney transplant, diabetes, hypertension, hyperlipidemia, gastroesophageal reflux disease (GERD), atrial fibrillation, obstructive sleep apnea, and hypothyroidism. He was living at home with his wife when he had a nighttime fall with loss of consciousness. The fall resulted in a lumbar spinal burst fracture that required spinal fusion surgery. His post-op course was complicated by delirium in the intensive care unit (ICU). He would become disoriented and agitated and throw himself from his bed to the floor. He was referred to geriatric psychiatry for consultation due to concerns about his agitated behavior since his arrival at hospital two weeks prior. He had poor nutritional intake with a 30-pound weight loss. This led to a PICC line placement for total parenteral nutrition (TPN). Before discharge TPN was stopped and Mr. S had a G-tube placed for nutritional support. He was in acute rehab for nine weeks before being transferred to long-term care.

The family reported that the patient was often irritable. He had increased confusion and agitation in the evening and continued to occasionally throw himself out of bed. He had had several urinary tract infections (UTIs) over the three months prior to long-term care.

The nursing staff informed his medical provider that the patient would yell at anyone involved in his care, including physical therapists and nurses. They said he would purposely throw himself out of his wheelchair or bed when his requests were not responded to promptly. He would not engage in social activities at the facility and complained of poor energy and always feeling tired.

Mr. S had no significant psychiatric history and had never been under the care of a psychiatrist before. His sleep was described as poor. He would sleep throughout the late morning and early afternoon and not sleep well at night. He still seemed to enjoy watching baseball games at times.

His mental status exam described his mood as sad, with poor eye contact and a mostly logical and linear thought process. He was also described as irritable during portions of the interview and cooperative at other times. He was oriented to person but was not oriented to place or time. He was unable to identify his wife's sister or name his two children.

The medical provider recommended routine bloodwork and a repeat urinalysis to check for potentially reversible causes of subtle delirium. He was put on trazodone 50 mg qhs for sleep and 25 mg twice daily as needed for anxiety or agitation.

At the time of follow-up two weeks later, Mr. S was found to be mostly unchanged. He continued with regular displays of agitation and aggression toward care staff and family members that seemed to become more pronounced in the late afternoon and early evening hours. His appetite continued to be poor and his mood was mostly described as irritable. He slept a bit better at night but would wake up in the early morning hours asking to get out of bed into his wheelchair, at which time he would be brought close to the nurse's station where he would often yell at staff.

The provider started the patient on sertraline 25 mg daily, which was soon increased to 50 mg daily. The physician recommended that the patient be brought out of his room and encouraged to participate in activities during the daytime instead of being allowed to stay in his room and sleep. Care staff were encouraged to bring Mr. S to the dining room for meals instead of allowing him to take his meals in his room. This was to encourage more socialization, combat boredom, and encourage the normalization of day/night cycles. Melatonin 5 mg qhs was also started.

At a four-week follow-up visit, Mr. S was found to be doing somewhat better. His mood was described as less irritable and he was more cooperative with care. His nutritional intake improved, and his weight loss started to level off. It was noted that care staff were taking the patient outdoors when the weather was good and he seemed to enjoy this. His family was pleased with his improvements in neuropsychiatric symptoms and encouraged by his increasing willingness to participate in therapies, with the goal of Mr. S being able to participate adequately enough in his care to potentially move back home with his family.

Teaching Points

"Sundowner syndrome" refers to a constellation of neuropsychiatric symptoms, usually accompanied by agitation that occurs late in the day in a patient with a major neurocognitive disorder (MNCD). In addition to agitation, anxiety, aggressiveness, increased confusion, and even visual or auditory hallucinations are common. Second only to wandering, sundowning is reported to be one of the most common disruptive behaviors in long-term care settings [1]. Symptoms usually emerge later in the day, classically in the late afternoon or early evening at the time of sunset. This neuropsychiatric syndrome can be very challenging for caregivers. Sundowning is a common reason for those with MNCDs to be moved from home to a long-term care facility. It is also one of the more common reasons for consultation with a geriatric psychiatrist in the long-term care setting.

Sundowning and delirium share some similarities with regard to underlying causes. Both are strongly associated with MNCDs. One key difference between sundowning and delirium is the time of day in which symptoms occur. Sundowning typically occurs and recurs in the late afternoon or evening hours whereas delirium can occur at any time of the day or night.

The treatment of delirium focuses on the identification and treatment of underlying medical issues or medications that may be contributing. In contrast, the treatment of sundowning focuses on altering environmental factors that can contribute to the condition.

The pathophysiology of sundowner syndrome is not fully understood, but there are several theories about the underlying mechanisms. These theories are not mutually exclusive.

One theory is that sundowning may be related to changes in the body's internal clock or circadian rhythm regulation. These rhythms are regulated by the suprachiasmatic nucleus (SCN), which responds to light and dark stimuli to help regulate sleep–wake cycles and other physiological processes. In individuals with dementia or other cognitive impairments, the SCN may be disrupted, leading to changes in sleep patterns and other circadian rhythms. This disruption may contribute to the development of sundowning symptoms in the late afternoon or evening.

Another theory is that sundowning may be related to pain or fatigue that becomes more pronounced in the late afternoon or evening. Individuals with dementia or other cognitive impairments may have difficulty communicating their discomfort, leading to increased agitation or confusion as a way of expressing their discomfort.

There is also evidence to suggest that sundowning may be related to changes in neurotransmitter levels, particularly concerning the neurotransmitter acetylcholine. Individuals with Alzheimer's disease or other forms of MNCD have a loss of acetylcholine-producing neurons in the brain, which contributes to changes in cognitive function and behavior [1].

Sensory deprivation can also play a role in sundowner syndrome. Seniors in long-term care are often lacking in stimulating daytime activities. A multidisciplinary approach to creating individualized care plans for seniors with MNCD is important. These care plans should allow seniors to have regular social interactions, physical activity, family-style mealtimes, time outdoors, and religious activities.

The treatment of sundowning depends on the acuity of symptoms. All patients should have a thorough examination of environmental factors that could be contributing to late-day confusion and agitation and changes made to improve those environmental factors. Medications that could be contributing to confusion should also be identified and removed.

At the time of this writing, there has been relatively recent approval from the US Food and Drug Administration (FDA) of the atypical antipsychotic brexpiprazole for treating agitation due to Alzheimer's disease[2]. There are several other pharmacologic options for the treatment of agitation in the setting of MNCDs. For mild symptoms, several studies have demonstrated improved outcomes for those with sundowner syndrome with melatonin [1]. Melatonin levels are deficient in those with MNCDs (especially Alzheimer's disease). Melatonin is generally well tolerated and may be worth trying in those with mild symptoms. In those patients with more severe symptoms, including severe agitation or psychosis, a trial of a second- or third-generation antipsychotic may be warranted [1]. Antipsychotics are used off-label and should be used with caution and in the smallest dose for the shortest possible duration. Regular efforts to decrease the dosage of antipsychotics are also needed once symptoms are controlled. Cholinesterase inhibitors such as donepezil are known to improve behavioral disturbances in patients with dementia but there are conflicting data on the effect of cholinesterase inhibitors on sundowner syndrome [1].

Take-Home Points

- Sundowner syndrome refers to a constellation of neuropsychiatric symptoms, usually accompanied by agitation that occurs late in the day in a patient with an MNCD. In addition to agitation, anxiety, aggressiveness, increased confusion, and even visual or auditory hallucinations are common.
- Mild symptoms may respond well to melatonin 5 mg in the late afternoon. In those patients with more severe symptoms, including severe agitation or psychosis, a trial of a second- or third-generation antipsychotic may be warranted.
- All patients should have a thorough examination of environmental factors that could be contributing to the late-day confusion and agitation and changes made to improve those environmental factors. Medications that could be contributing to confusion should also be identified and removed.

- Antipsychotics are used off-label and should be used with caution and in the smallest dose for the shortest possible duration. Regular efforts to decrease the dosage of antipsychotics are also needed once symptoms are controlled.

References

1. Canevelli, M., Valletta, M., Trebbastoni, A., Sarli, G., Tariciotti, L., & Bruno, G. (2015). Sundowning in dementia: Clinical relevance, pathophysiological determinants, and therapeutic approaches. *Frontiers in Medicine*, 3. https://doi.org/10.3389/fmed.2016.00073

2. Grossberg, G. T., Kohegyi, E., Mergel, V., Josiassen, M. K., Meulien, D., Hobart, M., Slomkowski, M., Baker, R. A., McQuade, R. D., & Cummings, J. L. (2020). Efficacy and safety of brexpiprazole for the treatment of agitation in Alzheimer's dementia: Two 12-week, randomized, double-blind, placebo-controlled trials. *The American Journal of Geriatric Psychiatry*, 28 (4), 383–400.

Further Reading

Ahmad, F., Sachdeva, P., Sarkar, J., & Izhaar, R. (2022). Circadian dysfunction and Alzheimer's disease: An updated review. *Aging Medicine*, 6 (1), 71–81. doi: 10.1002/agm2.12221. PMID: 36911088; PMCID: PMC10000289.

Carrarini, C., Russo, M., Dono, F., Barbone, F., Rispoli, M. G., Ferri, L., Pietro, M. D., Digiovanni, A., Ajdinaj, P., Speranza, R., Granzotto, A., Frazzini, V., Thomas, A., Pilotto, A., Padovani, A., Onofrj, M., Sensi, S. L., & Bonanni, L. (2020). Agitation and dementia: Prevention and treatment strategies in acute and chronic conditions. *Frontiers in Neurology*, 12. https://doi.org/10.3389/fneur.2021.644317

Desai, A., & Grossberg, G. (2018). *Psychiatric Consultation in Long-Term Care. A Guide for Healthcare Professionals.* 2nd ed. (Cambridge University Press.)

Guu, W., & Aarsland, D. (2022). Light, sleep–wake rhythm, and behavioural and psychological symptoms of dementia in care home patients: Revisiting the sundowning syndrome. *International Journal of Geriatric Psychiatry*, 37 (5). https://doi.org/10.1002/gps.5712

Lin, L., Huang, Q. X., Yang, S. S., Chu, J., Wang, J. Z., & Tian, Q. (2013). Melatonin in Alzheimer's disease. *International Journal of Molecular Sciences*, 14 (7), 14575–14593. doi: 10.3390/ijms140714575. PMID: 23857055; PMCID: PMC3742260.

Menegardo, C. S., Friggi, F. A., Scardini, J. B., Rossi, T. S., Vieira, S., Tieppo, A., & Morelato, R. L. (2019). Sundown syndrome in patients with Alzheimer's disease dementia. *Dementia & Neuropsychologia*, 13 (4), 469–474. https://doi.org/10.1590/1980-57642018dn13-040015

Sharma, A., Sethi, G., Tambuwala, M. M. A., Aljabali, A. A., Chellappan, D. K., Dua, K., & Goyal, R. (2021). Circadian rhythm disruption and Alzheimer's disease: The dynamics of a vicious cycle. *Current Neuropharmacology*, 19 (2), 248–264. https://doi.org/10.2174/1570159X18666200429013041

Todd, W. D. (2019). Potential pathways for circadian dysfunction and sundowning-related behavioral aggression in Alzheimer's disease and related dementias. *Frontiers in Neuroscience*, 14. https://doi.org/10.3389/fnins.2020.00910

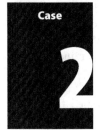

"I Think I Hit My Head"
MNCD Secondary to Alcohol Use Disorder

Mr. T is a 62-year-old gentleman recently admitted to long-term care after a two-week stay in acute rehab. This stay in acute rehab followed a week-long hospital stay. Mr. T presented to the hospital after being found on the floor of his home by a concerned neighbor who had not seen him on his front porch for two days. Mr. T was well known to be found on his front porch each afternoon and evening either yelling or waving at passersby.

Mr. T's neighbor let herself into the unlocked home and he was found on the floor, not able to put more than one or two words together other than, "I think I hit my head." He was at the base of a staircase with a large hematoma and dried blood on his scalp. The concerned neighbor called 911 and paramedics brought Mr. T to the local emergency department. Medical workup was significant for dehydration and mild renal failure. Blood counts showed mild anemia with mild thrombocytopenia and macrocytosis. A head CT showed a fresh subdural hematoma over the left parietal area and evidence of another more chronic subdural hematoma overlying the right frontal lobe. The head CT also showed some mild to moderate cerebral atrophy with enlarged ventricles and prominent widening of cerebral sulci.

Mr. T was admitted to hospital. Neurosurgery did an urgent craniotomy with evacuation of the subdural hematoma and he was treated in the ICU for three to four days. Mr. T's alertness was described as varying between stuporous and lethargic and at other times restless and agitated. His mental status did not improve despite the treatment for dehydration. A repeat head CT showed no unexpected findings or recurrence of the intracerebral bleeding.

On day three in hospital the ICU physician and social services successfully tracked down the patient's daughter, who lived several states away. The patient's daughter said she had not had much contact with her father in the years following the death of her mother. She said she was never very close to her father as he was often verbally and sometimes physically abusive to both her and her mother growing up. He was described as a heavy drinker.

With this new knowledge, the hospital team started treatment for alcohol withdrawal-related delirium with regularly scheduled IV lorazepam. He became calmer and gradually his alertness and orientation improved. He was moved out of the ICU. Physical therapy and occupational therapy evaluations showed that Mr. T had significant problems in multiple areas of mobility and self-care, and he was sent from the hospital to acute rehab.

The patient's physician in acute rehab found Mr. T to be generally pleasant but often confused. His therapy was slowed by difficulty following more complex instructions and retaining knowledge from one therapy session to another. Mr. T scored 18 out of 30 on his Saint Louis University mental status (SLUMS) exam. He was also found to have significant peripheral neuropathy in his feet and legs. Over the course of the next several weeks, it became clear that Mr. T was not going to be able to return to an independent living situation. Mr. T's daughter assisted social services in making arrangements for long-term care.

Mr. T's long-term care provider felt that Mr. T's MNCD was related to chronic alcohol use disorder (AUD).

Teaching Points

The majority of cases of MNCDs can be classified as related to Alzheimer's disease, vascular mechanisms, or Lewy Body dementia. Major neurocognitive disorders related to chronic alcohol use may be underrecognized as there are no definitive diagnostic criteria. The prevalence of the condition varies largely depending on the demographics of the population being studied, as alcohol consumption patterns vary based on social and ethnic patterns of alcohol use. It is estimated that 10–24% of those who have chronic AUD will develop dementia [1]. Studies have shown that alcohol-related dementia (ARD) is responsible for about 10% of early-onset dementia and about 1% of late-onset MNCDs [2].

The pathophysiology of ARD is complex and at present not well understood. Suggested factors likely to be involved include direct neurotoxicity of alcohol, chronic oxidative stress, neuroinflammation, vitamin deficiencies, alcohol-related impacts on neurotransmitter pathways, and vascular effects [3]. See Box 2.1.

There are psychosocial comorbidities to AUD that likely influence the development of dementia at a younger age than in non-alcohol-abusing cohorts. Those with AUD often experience social isolation, financial difficulties, relationship problems, and

---

Box 2.1 Suggested mechanisms influencing the development of MNCD in chronic AUD

1. Direct neurotoxicity of alcohol. Alcohol can disrupt cell membrane integrity and alter ionic balance within neurons. This can lead to cell damage or death [3].
2. Oxidative stress related to alcohol. The metabolism of alcohol creates reactive oxygen species as byproducts such as superoxide radicals and hydrogen peroxide. Heavy production of these substances can overwhelm antioxidant defense mechanisms and cause oxidative damage to cell membranes, intracellular proteins, and DNA.
3. Alcohol-related neuroinflammation. Alcohol can activate immune cells in the central nervous system (CNS) and lead to the release of pro-inflammatory cytokines, which can cause damage to cells within the CNS [4].
4. Vitamin deficiencies. Chronic heavy alcohol use can lead to deficiencies of thiamine, folate, and pyridoxine. These deficiencies can lead to dysfunctional cellular energy metabolism, impaired DNA synthesis and repair, and neurotransmitter synthesis.
5. Alcohol-related effects on neurotransmitter pathways. Alcohol negatively alters some key neurotransmitter systems.
6. Central nervous system vascular dysfunction related to chronic alcohol use. Chronically high levels of alcohol use can cause disruptions of the blood–brain barrier, cerebral blood flow irregularities, endothelial dysfunction, and hypertension-related small vessel disease of the brain [5].

Box 2.2 Common medical comorbidities seen in those with AUD

1. Liver disease. This can include alcoholic fatty liver, alcoholic hepatitis, and cirrhosis.
2. Cardiovascular disease. Those with AUD show higher rates of hypertension, cardiomyopathy, arrhythmia, and increased risk of stroke and heart attack.
3. Gastrointestinal disorders. Those with AUD are known to have higher incidences of gastritis, pancreatitis, and gastrointestinal (GI) bleeding.
4. Malnutrition and vitamin deficiencies (particularly B vitamins).
5. Neurologic disorders. These can include peripheral neuropathy, Wernicke–Korsakoff syndrome, and alcohol-related brain damage.
6. Alcohol-influenced psychiatric disorders. These can include depression, anxiety, and post-traumatic stress disorder (PTSD).
7. Respiratory complications. Those with chronic alcoholism are at increased risk of pneumonia secondary to immunosuppression and increased risk of aspiration.
8. Bone disorders. Those with AUD have a higher incidence of osteoporosis and risk of fracture.
9. Endocrine abnormalities. Men can show alcohol-related hypogonadism and both men and women can have adrenal insufficiency.
10. Metabolic syndrome. Those with chronic AUD have a higher risk of metabolic syndrome (a combination of obesity, insulin resistance, high blood pressure, and dyslipidemia) [6].

housing insecurity that may contribute to earlier cognitive decline. Those with AUD are less likely to adhere to medical treatments for conditions such as hypertension, diabetes, and cerebrovascular disease, causing earlier CNS-related complications of these conditions. Those with AUD are also much more likely to have alcohol-related head injuries from falls, which is known to increase the risk of early progressive cognitive impairment.

Unlike some other MNCDs, there are no specific cerebrospinal fluid (CSF) or imaging findings that are definitive for alcohol-related MNCD. Diagnosis is usually clinical. Those with AUD-related MNCD are more likely to have an earlier onset of dementia and the cognitive impairment will be in the setting of multiple other associated medical and psychosocial comorbidities of AUD [1]. Some other common conditions associated with chronic AUD are shown in Box 2.2.

Although uncommon, providers may be faced with the situation of a patient in long-term care who continues to intermittently abuse alcohol. Cravings for alcohol may remain long after admission and those patients with relatively preserved cognition and/or help from enabling friends or family may have access to alcohol while there. Naltrexone provides a generally well-tolerated pharmacologic option for blunting the pleasurable effects of alcohol in those with AUD. It acts through blockade of the mu-opioid receptors and therefore should not be administered to those who require opiate medications. Acamprosate is a good pharmacologic alternative for those patients who require intermittent or regular opiate use [7].

There are no specific pharmacologic treatments for alcohol-related MNCD. Clinical trials exploring the efficacy of cholinesterase inhibitors specifically in ARD are limited, and the existing data on their effectiveness on this condition are inconclusive. Treatment is largely symptomatic and focuses on the often-seen medical and psychiatric comorbidities that are seen with the condition. Abstinence from alcohol is the most critical factor in slowing the further decline in alcohol-related MNCD. By the time a patient ends up in long-term care, they have often been abstaining from alcohol for some time due to a lack of access from being in a highly controlled care setting. Cognitive rehabilitation with occupational therapy or speech therapy can produce some improvements in functionality and nutritional support is important. Those with ARD may have a long history of very poor nutrition. Psychiatric comorbidities such as depression and anxiety are common and should be treated similarly to those without a history of AUD. Social support and engagement can improve the quality of life in these patients.

The prognosis of ARD can be difficult to predict as there are many confounding variables that may influence outcomes. Those who have early recognition of the condition with early interventions are likely to fare better than those who present with more severe cognitive impairment in a later stage of the disease. Conversely, those who present with severe cognitive impairment at a younger age are more likely to have more aggressive cognitive decline. Those who cease consumption of alcohol clearly do better than those who continue to abuse alcohol and patients with fewer medical comorbidities have a longer life expectancy. In addition, those in a more controlled and supportive environment such as long-term care or assisted living with greater support of healthy living and less availability of alcohol are likely to have improved outcomes.

There are certain difficult situations that may arise in the care of those with early ARD in the assisted living or long-term care environment. Those with less severe cognitive impairments are often still able to direct their own care and may have the ability to obtain alcohol independently or via the help of others. Balancing the autonomy of the resident to potentially make bad choices with a facility's responsibility to provide a safe and healthy environment for the resident and other residents can be a difficult tightrope to navigate. The consequences of continued heavy alcohol use in one already experiencing cognitive and health declines will often progress to the point where the individual will need a surrogate decision-maker to facilitate placement in a more controlled environment, such as long-term care or memory care. Once active drinking has stopped, these patients may maintain relative medical and cognitive stability or experience only slow continued declines in cognitive abilities.

Take-Home Points

- Chronic heavy alcohol use is toxic to the brain via multiple mechanisms.
- Labs and imaging are not specific for alcohol-related MNCD. Diagnosis is usually via history and clinical findings.
- Alcohol-induced MNCD can be partially reversible with abstinence, but the degree of reversibility depends on the severity of pathology.
- Once alcohol use has stopped there can be a long period of cognitive stability.

References

1. Ritchie, K., & Villebrun, D. (2008). Epidemiology of alcohol-related dementia. *Handbook of Clinical Neurology*, 89, 845–850.

2. Cheng, C., Huang, C. L., Tsai, C. J., Chou, P. H., Lin, C. C., & Chang, C. K. (2017). Alcohol-related dementia: A systemic review of epidemiological studies. *Psychosomatics*, 58 (4), 331–342.

3. Zhang, K., & Luo, J. (2019). Role of MCP-1 and CCR2 in alcohol neurotoxicity. *Pharmacological Research*, 139, 360. https://doi.org/10.1016/j.phrs.2018.11.030

4. King, J. A., Nephew, B. C., Choudhury, A., Poirier, G. L., Lim, A., & Mandrekar, P. (2020). Chronic alcohol-induced liver injury correlates with memory deficits: Role for neuroinflammation. *Alcohol (Fayetteville, N.Y.)*, 83, 75–81. https://doi.org/10.1016/j.alcohol.2019.07.005

5. Sachdeva, A., Chandra, M., Choudhary, M., Dayal, P., & Anand, K. S. (2016). Alcohol-related dementia and neurocognitive impairment: A review study. *International Journal of High-Risk Behaviors & Addiction*, 5 (3), e27976 https://doi.org/10.5812/ijhrba.27976

6. MacKillop, J., Agabio, R., Feldstein-Ewing, S., Heilig, M., Kelly, J. F., Leggio, L., Lingford-Hughes, A., Palmer, A., Parry, C., Ray, L., & Rehm, J. (2022). Hazardous drinking and alcohol use disorders. *Nature Reviews. Disease Primers*, 8 (1), 80. https://doi.org/10.1038/s41572-022-00406-1

7. Murphy, C. E., Wang, R. C., Montoy, J. C., Whittaker, E., & Raven, M. (2022). Effect of extended-release naltrexone on alcohol consumption: A systematic review and meta-analysis. *Addiction*, 117 (2), 271–281. https://doi.org/10.1111/add.15572

Further Reading

Kaldy, J. (2023). Alcohol use in long-term care communities: Juggling choice and safety. *Caring for the Ages*, 24 (1), 1. https://doi.org/10.1016/j.carage.2022.12.013

Lohoff, F. W. (2020). Pharmacotherapies and personalized medicine for alcohol use disorder: A review. *Pharmacogenomics*, 21 (15), 1117–1138. https://doi.org/10.2217/pgs-2020-0079

Sullivan, E. V., & Pfefferbaum, A. (2019). Brain-behavior relations and effects of aging and common comorbidities in alcohol use disorder: A review. *Neuropsychology*, 33 (6), 760. https://doi.org/10.1037/neu0000557

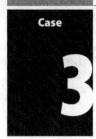

"It's like She's a Different Person"
Neuropsychiatric Complications of TBI

Mrs. S was a 78-year-old resident of a medium-sized skilled nursing facility. She had been a resident of the facility for four years following a fall at home. Nursing staff at the facility requested that the consulting psychiatrist see the patient after she had returned from hospital where she was evaluated after a fall with a scalp laceration. Since returning from the emergency department Mrs. S had not been acting as usual. She had been showing personality changes. Prior to her fall, she could be described as fairly quiet but pleasant. She enjoyed social functions in the nursing facility and was generally liked by other residents and nursing staff alike. She had a particular affinity for music and her favorite activities involved musical performers who would come to the facility once or twice a week. Mrs. S loved to play the piano and would often entertain others in the facility after evening meals with her piano playing and singing.

After her return from the emergency room following her fall three weeks prior, Mrs. S seemed to have little interest in social activities. She had stopped attending most musical activities and had stopped playing music for other residents even after much encouragement from her friends. Her friends and staff members had noted that Mrs. S was now described as often short-tempered and irritable with others. Mrs. S's daughter was also concerned about these changes. "It's like she's a different person, what happened to my mom!" her daughter exclaimed during the provider's first visit with the patient.

On review of Mrs. S's chart before the meeting, it was noted that she had a history of obesity class 3 (BMI 43), impaired mobility, hypertension, hyperlipidemia, and psoriasis. She had polio as a young girl which left her with shortening of her left lower extremity, scoliosis, and lifelong issues with impaired mobility. For most of her life, she was fully mobile with a cane or bilateral hand crutches but as she reached her 50s and 60s she began gaining weight. Her weight gain led to a slow steady decline in mobility. Prior to her most recent fall, she was dependent mostly on a motorized scooter for mobility but was still able to self-transfer from her bed to her scooter with the aid of her hand crutches.

A review of her chart also indicated that Mrs. S had several hospital visits for falls in the past year alone. None had resulted in serious injury, only scalp contusions or lacerations. The nursing staff mentioned that Mrs. S may have lost consciousness for "a while" after her most recent fall. Her falls always happened when she tried to transfer herself to her motorized scooter or while transferring on and off the commode. She had a CT brain scan after her latest fall that showed only mild age-related small vessel ischemic changes. There was no comment on atrophy or subdural hematoma. A review of recent labs indicated that the patient's comprehensive metabolic panel (CMP), complete blood count (CBC), thyroid studies, b12, and folate levels were all within normal limits.

Mrs. S's daughter was happy to be present during the initial psychiatric examination. Mrs. S was not very forthcoming during the interview. She could answer simple direct questions, but her daughter was forced to give most of the history. Mrs. S had no history of mental health issues. She was described as only mildly forgetful at times, but this had changed in recent weeks. Mrs. S now seemed unable to remember visits with her daughter from one week to the next and had little interest in gossiping about her extended family members or discussing her favorite soap operas as she used to do. She seemed to still be eating well. She slept well at night and indeed seemed to be sleeping more during the day as well.

Mrs. S scored a two out of a possible five on a mini-cog exam. Her mental status exam revealed her to be awake and alert. She was oriented to person and place but not to month or year. Her hygiene was fair to poor, her hair was disheveled, and she was wearing her nightgown that was littered with food stains at 2 p.m. Her mood seemed somewhat depressed and mildly irritable. Her affect was flat. She did not show any signs of hallucinations and denied feeling suicidal. Her behavior was calm. Her neurologic exam was consistent with her history of post-polio syndrome with weakness in her left leg, but no other focal findings were seen.

The patient and her daughter were counseled on the topic of neuropsychiatric complications of traumatic brain injury (TBI). They were informed that the diagnosis was that of depression following a TBI sustained during her last fall. It was recommended that the patient begin an antidepressant in hopes of improving her mood, energy, and social withdrawal. She started on fluoxetine 10 mg daily which was increased to 20 mg daily after two weeks. On a six-week follow-up visit, Mrs. S was doing somewhat better. Her daughter stated that Mrs. S was more pleasant and getting involved in more day-to-day activities at the facility. Her ability to play the piano had not quite returned to her pre-fall baseline; she would sit down at the piano and become frustrated after five or ten minutes when she could not seem to remember the songs that she had been playing for many years. Despite this, she still enjoyed listening to the volunteer musicians from the community who played at the facility. Mrs. S was finishing a course of physical and occupational therapy that included some cognitive retraining. Her cognition and ability to transfer seemed to be improving.

Teaching Points

Traumatic brain injury is more common in older adults than in any other age group. It is the most common fall-related injury among adults over the age of 65 [1]. Hospitalization rates for TBI increase exponentially with age. Rates of hospitalization for TBI are three times higher in those over 75 when compared to patients 65–74 years of age [1]. Traumatic brain injury is not only considered an acute condition but a chronic one as well. Most TBIs in low- to moderate-income countries are attributed to road traffic accidents while the highest numbers of TBIs in the US and other high-income countries are due to falls, especially in those over the age of 65. Older patients are generally considered to have poorer outcomes with more severe cognitive and functional impairments from TBI than younger patients [2].

The pathogenesis of TBI involves both primary and secondary injury mechanisms. Primary mechanisms involve mechanical injury that occurs from the physical forces that occur during the fall, including acceleration, deceleration, and direct impact. These can

> **Box 3.1** Some secondary mechanisms of TBI
>
> Ischemia and hypoxia: Reduced blood flow (ischemia) and oxygen supply (hypoxia) to brain tissue can occur due to blood vessel damage or swelling, leading to cell damage and death.
>
> Cerebral edema: Swelling of brain tissue, either cytotoxic (intracellular) or vasogenic (extracellular), can increase intracranial pressure and further damage brain cells.
>
> Excitotoxicity: Excessive release of neurotransmitters, such as glutamate, can lead to overstimulation of neurons, causing cell damage and death.
>
> Inflammatory response: The brain's immune response can be activated by TBI. This results in the release of proinflammatory cytokines and the recruitment of immune cells, which can contribute to brain tissue damage.
>
> Blood–brain barrier disruption: The integrity of the blood–brain barrier can be compromised, allowing harmful substances to enter the brain, further exacerbating inflammation and damage.
>
> Cerebral herniation: As intracranial pressure increases, the brain can be pushed against the skull, leading to displacement (herniation) of brain structures, which can be life-threatening.
>
> Oxidative stress: Increased production of reactive oxygen species can damage brain cells and further worsen injury.

cause contusions of brain tissues and surrounding structures. These mechanical forces also cause diffuse axonal injury from widespread damage to axons caused by shearing forces from acceleration and deceleration. These acute injuries often lead to short-term brain dysfunction resulting in concussion. Secondary injury mechanisms are the subsequent processes that follow the primary injury and can exacerbate damage to the brain. These mechanisms can evolve, sometimes hours to days after the initial trauma. Box 3.1 lists some of the secondary injury mechanisms of TBI [3].

Older adults are at higher risk of worse outcomes following traumatic brain injuries. Older adults are known to have age-related changes in brain structure such as brain atrophy and reduced blood flow, which make them more susceptible to injury. These changes can result in a decreased ability to recover from brain trauma. Older adults also often have pre-existing medical conditions which can complicate recovery from TBI. These comorbidities include higher incidences of hypertension, diabetes, and cerebrovascular disease. Medications more likely to be utilized in older adults can also increase the risk of TBI. These include medications that can increase the risk of intracerebral hemorrhage or microhemorrhages after injury. Older adults generally have slower healing following injury and may have a lower cognitive reserve, which lowers their ability to cognitively compensate for the effects of brain injury. The prevalence of coexisting neuropsychiatric disorders such as depression, anxiety, and neurodegenerative diseases is also higher in older adults. These comorbidities can complicate recovery. Seniors may have more limited access to post-injury specialized care. The increasing frailty of older adults can affect their ability to tolerate the physical and emotional stress of a TBI and its associated rehabilitation [3,4].

The treatment of traumatic brain injuries in older adults should consider the unique needs and challenges of this population. Hospital-level care focuses on stabilization and treating any acute issues such as bleeding or swelling of the brain. Rehabilitation is a critical component of TBI treatment for older adults. This includes physical therapy, occupational therapy, and speech therapy to address deficits in mobility, functional independence, and cognitive function. Rehabilitation aims to improve physical and cognitive abilities, enhance independence, and promote quality of life. Medications can be important to control mid-term and long-term complications of TBI including pain, agitation, depression, and sleep disturbances. Cognitive rehabilitation can help older adults regain cognitive function, memory, and executive skills that may have been negatively impacted by a TBI. Finally, those with TBI are more likely to suffer future TBI from falls and fall prevention strategies are essential to reduce further risk. Fall prevention strategies may include home modification, balance training, and exercise programs.

Traumatic brain injuries can lead to a wide range of neuropsychiatric symptoms and diagnoses both in the acute and long term. Box 3.2 lists some of the more common neuropsychiatric conditions that may result from TBI [5,6].

The prognosis of TBI in older adults is generally worse when compared to younger adults with similar injuries. Older adults are known to have slower recovery and on average have worse functional, cognitive, and psychosocial outcomes in the months or years post-injury.

Traumatic brain injuries are unfortunately quite common in the older adult long-term care population. The importance of TBIs in older adults lies in their vulnerability, the potential for worse outcomes, and the need for tailored care and prevention strategies to address the unique challenges of this population.

Box 3.2 Common neuropsychiatric conditions that may result from TBI

Post-concussion Syndrome:

- Post-concussion syndrome (PCS) is a common diagnosis following mild to moderate TBIs. It is characterized by a constellation of symptoms, including headaches, dizziness, fatigue, irritability, memory problems, and difficulty concentrating.

Mood Disorders:

- Depression: TBI can trigger depressive symptoms, which may include persistent sadness, loss of interest in activities, changes in appetite, and sleep disturbances.
- Anxiety: Generalized anxiety, panic disorder, and specific phobias may develop or worsen after TBI.
- Bipolar disorder: Some patients may experience mood swings and manic or hypomanic episodes following TBI.

Post-traumatic Stress Disorder:

- Post-traumatic stress disorder can develop after a TBI, especially if the injury results from a traumatic event, such as a car accident.

Aggression and Irritability:

- TBI can lead to increased irritability, impulsivity, and aggression. This is often referred to as "TBI-related aggression."

Substance Use Disorders:

- Some individuals may turn to alcohol or drugs as a way to cope with the physical and emotional challenges of TBI.

Box 3.2 *(cont.)*

Cognitive Impairments:

- TBI can result in deficits in memory, attention, processing speed, and executive function, which may lead to a cognitive disorder diagnosis.

Psychotic Disorders:

- In some cases, TBI can trigger or exacerbate psychotic symptoms, leading to a diagnosis of schizophrenia or other psychotic disorders.

Personality Changes:

- TBI can lead to alterations in personality, such as apathy, reduced impulse control, and diminished empathy.

Sleep Disorders:

- Insomnia, excessive daytime sleepiness, and sleep-related breathing disorders can develop or worsen after TBI.

Neurodegenerative Disorders:

- One study showed that TBI in older adults is associated with a 44% increased risk of Parkinson's disease and a 26% increase of MNCDs in general [7].

Take-Home Points

- Traumatic brain injury is more common in older adults than in any other age group. It is the most common fall-related injury among adults over the age of 65.
- The pathogenesis of TBI involves both primary and secondary injury mechanisms. Older adults are at higher risk of worse outcomes following traumatic brain injuries.
- Traumatic brain injuries can lead to a wide range of neuropsychiatric symptoms and diagnoses both in the acute and long term. These can include mood disorders, cognitive impairment, and increased risk of MNCD and Parkinson's disease.
- The severity of TBI in older adults lies in their vulnerability, the potential for worse outcomes, and the need for tailored care and prevention strategies to address the unique challenges of this population.

References

1. Albrecht, J. S., & Gardner, R. C. (2023). Traumatic brain injury in older adults: Epidemiology, management, outcomes. Unique features of traumatic brain injuries in older adults and the current landscape of treatment and management options. *Practical Neurology*, 22–24.

2. Gardner, R. C., Dams-O'Connor, K., Morrissey, M. R., & Manley, G. T. (2018). Geriatric traumatic brain injury: Epidemiology, outcomes, knowledge gaps, and future directions. *Journal of Neurotrauma*, 35 (7), 889–906. doi: 10.1089/neu.2017.5371. Epub 2018 Feb 15. PMID: 29212411; PMCID: PMC5865621.

3. Gibbons, L. E., Landau, A., Larson, E. B., & Crane, P. K. (2016). Health problems precede traumatic brain injury in older adults. *Journal of the American Geriatrics Society*, 64 (4), 844–848. https://doi.org/10.1111/jgs.14014

4. Chauhan, A. V., Guralnik, J., Sorkin, J. D., Badjatia, N., & Albrecht, J. S. (2022). Repetitive traumatic brain injury among older adults. *The Journal of Head Trauma Rehabilitation*, 37 (4), E242. https://doi.org/10.1097/HTR.0000000000000719

5. Brett, B. L., Kramer, M. D., Whyte, J., McCrea, M. A., Stein, M. B., Giacino, J. T., Sherer, M., Markowitz, A. J., Manley, G. T., Nelson, L. D., Investigators, T., Adeoye, O., Badjatia, N., Boase, K., Barber, J., Bodien, Y., Bullock, M. R., Chesnut, R., Corrigan, J. D., & Zafonte, R. (2021). Latent profile analysis of neuropsychiatric symptoms and cognitive function of adults 2 weeks after traumatic brain injury: Findings from the TRACK-TBI study. *JAMA Network Open*, 4 (3), e213467. https://doi.org/10.1001/jamanetworkopen.2021.3467

6. Ahmed, S., Venigalla, H., Mekala, H. M., Dar, S., Hassan, M., & Ayub, S. (2017). Traumatic brain injury and neuropsychiatric complications. *Indian Journal of Psychological Medicine*, 39 (2), 114–121. https://doi.org/10.4103/0253-7176.203129

7. Gardner, R. C., Burke, J. F., Nettiksimmons, J., Goldman, S., Tanner, C. M., & Yaffe, K. (2015). Traumatic brain injury in later life increases risk for Parkinson's disease. *Annals of Neurology*, 77, 987–995.

Further Reading

Cash, A., & Theus, M. H. (2020). Mechanisms of blood–brain barrier dysfunction in traumatic brain injury. *International Journal of Molecular Sciences*, 21 (9). https://doi.org/10.3390/ijms21093344

Perry, D. C., Sturm, V. E., Peterson, M. J., Pieper, C. F., Bullock, T., Boeve, B. F., Miller, B. L., Guskiewicz, K. M., Berger, M. S., Kramer, J. H., & Welsh-Bohmer, K. A. (2016). Association of traumatic brain injury with subsequent neurological and psychiatric disease: A meta-analysis. *Journal of Neurosurgery*, 124 (2), 511–526. https://doi.org/10.3171/2015.2.JNS14503

Torregrossa, W., Raciti, L., Rifici, C., Rizzo, G., Raciti, G., Casella, C., Naro, A., & Calabrò, R. S. (2023). Behavioral and psychiatric symptoms in patients with severe traumatic brain injury: A comprehensive overview. *Biomedicines*, 11 (5), 1449. https://doi.org/10.3390/biomedicines11051449

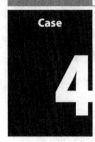

"I Am Tired All the Time"
Dementia with Lewy Bodies

Ms. S, a 79-year-old woman residing in a nursing home, was referred to psychiatry for evaluation of suspected depression. She had a history of memory problems, disorientation at times, recurrent falls, and sleep disturbances beginning two to three years ago and had been progressively getting worse. Her most recent fall caused her to have a bruise on her face but no fracture, and for two weeks she was increasingly withdrawn, staying in her room with mild impairment in appetite. On evaluation, the resident's main complaint was fatigue; she stated, "I am tired all the time." Her medical history was positive for hypertension, peripheral vascular disease, osteoarthritis of the knees, and carpal tunnel syndrome.

A review of systems revealed dysuria. She presented mentally slowed, with flat affect, and moderately disoriented to time and place. Her SLUMS score was 12/30. Physical examination revealed a low-frequency tremor of the arms and a slow gait. Laboratory results were within normal range and urinalysis revealed a bladder infection, which was treated with antibiotics. Ms. S was taking amlodipine, acetaminophen, and lorazepam 0.5 mg three times a day. To rule out chronic subdural hematoma, the physician recommended an emergency CT scan of the head, which showed old diffuse ischemic white matter changes and mild cortical atrophy. The lorazepam was gradually tapered and discontinued over two weeks. Ms. S was started on donepezil 5 mg once daily. Family and staff were counseled to have her walk regularly, as she had always enjoyed walking. After one month, she was sleeping better and her dysuria had cleared up, but she still complained of fatigue. She had tolerated donepezil well so far without developing any nausea or vomiting and her tremor had not worsened. The donepezil was increased to 10 mg daily. Water painting was added to her activity schedule, as Ms. S had shown interest in this activity when she was in an adult day program. After another month, she appeared to be doing much better. She still complained of fatigue, but less often. Her family felt she was more alert and interactive. Her repeat SLUMS score was 15. Final diagnosis of probable dementia with Lewy bodies (DLB) was given.

Teaching Points

It is important to note that adverse effects of benzodiazepines, such as fatigue, may take several weeks to improve after the drug is discontinued. Also, a UTI may manifest as fatigue, depression, and/or increased confusion. Often, there are multiple causes of symptoms and disability, with untreated MNCD being one of them. In this case, treatment of the UTI, discontinuation of lorazepam, the institution of cholinesterase inhibitor (ChEi) therapy, and aggressive use of strength-based personalized psychosocial sensory spiritual environmental initiatives with creative engagement helped improve the resident's quality of life.

Dementia with Lewy bodies is a neurodegenerative disorder characterized by the presence of Lewy bodies, which are abnormal protein deposits, in certain areas of the brain. These Lewy bodies are composed mainly of alpha-synuclein protein and their accumulation in the brain leads to the death of brain cells, causing a decline in cognitive and motor functions. Dementia with Lewy bodies is the second most common form of dementia after Alzheimer's disease, accounting for about 15% of all dementia cases. The accumulation of Lewy bodies (α-synuclein neuronal inclusions) and cell death is also the key pathophysiologic finding in Parkinson's disease. Up to 80% of those diagnosed with Parkinson's disease go on to develop DLB.

The symptoms of DLB can be variable and fluctuate from day to day, making it challenging to diagnose. The most common symptoms include cognitive impairment, such as difficulties with attention, memory, and problem-solving, as well as visual hallucinations, fluctuations in alertness and attention, and motor symptoms, such as muscle rigidity, tremors, and difficulty with balance and gait. Some individuals with DLB may also experience sleep disturbances, depression, and anxiety.

Dementia with Lewy bodies can be difficult to diagnose because there is a great deal of overlap with other neurodegenerative disorders such as vascular dementia, Parkinson's disease, and Alzheimer's disease. As with all potentially new MNCD diagnoses, a thorough medical history, physical exam, and neurologic testing are important in making a diagnosis. Imaging modalities such as MRI and dopamine active transporter (DAT) positron emission tomography (PET) scans can be helpful in making an accurate diagnosis and ruling out other possible causes of cognitive impairment.

There are central features, core features, suggestive features, and supportive features that can be used to aid in the diagnosis of DLB. Central features are required for possible or probable diagnosis of DLB. These include progressive dementia severe enough to interfere with normal social or occupational function and deficits on tests of attention, executive function, and visuospatial ability. Core features include fluctuating cognition, recurrent visual hallucinations, and spontaneous Parkinsonism. Two core features are required for probable DLB and one for possible diagnosis. Suggestive features of DLB include rapid eye movement (REM) sleep behavior disorder, severe sensitivity to anti-psychotics, and low dopamine transporter uptake in the basal ganglia. Any suggestive feature with at least one core feature defines probable DLB. Any suggestive feature in the absence of core features defines possible DLB. Supportive features can be commonly seen in DLB but do not have specificity for the disease. These features can include severe autonomic dysfunction, systematized delusions, depression, and unexplained loss of consciousness, among others.

REM sleep behavior disorder (RBD) is common in DLB and Parkinson-related dementia. It is a sleep disorder in which a person physically acts out their dreams during the REM stage of sleep. Normally, during REM sleep, the body's muscles are temporarily paralyzed, preventing movement during dreams. However, in individuals with RBD, this muscle paralysis is incomplete or absent, leading to physical movements and vocalizations during sleep. The movements associated with RBD can range from the simple, such as kicking or punching, to the complex and potentially dangerous, such as jumping out of bed or running around the room. This can pose a risk of injury to the person with RBD as well as their bed partner.

Distinguishing DLB from Parkinson's disease dementia is considered by some to be more of an academic distinction as it is thought that these two diagnoses exist on a continuum. In DLB, dementia develops one year or more prior to Parkinsonism. Parkinson's disease dementia develops in the context of established Parkinson's disease.

Unfortunately, there are no curative treatments for DLB, and treatment is mostly symptomatic. Medications like cholinesterase inhibitors can provide benefits and help improve cognition and reduce hallucinations in some individuals with DLB. In fact, cholinesterase inhibitors may be more effective in DLB than in patients with Alzheimer's disease. The acetylcholinesterase inhibitor rivastigmine has the most convincing data and should probably be the preferred acetylcholinesterase inhibitor. As DLB progresses there can be development of Parkinsonian symptoms such as resting tremor, bradykinesia, stiffness, impaired balance, and sleep disturbances, among others. Neuropsychiatric symptoms are common in DLB and may include hallucinations, delusions, depression, anxiety, apathy, agitation, and sleep disturbances. The treatment of these symptoms is more challenging as patients with DLB are often very sensitive to the negative effects of antipsychotic medications. For this reason every effort should be made to address neuropsychiatric symptoms in DLB without the use of antipsychotics.

Second- or third-generation antipsychotics are much preferred over first-generation antipsychotics in those with DLB. Quetiapine is probably the best choice if an antipsychotic is needed for neuropsychiatric symptoms in patients with DLB. Quetiapine has a relatively low affinity for dopamine receptors, which makes it less likely to exacerbate movement-related problems at low doses. Clozapine has been shown to be effective in treating psychosis related to DLB or Parkinson-related dementia but has other challenges related to its use. One promising newer drug is pimavanserin, a selective serotonin 5-HT2A inverse agonist, which significantly reduced psychotic symptoms in patients with Parkinson's disease and was well tolerated in a randomized controlled trial. A recent study published in the *New England Journal of Medicine* in 2020 evaluated the effectiveness of pimavanserin in patients with dementia related to Parkinson's disease (PD-D). The study included 392 participants with PD-D and symptoms of psychosis, including hallucinations and delusions.

The participants were randomly assigned to receive either pimavanserin or a placebo (inactive treatment) for 12 weeks. The study found that treatment with pimavanserin resulted in a significant improvement in psychosis symptoms compared to the placebo, as measured by the Scale for the Assessment of Positive Symptoms – Hallucinations and Delusions subscale (SAPS–H+D).

The study also found that pimavanserin was generally well tolerated, with few serious adverse events reported.

Nonpharmacologic therapies are important for those with DLB. Occupational therapy, physical therapy, and speech therapy can help to optimize function in those with DLB and associated Parkinsonian symptoms.

The natural history of the disease is generally a slow progression in neuropsychiatric symptoms and motor functions over time. Some patients may experience a more rapid decline than others. Many patients with advanced DLB will need more specialized care in a memory care unit of a long-term care facility.

Take-Home Points

- Dementia with Lewy bodies is a neurodegenerative disorder characterized by the presence of Lewy bodies, which are abnormal protein deposits, in certain areas of the brain. It is the second most common form of MNCD after Alzheimer's disease, accounting for about 15% of all dementia cases.
- Unfortunately, there are no curative treatments for DLB, and treatment is mostly symptomatic. Medications such as cholinesterase inhibitors can provide benefits and help improve cognition and reduce hallucinations in some individuals with DLB.
- There are central features, core features, suggestive features, and supportive features that can be used to aid in the diagnosis of DLB.
- Second- or third-generation antipsychotics are preferred over first-generation antipsychotics in those with DLB. Quetiapine is probably the best choice if an antipsychotic is needed for neuropsychiatric symptoms in patients with DLB.

Further Reading

American Psychiatric Association. (2022). *Diagnostic and Statistical Manual of Mental Disorders*. 5th ed. text rev. (American Psychiatric Association Publishing).

Cummings, J., Isaacson, S., Mills, R., Williams, H., Chi-Burris, K., Corbett, A., Dhall, R., & Ballard, C. (2014). Pimavanserin for patients with Parkinson's disease psychosis: A randomized, placebo-controlled phase 3 trial. *Lancet*, 383, 533–540.

Desai, A., & Grossberg, G. (2018). *Psychiatric Consultation in Long-Term Care. A Guide for Healthcare Professionals*. 2nd ed. (Cambridge University Press). pp. 51–53.

Emre, M., Aarsland, D., Brown, R., Burn, D. J., Duyckaerts, C., Mizuno, Y., Broe, G. A., Cummings, J., Dickson, D. W., Gauthier, S., Goldman, J., Goetz, C., Korczyn, A., Lees, A., Levy, R., Litvan, I., McKeith, I., Olanow, W., Poewe, W., Quinn, N., Sampaio, C., Tolosa, E., & Dubois, B. (2007). Clinical diagnostic criteria for dementia associated with Parkinson's disease. *Movement Disorders*, 22 (12), 1689–1707; quiz 1837. doi: 10.1002/mds.21507. PMID: 17542011.

Haider, A., Spurling, B. C., & Sánchez-Manso, J. C. (2023). Lewy body dementia. [Updated February 12]. In StatPearls [Internet]. Treasure Island, FL: StatPearls Publishing. www.ncbi.nlm.nih.gov/books/NBK482441/

Outeiro, T. F., Koss, D. J., Erskine, D., Walker, L., Kurzawa-Akanbi, M., Burn, D., Donaghy, P., Morris, C., Taylor, J. P., Thomas, A., Attems, J., & McKeith, I. (2019). Dementia with Lewy bodies: An update and outlook. *Molecular Neurodegeneration*, 14 (1), 5. doi: 10.1186/s13024-019-0306-8. PMID: 30665447; PMCID: PMC6341685.

Smith, G. E., Boeve, B., Pankratz, S., Jacobson, K., Aakre, J., & Tanis, F. (2009). Time course of diagnostic features of Lewy body disease. *Neurology*, 72 (11), A246–A246, 530.

Tariot, P. N., Cummings, J. L., Soto-Martin, M. E., Ballard, C., Erten-Lyons, D., Sultzer, D. L., Devanand, D. P., Weintraub, D., McEvoy, B., Youakim, J. M., Stankovic, S., & Foff, E. P. (2021). Trial of pimavanserin in dementia-related psychosis. *New England Journal of Medicine*, 385 (4), 309–319. doi: 10.1056/NEJMoa2034634. PMID: 34289275.

Vann Jones, S. A., & O'Brien, J. T. (2014). The prevalence and incidence of dementia with Lewy bodies: A systematic review of population and clinical studies. *Psychological Medicine*, 44 (4), 673–683. doi: 10.1017/S0033291713000494. Epub 2013 Mar 25. Erratum in: Psychol Med. 2014 Mar;44(4):684. PMID: 23521899.

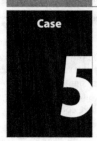

"I Am Okay"
Frontotemporal Dementia

Mr. C, a 55-year-old male, became socially withdrawn, developed poor decision-making ability, and had a significant weight gain over two years. He entered a long-term care facility for rehabilitation after surgery for a hip fracture. Mr. C seemed not to be bothered by the hip fracture and needed encouragement during physical therapy. He was diagnosed with depression and tried various antidepressants without success. He was then referred to a psychiatrist for a trial of electroconvulsive therapy (ECT).

Mr. C told the psychiatrist during the interview, "I am okay," and did not endorse depressive symptoms. The psychiatrist felt this was a new-onset apathy syndrome and ordered an MRI of the brain to rule out any neurological cause. Mr. C had no history of depression before the two-year period of weight gain and there was no family history of depression. Mr. C had a vague history of possible transient ischemic attack.

An MRI revealed right temporal, frontal, and parietal atrophy. The psychiatrist referred Mr. C to a neurologist at a local memory and aging disorder clinic at an academic institution for evaluation of possible frontotemporal dementia (FTD). Mr. C underwent a comprehensive evaluation, including neuropsychological testing, and was diagnosed with probable behavioral variant (bv)FTD. Mr. C's socially withdrawn behavior was thought to reflect apathy more than depression and all antidepressants were discontinued without any worsening of clinical symptoms. The family and staff at the long-term care facility were educated about the diagnosis. Strength-based, personalized, psychosocial sensory spiritual environmental initiatives and creative engagement (SPPEICE) were identified and initiated to address apathy. Mr. C passed away six years after the diagnosis of FTD due to complications related to advanced stages of FTD. A brain autopsy was performed and the pathological diagnosis of FTD (ubiquitin-positive) was given.

Teaching Points

Frontotemporal dementia is the name of a group of dementias that primarily involve the frontal and temporal lobes of the brain. They are progressive neurodegenerative disorders that are typically diagnosed in individuals under the age of 65. Major declines in cognition, behavior, and language are seen. Frontotemporal dementias and their variants are the second most common type of dementia diagnosed in those under 65 years of age and the third most common type of MNCD overall, behind Alzheimer's disease and dementia with Lewy bodies. Different epidemiologic studies have shown relatively wide differences in estimations of the prevalence of the disease. Estimating the prevalence of

FTD can be difficult as there is a good deal of overlap in symptomatology between FTD and other forms of major neurocognitive disorders.

There are six subtypes of the disease. The behavioral variant (bvFTD) can be described by noted changes in behavior, personality, and social functioning. Symptoms may include apathy, lack of empathy, socially inappropriate behavior, and a decline in personal hygiene. The semantic variant primary progressive aphasia (svPPA) is a subtype characterized by a progressive decline in language functioning, including difficulty with word finding, word comprehension, and loss of knowledge of word meanings. These patients may eventually lose the ability to speak altogether. Progressive nonfluent variant primary progressive aphasia (PNFA) is a rare form of FTD that also affects language and speech production. Patients have speech that can be described as difficult, halting, with grammatical errors and difficulty with word retrieval. There are three subtypes of FTD that have prominent motor symptoms. These include corticobasal degeneration (CBD), progressive supranuclear palsy (PSP), and FTD with motor neuron disease amyotrophic lateral sclerosis (ALS).

Symptoms of FTD are variable and depend on the subtype of the disease but most show some changes in behavior, personality, language, and movement. Movement disorders such as Parkinsonism may also occur in some subtypes of FTD. The initial presentation of FTD is often mistaken for depression and accurate diagnosis requires a high index of suspicion. A history of insidious onset of apathy and lack of concern for self should raise the possibility of FTD and we strongly recommend referral to a geriatric psychiatrist or a neurologist for early accurate diagnosis.

The exact causes of FTD are not yet fully understood, but genetic mutations have been identified as a significant risk factor. Familial FTD accounts for approximately one-third to one-half of all FTD cases and presents more commonly as bvFTD than other FTD subtypes [1]. Mutations in microtubule-associated protein tau (MAPT), progranulin (PGRN), and chromosome 9 open reading frame 72 (C9orf72) expansion mutations have been found to be the most common causes of familial FTD. In addition, abnormal protein deposits in the brain (tau, TDP-43, and FUS) have also been implicated in the development of FTD. The abnormal accumulation of tau and TDP-43 proteins causes damage to the nerve cells in the brain, leading to cell death and eventually symptoms of FTD.

Diagnosis of FTD involves a comprehensive neurological evaluation, including labs and MRI or CT, as well as neuropsychological testing to assess cognitive and language function. In some cases, genetic testing may also be recommended. Definitive serum or csf biomarkers for FTD have been elusive.

Possible, probable, and definitive diagnosis of bvFTD can be made using the following criteria developed by the International Behavioral Variant FTD Criteria Consortium in 2011. Patients must all show a progressive decline in behavior as observed by a reliable caregiver.

Possible bvFTD is diagnosed if three or more of the following are present: (a) early behavioral disinhibition described as socially inappropriate behavior, loss of manners/decorum, impulsivity, and rash actions; (b) early apathy or inertia; (c) early loss of empathy or sympathy, including diminished response to other people's needs or sympathies, and diminished social interest; (d) early perseverative or compulsive/ritualistic behavior, (i.e. simple repetitive movements, complex, compulsive, or ritualistic behavior, stereotypy of speech); (e) hyperorality and dietary changes, including altered food preferences, binge eating, increased consumption of alcohol and cigarettes, oral exploration or consumption of inedible objects; (f) neuropsychological profile demonstrates deficits in executive functioning and relative sparing of episodic memory and visuospatial functioning.

Probable bvFTD diagnosis would need to meet the criteria for possible bvFTD, but also includes imaging with frontal or anterior atrophy on MRI or CT. Alternatively, PET or single-photon emission computed tomography (SPECT) imaging demonstrating hypometabolism in the frontal or anterior temporal regions could be used to diagnose probable bvFTD.

Definitive diagnosis of bvFTD requires the patient to meet the criteria for possible or probable bvFTD but must also include histopathological evidence of FTD on biopsy or at post mortem or the presence of a known pathogenic mutation.

The diagnosis of the PPA variant of FTD is made when clinician evaluation shows a patient to have prominent and progressive difficulty with language as the primary source of impairment in daily activities. Aphasia not otherwise attributed to another neuropsychiatric disorder is the most notable language deficit noted. There are several variants to the PPA variant of FTD [2].

There is no cure for the disease. Speech and language therapy can be useful in patients to help them maintain social and language functions and physical therapy can be used to help maintain motor functions in those with variants that have prominent motor symptoms. Patient-centered nonpharmacologic interventions focused on decreasing triggers of problematic behaviors should be attempted prior to or concurrent with pharmacologic interventions. There have been studies that have reported improvements in behavioral symptoms with selective serotonin reuptake inhibitors and stimulants have been tried with some success to address disinhibition, apathy, and risk-taking behavior. Studies with memantine and cholinesterase inhibitors have shown no benefit.

Antipsychotics are options for the treatment of agitation and psychosis but should be used with extra caution. Riluzole is FDA-approved for the treatment of the ALS variant of FTD and has been shown to have modestly prolonged survival. Its mechanism is to reduce the release of glutamate, an excitatory transmitter that is involved in the degeneration of motor neurons in ALS.

Take-Home Points

- Frontotemporal dementia is the name of a group of dementias that primarily involve the frontal and temporal lobes of the brain. They are progressive neurodegenerative disorders that are typically diagnosed in individuals under the age of 65.
- Diagnosis of FTD involves a comprehensive neurological evaluation, including labs and MRI or CT, as well as neuropsychological testing to assess cognitive and language function. In some cases, genetic testing may be recommended.
- Symptoms of FTD are variable and depend on the subtype of disease but most show some changes in behavior, personality, language, and movement. A history of insidious onset of apathy and lack of concern for self should raise the possibility of FTD.
- There is no cure for the disease. Speech and language therapy can be useful in patients to help them maintain social and language functions. Physical therapy can be used to help maintain motor functions in those with variants that have prominent motor symptoms.

References

1. Onyike, C. U., & Diehl-Schmid, J. (2013). The epidemiology of frontotemporal dementia. *International Review of Psychiatry*, 25 (2), 130–137.

2. Gorno-Tempini, M. L., Dronkers, N. F., Rankin, K. P., Ogar, J. M., Phengrasamy, L., Rosen, H. J., & Miller, B. L. (2004). Cognition and anatomy in three variants of primary progressive aphasia. *Annals of Neurology: Official Journal of the American Neurological Association and the Child Neurology Society*, 55 (3), 335–346.

Greaves, C. V., & Rohrer, J. D. (2019) An update on genetic frontotemporal dementia. *Journal of Neurology*, 266 (8), 2075–2086. doi: 10.1007/s00415-019-09363-4. Epub 2019 May 22. PMID: 31119452; PMCID: PMC6647117.

Rascovsky, K., Hodges, J. R., Knopman, D., Mendez, M. F., Kramer, J. H., Neuhaus, J., & Miller, B. L. (2011). Sensitivity of revised diagnostic criteria for the behavioural variant of frontotemporal dementia. *Brain*, 134 (9), 2456–2477.

Further Reading

Desai, A., & Grossberg, G. (2018). *Psychiatric Consultation in Long-Term Care. A Guide for Healthcare Professionals.* 2nd ed. (Cambridge University Press.)

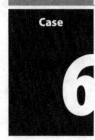

"Leave Me Alone"
Agitation in MNCD

For several weeks, Mrs. L, who has MNCD due to probable Alzheimer's disease in a moderate stage, had been growing agitated in the afternoon and evening and was attempting to leave the long-term care facility. She would become physically aggressive when prevented from leaving and often yelled, "Leave me alone, let me go."

Mrs. L was taking citalopram 20 mg daily, donepezil 10 mg daily in the morning, and memantine 10 mg twice daily for MNCD and anxiety symptoms. These medications had helped decrease Mrs. L's agitation to some extent, but she continued to have at least one incident a week of physical aggression toward staff.

Mrs. L was referred to a consultant psychiatrist for potential medication changes to "control her aggression." After a comprehensive psychiatric evaluation with team discussion, the psychiatrist ruled out easily correctable causes (e.g. anticholinergic medication, medical conditions). The psychiatrist met with the team members (Mrs. L's family, a certified nursing assistant, licensed practical nurse, and social worker) and discussed various potential SPPEICE that could be instituted. Mrs. L's daughter mentioned that her mother had always loved to work in the house rather than watch TV or play games. Mrs. L had never had pets and did not like them and had never been a regular listener of music.

The team decided to give Mrs. L simple tasks, such as setting the table, folding napkins, and putting letters in envelopes. Other interventions, such as pets or music groups, were not selected. After two weeks of implementing these person-centered approaches, Mrs. L had become significantly less distressed, as shown by a reduction in agitated behaviors, and was more easily reassured and redirected.

Teaching Points

Agitation is a neuropsychiatric syndrome that is commonly seen in those with MNCDs. Those demonstrating agitation can show an increase in motor activity, restlessness, emotional distress, and physical or verbal aggressiveness. The estimated prevalence of agitation in those with MNCD is estimated to be 30–50% of those with Alzheimer's disease, 30% of those with DLB, 40% in FTD, and 40% in vascular dementia. It is the third most common neuropsychiatric symptom in dementia after apathy and depression. Up to 80% of people with dementia experience some degree of agitation at some point during the course of their illness.

Agitation in dementia can take many forms such as restlessness, pacing, verbal or physical aggression, and resistance to care. It can be triggered by a variety of factors, including pain, discomfort, environmental changes, and communication difficulties.

Collectively, agitation in those with MNCD produces a very high burden to the health-care system. Agitation increases caregiver burnout, the need for hospital admissions, and medication burden, and even increases mortality.

Assessing agitation can be somewhat subjective but this can be aided by the use of rating scales such as the Pittsburgh agitation scale [1]. The Cohen-Mansfield Agitation Inventory is a rating scale filled out by caregivers that can help assess the degree of agitation and response to treatment [2].

There are several possible overlapping causes or triggers of agitation in MNCD. Agitation is likely related to degenerative changes in the brain that regulate mood and behavior, more specifically, pathology in the function of the anterior cingulate cortex and orbitofrontal cortex. Increased sensitivity to noradrenergic signaling has been described, which is possibly due to a frontal lobe upregulation of adrenergic receptors that happens as a reaction to the depletion of noradrenergic neurons within the locus coeruleus. This might explain the abnormal reactivity to weak stimuli and global arousal found in many patients with MNCDs.

Agitation can be a normal response for those with MNCD when they are experiencing physical discomfort or pain and seemingly innocuous changes in the environment can also be triggers. Examples include changes in routine, moving to a new room or facility, surroundings that are too warm or cool, hunger, or an increase in ambient noise. Agitation can also be seen in dysfunction in social interactions such as those seen with caregiver stress and loneliness.

Prevention of agitation is the goal. Knowing a resident well includes knowing a resident's personality, favorite people, preferences for activities, preferences for foods, personal and family history, and a wide variety of other factors. Long-term care facilities often make a point of including pages of intake information when admitting a new resident in an effort to provide a more comfortable environment for them.

In regard to the case of Mrs. L, attempts were made to get to know the patient better. Knowing the resident well (including the resident's role in life before entering long-term care, the resident's daily interests, and what activities give the resident meaning in life [life history]) is key to significantly improving the success rate of SPPEICE. If the team had not tried to address Mrs. L's underlying need to feel useful and engage in activities that gave meaning to her life, her agitation and aggression could have continued and she may even have been prescribed antipsychotic medication, putting her at risk of accelerated cognitive and functional decline.

It is good to note that nonpharmacologic interventions are often key to minimizing episodes of agitation in those with MNCD. Environmental interventions focus on changing the living environment to reduce agitating triggers and create a calmer atmosphere. Reducing ambient noise levels, providing adequate lighting, ensuring a comfortable temperature, and trying to create a home-like environment as much as possible can be helpful environmental interventions.

Sensory interventions focus on reducing sensory inputs that can trigger agitation and increasing sensory inputs that can improve relaxation. Making sure that residents have a favorite comfortable chair to sit in and a comfortable warm bed to sleep in is key. Shower times can be easier when a resident is not exposed to water that they may find too hot or cold. Washing one body area at a time while others are kept covered can also lead to more comfort and dignity. Living areas that are quieter and more private can allow residents to have some quiet time to themselves. Patient-tailored sensory interventions that can be helpful also include massage therapy, music therapy, aromatherapy, and therapeutic touch. The utilization of music in long-term care settings has received particularly favorable attention in the literature [3].

Psychosocial interventions focus on addressing the underlying psychological and emotional needs of the patient that may contribute to agitation. Interventions can include providing social interactions with other residents such as "mocktail" hour, games, and group entertainment. Some patients may respond positively to being involved in simple "chores" that can help them feel more useful and less bored. Pet therapy is becoming more common in long-term care settings and can provide emotional comfort and a way to connect with others. Exercise programs not only provide an opportunity for maintaining strength and agility but can also provide another venue for interacting with peers.

Social interventions should be tailored to the individual needs and preferences of the patient. What works for one patient may not work for another, so it is important to involve the patient and their caregivers in the intervention planning process. Additionally, social interventions should be implemented in conjunction with other treatments, such as medication or medical interventions, as appropriate.

The pharmacologic management of agitation in those with MNCDs is complex and many studies have shed light on the topic. The treatment may depend on the acuity of the agitated behaviors and the underlying subtype of MNCD. In those with Alzheimer's disease, selective serotonin reuptake inhibitors (SSRIs), trazodone, mirtazapine, prazosin, and low-dose atypical antipsychotics can be trialed. At the time of writing, brexpiprazole had recently been FDA approved for the treatment of agitation in Alzheimer's disease [4]. Rivastigmine can be trialed in those with DLB or PD-D [5].

Agitation can also be related to dopaminergic drugs such as carbidopa/levodopa, particularly when combined with SSRIs or serotonin–norepinephrine reuptake inhibitors (SNRIs). If an atypical antipsychotic is thought to be warranted, an agent with low D2 receptor affinity such as quetiapine is probably preferred. Trazodone, SSRIs, and atypical antipsychotics can be tried for patients with agitation related to frontotemporal dementia. Those with vascular dementia may respond well to SSRI with second- or third-generation antipsychotics being preferred in more significant agitation or agitation with psychosis.

Take-Home Points

- Agitation is a neuropsychiatric syndrome that is commonly seen in those with MNCDs. Those demonstrating agitation can show an increase in motor activity, restlessness, emotional distress, and physical or verbal aggressiveness.
- Agitation in dementia can take many forms such as restlessness, pacing, verbal or physical aggression, and resistance to care.
- Agitation is the third most common neuropsychiatric symptom in dementia after apathy and depression. Up to 80% of people with dementia experience some degree of agitation at some point during the course of their illness.
- The pharmacologic management of agitation in those with MNCDs is complex and many studies have shed light on the topic. At the time of writing brexpiprazole had recently been FDA approved for the treatment of agitation in Alzheimer's disease.

References

1. Rosen, J., Burgio, L., Kollar, M., Cain, M., Allison, M., Fogleman, M., & Zubenko, G. S. (1994). The Pittsburgh Agitation Scale: A user-friendly instrument for rating agitation in dementia patients. *The American Journal of Geriatric Psychiatry*, 2 (1), 52–59.

2. Cohen-Mansfield, J., & Libin, A. (2004). Assessment of agitation in elderly patients with dementia: Correlations between informant rating and direct observation. *International Journal of Geriatric Psychiatry*, 19 (9), 881–891.

3. Pedersen, S. K., Andersen, P. N., Lugo, R. G., Andreassen, M., & Sütterlin, S. (2017). Effects of music on agitation in dementia: A meta-analysis. *Frontiers in Psychology*, 8, 742.

4. Grossberg, G. T., Kohegyi, E., Mergel, V., Josiassen, M. K., Meulien, D., Hobart, M., Slomkowski, M., Baker, R. A., McQuade, R. D., & Cummings, J. L. (2020). Efficacy and safety of brexpiprazole for the treatment of agitation in Alzheimer's dementia: Two 12-week, randomized, double-blind, placebo-controlled trials. *American Journal of Geriatric Psychiatry*, 28 (4), 383–400. doi: 10.1016/j.jagp.2019.09.009. Epub 2019 Oct 1. PMID: 31708380.

5. Hershey, L. A., & Coleman-Jackson, R. (2019). Pharmacological management of dementia with Lewy bodies. *Drugs Aging*, 36 (4), 309–319. doi: 10.1007/s40266-018-00636-7. PMID: 30680679; PMCID: PMC6435621.

Further Reading

Desai, A., & Grossberg, G. (2018). *Psychiatric Consultation in Long-Term Care. A Guide for Healthcare Professionals.* 2nd ed. (Cambridge University Press.)

Gitlin, L. N., Kales, H. C., & Lyketsos, C. G. (2012). Nonpharmacologic management of behavioral symptoms in dementia. *JAMA*, 308 (19), 2020–2029. doi: 10.1001/jama.2012.36918. PMID: 23168825; PMCID: PMC3711645.

Haight, R. J., Di Polito, C. N., Payne, G. H., Bostwick, J. R., Fulbright, A., Lister, J. F., & Williams, A. M. (2023). Psychotropic stewardship: Advancing patient care. *Mental Health Clinician*, 13 (2), 36–48. doi: 10.9740/mhc.2023.04.036. PMID: 37063939; PMCID: PMC10094994.

Keszycki, R. M., Fisher, D. W., & Dong, H. (2019). The hyperactivity–impulsivity–irritiability–disinhibition–aggression–agitation domain in Alzheimer's disease: Current management and future directions. *Frontiers in Pharmacology*, 10, 1109. doi: 10.3389/fphar.2019.01109. PMID: 31611794; PMCID: PMC6777414.

Salzman, C., Jeste, D. V., Meyer, R. E., Cohen-Mansfield, J., Cummings, J., Grossberg, G. T., Jarvik, L., Kraemer, H. C., Lebowitz, B. D., Maslow, K., Pollock, B. G., Raskind, M., Schultz, S. K., Wang, P., Zito, J. M., & Zubenko, G. S. (2008). Elderly patients with dementia-related symptoms of severe agitation and aggression: Consensus statement on treatment options, clinical trials methodology, and policy. *Journal of Clinical Psychiatry*, 69 (6), 889–898. doi: 10.4088/jcp.v69n0602. PMID: 18494535; PMCID: PMC2674239.

Testad, I., Corbett, A., Aarsland, D., Lexow, K., Fossey, J., Woods, B., & Ballard, C. (2014). The value of personalized psychosocial interventions to address behavioral and psychological symptoms in people with dementia living in care home settings: A systematic review. *International Psychogeriatrics*, 26 (7), 1083–1098. doi:10.1017/S1041610214000131

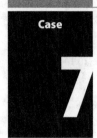

Case

"I Am Fine"
Apathy Syndrome

Mr. L, an 80-year-old married, retired business entrepreneur, moved to an assisted living (AL) home after experiencing difficulty managing day-to-day activities and an inability to take care of his home. He was also forgetting to take his medications. His wife of 48 years also moved with him, as Mr. L would not move otherwise. She was experiencing severe stress from caregiving and could not continue to care for Mr. L at home. She also had her own health problems, including severe rheumatoid arthritis.

Over six months, Mrs. L had noticed that Mr. L had stopped initiating conversation, avoided going to social gatherings, and became irritated when she insisted that they attend at least some of the family functions that they had been attending for more than four decades. Mr. L would spend a major part of the day watching TV and avoid changing clothes, only taking baths when Mrs. L became adamant that he do so. Mrs. L was concerned that her husband was depressed and requested a psychiatric consultation.

Mrs. L told the psychiatrist that her husband had always enjoyed company, had many interests that he shared with friends and family (such as golf and hunting), and had always looked forward to family events. She related that Mr. L had bypass surgery in the previous year and had experienced a slow recovery. Some of the symptoms of lack of motivation may have started a month or two after the surgery, but Mrs. L noticed that in the six months before the consultation, Mr. L was "definitely not himself." Mr. L did not mind being interviewed by the psychiatrist, stated, "I am fine," and did not understand his wife's concerns. Mr. L had neither a personal nor a family history of depression, answered all of the psychiatrist's questions in short sentences, and did not initiate any conversation. He denied feeling down, reported that he was content with his life, denied any problems with sleep or appetite, feeling pessimistic or hopeless, and did not feel he was a burden to others. He denied feeling that life was not worth living. He said that he had several interests but that he was "too old" for golf and hunting and enjoyed watching TV. His SLUMS score was 21 and a head CT showed lacunae in the right basal ganglia and pons. All other laboratory tests were normal.

The psychiatrist diagnosed apathy in the context of mild, vascular type MNCD (vascular dementia [VaD]). Neuropsychological testing confirmed significant frontal lobe dysfunction (as indicated by severe executive dysfunction). Mr. L's wife was educated about apathy and how it differed from depression. The psychiatrist also explained various treatment options. Mrs. L preferred nondrug interventions as opposed to experimental medication trials. Mr. L had always loved music and agreed to see a music therapist once a week on an individual basis. He also agreed to help his great-grandson with a life history project that would involve reminiscing about

Mr. L's successful professional career. The psychiatrist counseled Mrs. L not to insist that Mr. L attend social and family events and to lower her expectations regarding daily bathing, becoming content with twice-weekly bathing. The psychiatrist also recommended that she see a social worker for individual counseling to address the stress of caregiving and the grief of losing parts of her husband's original personality. After 12 weeks, Mrs. L's depression had decreased significantly, and Mr. L showed mild interest in music therapy and in his life history project. He was agreeable to continuing these activities.

Teaching Points

Apathy syndrome is a frequently observed condition among older adults, particularly in long-term care environments, and its prevalence varies depending on the specific population under study. Estimates suggest that up to 70% of individuals with Alzheimer's disease, 40% of those with Parkinson's disease, and 38% of those with late-life depression may experience symptoms of apathy [1]. It is also commonly seen in those with a history of TBI and stroke but can be seen in virtually any neurodegenerative disease.

Apathy syndrome is a clinical condition characterized by a lack of motivation, interest, or emotional responsiveness. It involves a reduced or diminished ability to initiate and sustain goal-directed behavior, leading to a general indifference or disinterest in one's surroundings, activities, or social interactions. Individuals with apathy syndrome may exhibit a lack of enthusiasm, initiative, or drive, often appearing uninterested or detached from their usual activities or responsibilities. They may display decreased involvement in hobbies, reduced social interaction, and diminished emotional expression. Apathy syndrome can significantly impact a person's daily functioning, productivity, and overall quality of life. Patients do not meet the criteria for apathy if symptoms can be better explained by other factors such as intellectual, physical, or motor disability, changes in level of consciousness, or the direct effect of substance use.

Depression is also common in neurocognitive disorders, making the need to distinguish between the two conditions more pertinent for those who regularly care for those in the long-term care setting. It is possible to have comorbid depression and apathy syndrome associated with the underlying neurocognitive disease. Co-occurrence rates of apathy and depression are estimated at 14–38% in those with neurocognitive disorders [2].

The Apathy Evaluation Scale was developed by Robert S. Marin, MD, and has several versions that can be self-administered or administered by a caregiver or clinician [3]. The problem does not come from the recognition of apathy syndrome, but in the treatment. Medical treatment should focus on optimizing treatment of the underlying condition, such as Alzheimer's or Parkinson's disease, or underlying neurocognitive disorder. Attention should be paid to rule out underlying psychiatric conditions such as depression. Apathy is common in depression, but straightforward apathy syndrome lacks the typical symptoms of depression such as sadness, helplessness, hopelessness, impaired sleep, changes in appetite, and so on.

Apathy is often most concerning to family members. Concerned caregivers will most often bring the symptoms of apathy to the attention of the clinician. Apathy is associated with a high degree of caregiver burden and distress.

There are no FDA-approved treatments for apathy syndrome. A study in 2018 of pharmacologic interventions for apathy in Alzheimer's disease revealed sparse evidence to support the use of antidepressants for this indication [4]. Despite the lack of efficacy, up to one-third of patients with apathy with no depression were found to be on antidepressants [5]. Differentiating accurately between apathy and depression is crucial due to the potential link between the use of SSRIs and higher rates of apathy. Among older adults without dementia, the utilization of SSRIs was a strong predictor of apathy, showing a higher occurrence when compared to non-SSRI antidepressants. The mechanism behind increased apathy in older adults treated with SSRIs is not well understood but it is thought that the elevated levels of serotonin might lead to alterations in dopamine and downregulation of dopaminergic receptors, thereby causing downregulation of responses to both rewarding and aversive stimuli and the development of apathy [6].

A study by Rosenberg et al. showed significant improvement in apathy in Alzheimer's disease with the use of methylphenidate [7]. Another study in 2021 by Mintzer et al. also showed efficacy in treating apathy in Alzheimer's disease with methylphenidate [8]. Therefore, methylphenidate at a dose of 10 mg bid may be a worthwhile intervention. Some clinicians may be hesitant to use a stimulant such as methylphenidate in frail older adult patients due to concerns over appetite suppression or increased cardiovascular complications. Stimulant use in older adults has been shown to have more of a positive effect on appetite. A study by Tadrous et al. in 2021 did find an increase of 40% in cerebrovascular events such as heart attack, stroke, and tachyarrhythmias at 30 days for those older adults prescribed stimulants when compared to those not using stimulants. This increased risk was not seen at 180 days or 365 days of stimulant use [9]. Box 7.1 gives a suggested approach to starting an older adult patient with apathy syndrome on methylphenidate.

It also may be worthwhile trialing one of several other medications that have been used with sporadic success in cases of severe apathy syndrome. These medications might

---

Box 7.1 Suggested approach to starting an older adult patient with apathy syndrome on methylphenidate

1. Identify a patient with potential apathy syndrome.
2. Rule out potential medical mimickers of apathy syndrome such as hypothyroidism, medication side effects, and depression.
3. Institute some nonpharmacologic interventions as listed in Table 2.
4. Take extra caution and gain informed consent from patients with apathy syndrome, a history of stroke, coronary artery disease, or tachyarrhythmias. Stimulants have shown an increased risk of adverse cerebrovascular and cardiac complications in older adults in the short term. These negative effects may attenuate with time.
5. Discuss the use of stimulant medication with the patient and surrogate. Explain the risks and benefits of the medication.
6. Initiate methylphenidate at 5 mg twice daily (morning and midday). Evaluate for effect and tolerability after 2–4 weeks.
7. Consider increasing the dose of methylphenidate to 10 mg twice daily if inadequate response to 5 mg bid dosing.
8. Re-evaluate after another 4–6 weeks. Consider discontinuing medication if no improvement in apathy syndrome is noted with methylphenidate 10 mg bid dosing.

Box 7.2 Nonpharmacologic interventions that may help with apathy syndrome

1. Consider being more authoritarian by initiating potentially pleasurable activities for those with apathy syndrome. For example, a statement such as, "It's time for our walk," may be better received than, "Would you like to go for a walk now?"
2. Establish routines for scheduled activities. A schedule that includes regular activities such as exercise, crafts, socializing, games, and outdoor activities can create positive momentum and help to combat apathy.
3. Make sure activities are appropriate to the level of function for those with minor or major neurocognitive disease. A short game of Yahtzee or bingo may be more well-received than an outing to the symphony, for example.
4. Gradually increase the level of engagement. Start with short, easy, pleasurable activities and gradually work up to those activities that may be more involved.
5. Create a living environment that is full of stimulating and interesting things.
6. Tie together activities that are less appealing to a patient with activities that are always appealing to a patient. For example, stopping for an ice cream cone after a visit to the pharmacy or a trip to the doctor's office.
7. Consider including exercise, music therapy, multisensory stimulation, and pet therapy in the regular schedule of a person with apathy syndrome.

include modafinil, bupropion, dopamine agonists such as pramipexole or amantadine, or cholinesterase inhibitors (donepezil, rivastigmine) [10].

Nonpharmacologic interventions are often more helpful than medications in apathy syndrome. Caregivers and clinicians should encourage social interactions, involvement in group activities, and maintaining social connections. This can help combat isolation and improve motivation. A long-term care environment that is structured, supportive, and stimulating can reduce apathy. Regular physical activity has been shown to improve apathy as well. See Box 7.2 for further recommendations on nonpharmacologic interventions that may be helpful for apathy syndrome.

Take-Home Points

- Apathy syndrome is a clinical condition characterized by a lack of motivation, interest, or emotional responsiveness. It involves a reduced or diminished ability to initiate and sustain goal-directed behavior, leading to a general indifference or disinterest in one's surroundings, activities, or social interactions.
- Apathy syndrome is a frequently observed condition among older adults, particularly in long-term care environments. Estimates suggest that up to 70% of individuals with Alzheimer's disease, 40% of those with Parkinson's disease, and 38% of those with late-life depression may experience symptoms of apathy.
- Some studies have shown improvement in apathy syndrome with methylphenidate. Initiate methylphenidate at 5 mg twice daily (morning and midday). Evaluate for effect and tolerability after 2–4 weeks. Consider increasing the dose of methylphenidate to 10 mg twice daily if inadequate response to 5 mg bid dosing.

References

1. Chen, P., Guarino, P. D., Dysken, M. W., Pallaki, M., Asthana, S., Llorente, M. D., & Sano, M. (2018). Neuropsychiatric symptoms and caregiver burden in individuals with Alzheimer's disease: The TEAM-AD VA cooperative study. *Journal of Geriatric Psychiatry and Neurology*, 31 (4), 177–185.

2. Lanctôt, K. L., Ismail, Z., Bawa, K. K., Cummings, J. L., Husain, M., Mortby, M. E., & Robert, P. (2023). Distinguishing apathy from depression: A review differentiating the behavioral, neuroanatomic, and treatment-related aspects of apathy from depression in neurocognitive disorders. *International Journal of Geriatric Psychiatry*, 38 (2). https://doi.org/10.1002/gps.5882

3. Marin, R. S., Biedrzycki, R. C., & Firinciogullari, S. (1991). Reliability and validity of the Apathy Evaluation Scale. *Psychiatry Research*, 38 (2), 143–162.

4. Ruthirakuhan, M. T., Herrmann, N., Abraham, E. H., Chan, S., & Lanctôt, K. L. (2018). Pharmacological interventions for apathy in Alzheimer's disease. *Cochrane Database of Systematic Reviews*, (5). DOI: 10.1002/14651858.CD012197.pub2

5. Benoit, M., Andrieu, S., Lechowski, L., Gillette-Guyonnet, S., Robert, P. H., & Vellas, B. (2008). Apathy and depression in Alzheimer's disease are associated with functional deficit and psychotropic prescription. *International Journal of Geriatric Psychiatry: A journal of the psychiatry of late life and allied sciences*, 23 (4), 409–414.

6. Ma, H., Cai, M., & Wang, H. (2021). Emotional blunting in patients with major depressive disorder: A brief non-systematic review of current research. *Frontiers in Psychiatry*, 12, 792960.

7. Rosenberg, P. B., Lanctôt, K. L., Drye, L. T., Herrmann, N., Scherer, R. W., Bachman, D. L., & Mintzer, J. E. (2013). Safety and efficacy of methylphenidate for apathy in Alzheimer's disease: A randomized, placebo-controlled trial. *The Journal of Clinical Psychiatry*, 74 (8), 810. https://doi.org/10.4088/JCP.12m08099

8. Mintzer, J., Lanctôt, K. L., Scherer, R. W., Rosenberg, P. B., Herrmann, N., Padala, P. R., Brawman-Mintzer, O., Porsteinsson, A. P., Lerner, A. J., Craft, S., Levey, A. I., Burke, W., Perin, J., & Shade, D. (2021). Effect of methylphenidate on apathy in patients with Alzheimer disease: The ADMET 2 randomized clinical trial. *JAMA Neurology*, 78 (11), 1–9. https://doi.org/10.1001/jamaneurol.2021.3356

9. Tadrous, M., Shakeri, A., Chu, C., Watt, J., Mamdani, M. M., Juurlink, D. N., & Gomes, T. (2021). Assessment of stimulant use and cardiovascular event risks among older adults. *JAMA Network Open*, 4 (10). https://doi.org/10.1001/jamanetworkopen.2021.30795

10. Desai, A., & Grossberg, G. (2018). *Psychiatric Consultation in Long-Term Care. A Guide for Healthcare Professionals*. 2nd ed. (Cambridge University Press.) pp. 148–151.

Further Reading

Dickson, S. S., & Husain, M. (2022) Are there distinct dimensions of apathy? The argument for reappraisal. *Cortex*, 149, 246–256. doi:10.1016/j.cortex.2022.01.001

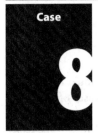

"Those Children Are Cute"
Cholinesterase Inhibitors and Memantine

Ms. L was an 84-year-old widow who had MNCD due to probable Alzheimer's disease and was admitted to an assisted living home because of increasing problems with agitation, incontinence, lack of self-care, and wandering. She had been in the AL home for more than six months. The family had noticed that, even when Ms. L had been living in her home, she talked about children coming into her house and bringing cats and dogs. Over four months, Ms. L was having periods of agitation and anxiety over "little children" going through her belongings. She was also complaining of being upset with the AL staff because they would allow cats and dogs to roam freely into her room. Ms. L was referred to the psychiatrist for the management of hallucinations.

On evaluation, she was not taking any medication that could have caused hallucinations, nor was she having any physical aggression or depressive symptoms. Ms. L was taking memantine 10 mg twice daily and donepezil 10 mg daily, as well as medications for hypertension (hydrochlorothiazide and atenolol) and hyperlipidemia (simvastatin). She did not complain of any new physical health problems, and family and staff reported that episodes of agitation and hallucination occurred once or twice a week. Staff reported that Ms. L participated in activities, slept well, and had a good appetite.

When the psychiatrist inquired how staff and family dealt with Ms. L's complaints, they reported that they would try to convince Ms. L that she was imagining things and that there were no children or animals coming to her room. Staff and family said that often this would agitate Ms. L even more. The psychiatrist inquired about Ms. L's personality before the MNCD, and the family reported that she had always been active and liked to be busy and "on the go."

During the interview, Ms. L denied having any problems, denied being in physical pain, reported feeling "fine," said "yes" to feeling bored and lonely, but reported good sleep and appetite. She stated that "those children are cute" and did not seem bothered by their presence in her room. Her mental status exam showed significant short-term memory loss (recall was 0/3), and her SLUMS score was 12.

The psychiatrist explained to the family and staff that visual hallucinations were a symptom of MNCD such as Alzheimer's disease and that current symptoms were best managed with SPPEICE [1]. The psychiatrist recommended that family and staff not correct or argue with Ms. L, but try to reassure and then distract her. The psychiatrist, together with family and staff, devised a daily activity schedule that would involve more activities that staff and family could engage Ms. L in (e.g. reminiscing with old photos, listening to preferred music, reading the Bible to Ms. L) and a short nap in the afternoon. Ms. L continued to have transient visual hallucinations but her agitation during those periods gradually decreased, and the staff became more adept at distracting Ms. L after reassuring her that they would "take care" of the problem promptly.

Teaching Points

Alzheimer's disease is the most common form of MNCD, causing gradual declines in many areas of cognition. Alzheimer's disease accounts for 60–70% of cases of dementia worldwide and causes a gradual deterioration of various cognitive domains, including decision-making, language, memory, learning, orientation, and judgment [2]. The exact pathophysiology of cognitive decline in dementia is still being intensely studied but one of the pillars of our understanding of Alzheimer's disease and some other dementias is a gradual development of acetylcholine deficiency in key neural pathways. Cholinesterase inhibitors such as donepezil, rivastigmine, and galantamine slow down the breakdown of acetylcholine within the synapses, thereby effectively increasing the available acetylcholine within neural pathways involved in cognition (Table 8.1).

Donepezil is a prototypical cholinesterase inhibitor (ChEi) and was approved for use in 1996. It is FDA-approved for the treatment of mild, moderate, or severe Alzheimer's disease and is considered a symptomatic treatment for Alzheimer's disease and some other dementias as it does little to alter the course of the disease. It may have benefits in cognition, mild neuropsychiatric symptoms, and possibly delay the need for transfer to a

Table 8.1 Medications commonly used in MNCD: Cholinesterase inhibitors and memantine.

Medication	Starting Dose and Dosing Schedule	Therapeutic Daily Dose (Range)
Donepezil	5 mg once a day after meals, may increase every four weeks by 5 mg to highest tolerated therapeutic daily dose	5–23 mg
Rivastigmine transdermal patch	4.6 mg/24-hour patch applied on a clean, dry, hairless part (upper back usually), may be increased every four weeks to the highest tolerated therapeutic daily dose	9.5–13.3 mg
Rivastigmine	1.5 mg twice daily after meals, may increase every four weeks by 3 mg/day to the highest tolerated therapeutic daily dose	6–12 mg
Galantamine extended release	8 mg once daily after meals, may increase every four weeks by 8 mg to the highest tolerated therapeutic daily dose	16–24 mg
Memantine extended release	7 mg once daily, may increase by 7 mg every seven days to the highest tolerated therapeutic daily dose	14–28 mg (7–14 mg for residents who have creatine clearance less than 30)
Memantine	5 mg once a day, may increase by 5 mg per week to the highest tolerated therapeutic daily dose	20 mg in two divided doses (5–10 mg for residents who have creatine clearance less than 30)

care facility for those with mild-to-moderate disease. The side effects of donepezil and other cholinesterase inhibitors are well-known and include possible insomnia, diarrhea, muscle cramps, nausea, and loss of appetite. Donepezil is usually dosed in the morning due to the risk of insomnia and should be avoided, along with other cholinesterase inhibitors, in those with known bradyarrhythmia or sick sinus syndrome.

When counseling patients and families on the use of cholinesterase inhibitors it is important to inform them that studies of these medications indicate that improvements in measures of cognition are generally modest. Side effects are also somewhat common and are usually GI-related. A trial of donepezil is warranted for nearly all patients with Alzheimer's disease. Rivastigmine is FDA-approved for Parkinson's dementia and is often used off-label for DLB. There is less support for the use of ChEis in vascular dementia and they are not indicated for FTD.

Dosing of donepezil usually starts at 5 mg daily. If a patient or caregiver notes improvement in cognition, it is appropriate to encourage the patient to continue with the medication and increase the dose to 10 mg daily if tolerated. If there are GI side effects to lower doses of donepezil, a few different approaches can be taken. A dose of donepezil can be taken at bedtime, which may help with the experience of GI side effects. Donepezil can also be switched to transdermal rivastigmine. Transdermal rivastigmine, although more costly, is known to have much lower GI side effects. A more complete list of strategies to deal with ChEi intolerance is presented in Box 8.1. If these strategies to improve tolerance of the medication are unsuccessful or there are other side effects or worsening of neuropsychiatric symptoms it is probably advisable to discontinue the medication.

Another medication that is FDA-approved for the treatment of moderate-to-severe Alzheimer's disease is memantine. It acts as an NMDA receptor antagonist within the CNS and thereby helps to blunt the excitotoxic effects of glutamate and potentially delay the progression of the disease. Memantine is generally well tolerated when titrated to a goal dose of 20 mg daily. Some patients may experience an exacerbation of neuropsychiatric symptoms with memantine, and this may be a reason for discontinuing the medication during the titration phase. Memantine is probably more effective as a disease-modifying agent than as a medication to improve symptoms of MNCD [3]. It can be used either alone or in combination with acetylcholinesterase inhibitors.

The use of a combination of cholinesterase inhibitor and memantine is recommended for all Alzheimer's disease patients if tolerated [4]. In December 2014, the FDA approved the

Box 8.1 Strategies to improve tolerance of ChEi donepezil

1. If nausea is encountered try moving the dose to bedtime.
2. Decrease the starting dose of donepezil to 2.5 mg and move to a bedtime schedule.
3. If symptoms are relatively mild it is appropriate to watch and wait. Side effects often decrease with time.
4. In patients that report nightmares or sleep disturbance consider changing the dosing schedule to morning dosing.
5. Discontinue the ChEi and start memantine. Donepezil or other ChEis may be better tolerated after a patient has been started on memantine. Some limited evidence suggests that memantine may make the initiation of ChEis better tolerated.
6. Consider switching oral donepezil, rivastigmine, or galantamine to a transdermal rivastigmine patch or a transdermal once weekly donepezil patch. The patch is likely to be better tolerated with reduced gastrointestinal side effects.

combination of donepezil and memantine extended release for patients with moderate-to-severe Alzheimer's disease. Combination therapy has been shown to provide benefits over ChEis alone and may postpone the need for admission to a skilled nursing facility. The increased cost of the fixed-dose combination donepezil/memantine formulation should be weighed against the lower cost of standard generic donepezil/memantine separate product dosing. The fixed-dose combination formulation may be useful for those who desire decreased pill burden and those with dysphagia as it can easily be sprinkled onto soft foods.

Once a ChEi has been started and seems well tolerated it may be a challenge to keep patients and caregivers motivated to continue the medication, especially as major neurocognitive disorders will invariably continue to produce cognitive and behavioral declines. In these cases, it can be helpful to remind caregivers that there are benefits to continuing medications for dementia even in light of continued decline. The advantages to maintaining the medication include continued slowing of the decline in cognition, delaying the need for a higher level of care, and potentially delaying the need for medications to address neuropsychiatric symptoms.

Another scenario to occasionally present itself to a provider who often cares for older adults is when to stop medications for dementia when the dementia is quite advanced. The stages of MNCD often progress in a stepwise fashion according to the Functional Assessment Staging (FAST) scale (see Figure 8.1). The FAST scale was developed by

Stage	Stage Name	Characteristic
1	Normal Aging	No deficits whatsoever
2	Possible Mild Cognitive Impairment	Subjective functional deficit
3	Mild Cognitive Impairment	Objective functional deficit interferes with a person's most complex tasks
4	Mild Dementia	IADLs become affected, such as bill paying, cooking, cleaning, traveling
5	Moderate Dementia	Needs help selecting proper attire
6a	Moderately Severe Dementia	Needs help putting on clothes
6b	Moderately Severe Dementia	Needs help bathing
6c	Moderately Severe Dementia	Needs help toileting
6d	Moderately Severe Dementia	Urinary incontinence
6e	Moderately Severe Dementia	Fecal incontinence
7a	Severe Dementia	Speaks 5-6 words during day
7b	Severe Dementia	Speaks only 1 word clearly
7c	Severe Dementia	Can no longer walk
7d	Severe Dementia	Can no longer sit up
7e	Severe Dementia	Can no longer smile
7f	Severe Dementia	Can no longer hold up head

Figure 8.1 FAST scale [5].

> **Box 8.2** Questions to address when considering discontinuing medications for dementia
>
> 1. What is the stage of dementia? In patients in the final stages of dementia, a reasonable argument can be made to consider discontinuing medications unlikely to continue to give meaningful improvements in quality of life.
> 2. What are the goals of care of the family/caregivers?
> 3. Is the patient showing potential signs and symptoms of becoming poorly tolerant of the medication, such as diarrhea, nausea, vomiting, weight loss, agitation from possible GI upset?
> 4. Has the patient had increased neuropsychiatric symptoms when tapering these medications in the past?
> 5. Is the patient having difficulty swallowing medications?

Dr. Barry Reisberg and his colleagues at the New York University School of Medicine's Aging and Dementia Research Center. The scale was designed to assess and stage the functional decline associated with Alzheimer's disease and other dementias. It provides a framework for tracking and describing the progression of functional impairment in individuals with dementia.

Those patients with FAST scores in the 7s are considered to be in the final stage of the disease. During this stage, there may be a question as to the continued benefit of dementia medications. Caregivers should be given enough information to make an informed shared decision with the clinician. On one hand, discontinuing ChEis in those who have taken them for some time can potentially lead to decreased cognitive function or an increase in neuropsychiatric symptoms. On the other hand, discontinuing these medications could lead to a decreased pill burden and potentially decreased side effects of the medication(s). It can be difficult for those with advanced dementia to voice concern for side effects and it can be reasonable to discontinue ChEis in those with suspicion of GI side effects (decreased appetite, nausea/vomiting, diarrhea, signs of abdominal discomfort). Questions to consider with caregivers when deciding when to discontinue medications for dementia are presented more fully in Box 8.2.

> **Take-Home Points**
>
> - Alzheimer's disease is the most common form of MNCD, causing a gradual decline in many areas of cognition. Alzheimer's disease accounts for 60–70% of cases of dementia worldwide.
> - Once a ChEi has been started and seems well tolerated it may be a challenge to keep patients and caregivers motivated to continue the medication, especially as MNCDs will invariably continue to produce cognitive and behavioral declines.
> - Donepezil is a prototypical ChEi and was approved for use in 1996. It is FDA-approved for the treatment of mild, moderate, or severe Alzheimer's disease and is considered a symptomatic treatment for Alzheimer's disease and some other dementias as it does little to alter the course of the disease.
> - The advantages of maintaining patients on ChEis include continued slowing of the decline in cognition, delaying the need for a higher level of care, and potentially delaying the need for medications to address neuropsychiatric symptoms.

References

1. Desai, A., & Grossberg, G. (2017). *Psychiatric Consultation in Long-Term Care (A Guide for Healthcare Professionals).* 2nd ed. (Cambridge University Press.)

2. Sharma, K. (2019). Cholinesterase inhibitors as Alzheimer's therapeutics. *Molecular Medicine Reports*, 20 (2), 1479–1487. https://doi.org/10.3892/mmr.2019.10374

3. Knorz, A. L., & Quante, A. (2022). Alzheimer's disease: Efficacy of mono- and combination therapy. A systematic review. *Journal of Geriatric Psychiatry and Neurology*, 35 (4), 475–486. https://doi.org/10.1177/08919887211044746

4. Deardorff, W. J., & Grossberg, G. T. (2015). A fixed-dose combination of memantine extended-release and donepezil in the treatment of moderate-to-severe Alzheimer's disease. *Drug Design, Development and Therapy*, 10, 3267–3279. https://doi.org/10.2147/DDDT.S86463

5. Reisberg, B. (1988). Functional assessment staging (FAST). *Psychopharmacology bulletin*, 24 (4), 653–659. PMID: 3249767.

Further Reading

Boer, D. D., Nguyen, N., Mao, J., Moore, J., & Sorin, E. J. (2021). A comprehensive review of cholinesterase modeling and simulation. *Biomolecules*, 11 (4). https://doi.org/10.3390/biom11040580

DeTure, M. A., & Dickson, D. W. (2019). The neuropathological diagnosis of Alzheimer's disease. *Molecular neurodegeneration*, 14 (1), 1–18.

Guo, J., Wang, Z., Liu, R., Huang, Y., Zhang, N., & Zhang, R. (2020). Memantine, donepezil, or combination therapy: What is the best therapy for Alzheimer's disease? A network meta-analysis. *Brain and Behavior*, 10 (11). https://doi.org/10.1002/brb3.1831

Kobayashi, H., Ohnishi, T., Nakagawa, R., & Yoshizawa, K. (2016). The comparative efficacy and safety of cholinesterase inhibitors in patients with mild-to-moderate Alzheimer's disease: A Bayesian network meta-analysis. *International Journal of Geriatric Psychiatry*, 31 (8), 892–904.

Walczak-Nowicka, Ł. J., & Herbet, M. (2021). Acetylcholinesterase inhibitors in the treatment of neurodegenerative diseases and the role of acetylcholinesterase in their pathogenesis. *International Journal of Molecular Sciences*, 22 (17). https://doi.org/10.3390/ijms22179290

Case

9

"Those Terrible Men Have Left"
Agitation in MNCD

Mrs. S was a 78-year-old woman who had DLB and was living in an AL home. Over several months, she had been expressing concerns that men were in her "home" telling her to do inappropriate acts like take down her pants. Mrs. S would typically start yelling at 3 pm that she can see "the man" in the trees looking into her room. She was not sleeping well, and she used foul language toward staff during personal care. Over a period of four weeks, Mrs. S had become physically aggressive toward staff, hitting, slapping, kicking, and biting them. Individualized activities and attention had initially been successful, but during those four weeks her behavior was not manageable. She was referred to the consulting psychiatrist for the management of aggression. On examination, the psychiatrist found that Mrs. S had mild muscle stiffness, restricted affect, and persecutory delusions. The medication review did not identify any medication as potentially being responsible. She was taking rivastigmine 3 mg twice daily with meals. She had a history of not tolerating a higher dose of rivastigmine and could not tolerate memantine. Laboratory tests were within normal limits and urine analysis was negative for infection.

Staff and family were counseled regarding the possibility of engaging in personalized activities and interventions to reduce Mrs. S's agitation. For example, one staff member would engage Mrs. S from 2 pm onward in a coloring activity and another staff member would close the curtains in her room so that when Mrs. S would go there she would not see trees outside her window. Additionally, only female staff were allowed to provide personal care.

The risk of stroke and premature death associated with the use of atypical antipsychotics was explained to the family, as well as the risks of not giving an antipsychotic at all. The family agreed to a trial of low-dose quetiapine. Mrs. S was started on quetiapine 12.5 mg in the morning and at bedtime daily. She developed daytime sedation and hence her quetiapine was shifted to 25 mg daily at bedtime. After one week, her sleep had improved but the agitation and aggression persisted, so the quetiapine was increased to 37.5 mg daily at bedtime and, after four days, to 50 mg daily at bedtime. She had mild daytime sedation, but it resolved over five days. Over the next two weeks, her agitation and aggression improved significantly, she allowed most activities of daily living (ADL) care, and stated, "I am so glad those terrible men have left," and felt relieved. She still expressed periodic concern that the men were coming and going through her suitcases and her drawers but could be reassured and distracted most of the time. After three months, the quetiapine was tapered and then discontinued over four weeks. Mrs. S did not show any worsening symptoms.

Teaching Points

This case highlights an important topic in the treatment of those with MNCD. Those with MNCD can demonstrate a wide variety of behaviors that may be considered disruptive and can be attributed to a patient's underlying neuropathology. Terms for the behavioral disturbances seen in MNCD have been referred to a number of ways, including behavioral disturbances, behavioral and psychological symptoms of dementia, responsive behaviors, biopsychosocial–spiritual distress (BPSD), and simple agitation. The term BPSD is the term this author prefers as it stresses that behavioral issues in MNCD are often contributed to by a patient's unmet needs.

The biological and psychological/emotional needs of those with MNCD are the same as those without. The needs of all persons were presented as a "hierarchy of needs" by Abraham Maslow in 1943 and his model is still a useful way of conceptualizing human needs today. Physiological or biological needs are considered the most basic and essential for life and include needs such as air, food, water, shelter, and sleep. Safety needs come next in importance and involve being in a safe, secure environment, free from the potential of harm. Needs for love and belonging come next and include the needs of a person to have friendships, love, intimacy, and social connectedness. Esteem needs are one step further up the pyramid and include maintaining dignity and having the respect of others. Self-actualization needs include a person's being able to grow and live up to one's full potential. See Box 9.1.

Biopsychosocial–spiritual distress can be experienced by anyone with unmet needs in any of the above areas. Those with MNCD may be unable to verbally describe their unmet needs but often give other clues as to their presence. Common behavioral signs of unmet biopsychosocial needs are shown in Box 9.2.

Identifying the behaviors of BPSD is the easiest part of the process of addressing them. These behaviors are usually first noted by caregivers or the family of the patient. The clinician should resist the urge to quickly turn to pharmacologic interventions for

---

Box 9.1 Maslow's hierarchy of needs

1. Biological needs.

   Food, water, shelter, acceptable ambient temperature, sleep.

2. Safety needs.

   Having a safe and secure environment free from the threat of physical or emotional harm. Being free of pain.

3. Needs for love and belonging.

   Having strong interpersonal relationships, a need for intimacy, being able to give and receive affection, and social connectedness.

4. Esteem needs.

   Maintaining dignity and having the respect of others.

5. Self-actualization needs.

   Being able to live up to one's full potential.

Box 9.2 Potential signs of BPSD in those with MNCD

Restlessness: The older adult may exhibit constant movement, pacing, or fidgeting.
Aggression: This may include hitting, kicking, biting, pinching, and so on. Verbal aggression includes behaviors such as shouting, cursing, or making threats to others.
Verbal outbursts: The individual may engage in continuous or repetitive vocalizations, such as yelling, screaming, or making nonsensical sounds.
Agitation during personal care: Bathing, dressing, or other routine activities may trigger agitation.
Agitation in the evening (sundowning): Increased restlessness, confusion, and agitation during the late afternoon or evening.
Wandering and exit seeking: The person may walk aimlessly or pace back and forth without a clear purpose or destination.
Irritability: The individual may become easily frustrated, impatient, or agitated in response to minor triggers or changes in routine.
Social withdrawal: Agitation can lead to a desire to isolate oneself, avoid social interactions, or become emotionally distant. Long-term care residents may be observed spending more time isolated in their rooms or participating less in group activities.
Repetitive behaviors: Engaging in repetitive movements or actions, such as hand-wringing, picking at clothing, or tapping surfaces, can be a sign of agitation.
Increased anxiety or restlessness: The person may appear anxious, exhibit signs of tension, or have difficulty staying still or focused.

behavioral disturbances. Studies suggest that nonpharmacologic interventions are under-utilized [1]. A simple five-minute conversation with a trusted caregiver may quickly identify the unmet biopsychosocial–spiritual needs that can be addressed prior to initiating pharmacologic interventions.

The potential causes of biopsychosocial distress are many and varied. Some are listed in Box 9.3. A true exploration of the possibility of unmet biopsychosocial–spiritual needs takes time. This is time that a busy provider may not have, but the rewards for a few extra minutes of detective work can be well worth it.

Sometimes reasonable consideration has been given to unmet biopsychosocial needs and no identifiable targets for change can be found. In this case, the clinician can turn to possible pharmacologic interventions for anxiety or agitation. At this time the potential of an undiagnosed or inadequately treated primary neuropsychiatric condition should be considered. Diagnosing primary anxiety or mood disorders can be quite difficult in those with MNCD. These patients may be unable to describe their feelings or symptoms and most clues may come from behavioral observations. Those with experience in the primary care or psychiatric care of older adults often develop a high index of suspicion for undertreated or unrecognized mood or anxiety disorders. A trial of an SSRI such as sertraline can be beneficial. Although starting doses are usually smaller for older adults, efforts to slowly increase the dose to one that is well within the therapeutic range will give a higher chance of success. Consider an SNRI such as duloxetine for those with a suspected mood or anxiety disorder with comorbid chronic pain. See Box 9.4 for therapeutic options for anxiety/agitation in older adults.

A few words should be said about the use of antipsychotics for the treatment of agitation and anxiety. The use of antipsychotics is generally reserved for those patients

Box 9.3 Potential unmet biopsychosocial needs in the long-term care setting

1. Loneliness. Is the resident lacking in meaningful connection with loved ones? Has there been a recent loss of a loved one? Potential interventions: Calling involved family members and encouraging visits. Is there a volunteer program to provide visits to those with MNCD? Is pet therapy available? Consider doll therapy for those with moderate–severe MNCD.
2. Boredom. Is there a lack of appropriate activities for the patient? Potential interventions: Ask the activities director and care staff to encourage the patient to participate in scheduled activities or explore new activities. Ask the family about the patient's interests prior to entering the long-term care facility.
3. Pain. Ask about any suspicion of a recent fall or injury, undertreated musculoskeletal pain, urinary tract infection, skin breakdown, or history of headaches, and so on. Potential interventions: Trial of scheduled acetaminophen to treat chronic pain. Trial of duloxetine for the treatment of chronic pain.
4. Hunger. Ask about eating habits. Is the patient eating a light meal or missing meals and becoming agitated prior to the next meal? Potential intervention: Offer appealing snacks in between meals.
5. Toileting issues. Is the resident wet due to infrequent changes? Is the resident guided to the bathroom on a regular basis for bowel movements? Is constipation possible?
6. Difficulty communicating needs. Those with MNCD may have difficulty expressing their needs and wants.
7. Medical interventions: Does the resident have any treatments that are potentially uncomfortable? Is there any room to deprescribe any potentially unnecessary medications that may be contributing to the cumulative side effect burden?
8. Changes in routine. Have there been any potentially anxiety-provoking changes in day-to-day routines?
9. Interpersonal conflicts. Are there any new relationships that could be anxiety-provoking to the resident? Sometimes the loss of a trusted caregiver or the introduction of an unfamiliar one can provoke signs of BPSD.
10. Staff issues. Are staff members overworked? Those with MNCD can sense the distress of others and may react in a like fashion.
11. Issues with other residents. Are there other residents with behavioral issues that may be creating a threatened sense of safety and security?

that are experiencing psychosis. Antipsychotic use should be limited due to the well-known black box status of these medications. It should also be kept in mind that psychosis may be more subtly demonstrated in those with MNCD and thereby more difficult to detect. These patients may not be able to describe their hallucinations or be willing to freely discuss delusions. Some more subtle signs of psychosis in those with MNCD are listed in Box 9.5.

The choice of antipsychotics in older adults with agitation and psychosis is a potentially complicated topic. A clinician would be well served by becoming comfortable with the use of one or two antipsychotics. Every attempt should be made to avoid first-generation antipsychotics as newer atypical antipsychotics are generally better tolerated. At the time of writing, the medication brexpiprazole had recently been FDA-approved for the treatment of agitation in Alzheimer's disease. Barriers to the use of this medication will undoubtedly be cost-related due to the medication's current brand name-only status.

Box 9.4 Potential therapeutic options for anxiety and agitation in those with MNCD

Consider:

1. SSRIs (sertraline, fluoxetine). Can be quite effective if suspicion of an underlying mood disorder. May take weeks for clinical response.
2. SNRIs (duloxetine/venlafaxine). Consider if underlying chronic pain. May take weeks for clinical response. Tapering can cause mild to moderately uncomfortable withdrawal syndrome.
3. Trazodone. Generally considered safe in older adults. Mild sedating effects of this antidepressant can be effective for anxiety. Results can be seen soon after the dose is given. Consider routine administration if there are regular signs and symptoms of anxiety. Can be given prn.
4. Buspirone. Can be effective. Often prescribed at an inadequate dose. The dose should be increased to at least 30 mg daily (divided). May take some weeks for a response.
5. Gabapentin. The anxiolytic effects can be brisk. Generally well tolerated at low to moderate doses. Avoid high doses in older adults due to side effects. Must be dosed 2–3 times daily due to short half-life.
6. Mirtazapine. Low doses of 7.5–15 mg have a mild sedative effect. Dosed at night. May help with nighttime anxiety and insomnia. Good appetite stimulant and may be a good choice if anxiety with comorbid malnutrition.
7. Propranolol. Small doses of propranolol (10 mg bid) can be helpful.

Avoid:

1. Benzodiazepines. Older adults can have worsening cognition and worsening disinhibited behaviors and increased falls with benzodiazepines. Risks usually outweigh benefits.
2. Antihistamines (hydroxyzine, diphenhydramine). Although well tolerated and effective in younger adults they should be avoided in older adults due to anticholinergic effects.
3. Antipsychotics (quetiapine, risperidone, olanzapine, aripiprazole). These should be reserved for those who may be experiencing psychotic symptoms.

Box 9.5 Potential signs of psychosis in those with MNCD

1. Screaming out as if afraid in the absence of threat.
2. Picking at the skin as if responding to bugs or other irritants.
3. Extreme agitation with personal care. The patient may be mistaking caregivers for strangers with ill intent during personal care.
4. Talking to oneself. This may be a sign that a patient is responding to internal stimuli/voices.
5. Signs of compulsive behaviors, repetitive maladaptive behaviors, or repetitive bizarre behaviors. Behaviors such as these can be a sign of psychosis.
6. Presence of paranoia. Patients with subtle psychosis may have persistent false beliefs that others are out to harm or steal from them. A common psychotic delusion in those with MNCD is the thought of spousal infidelity or that loved ones are stealing money or treasured belongings.

If antipsychotics are indicated, they must be prescribed "off label" (all but brexpiprazole). For this reason, the provider should clearly document the indication of the need for the antipsychotic. The suspicion or observations of psychotic behaviors should be documented in the medical record as it should be clear to any interested party why these potentially high-risk medications were needed.

Special note should also be made when considering antipsychotic choices in those with MNCD due to Parkinson's disease or related DLB. These patients are almost universally sensitive to the D2-blocking effects of nearly all antipsychotics. The best medications for psychosis in these conditions are clozapine (should probably be prescribed after consulting with a psychiatrist), quetiapine (due to lower affinity for D2 receptors/lower side effects), and pimavanserin (does not bind to D2 receptors). Pimavanserin is an excellent choice but can be limited by cost and insurance coverage.

It is great when a course of antipsychotic medication is successful in controlling anxiety or agitation related to psychosis in those with MNCD. Within a relatively brief period (weeks or months) the provider should consider tapering the medication off or to the lowest effective dose possible. Although these medications can be quite effective, the side effects of increased risk of falls and potentially increased cardiovascular complications warrant limiting their use to the lowest dose possible for the shortest length of time clinically indicated.

Take-Home Points

- Biopsychosocial–spiritual distress, also known as agitation, can be experienced by anyone with unmet biological needs, safety needs, need for love and belonging, and need for self-actualization.
- Common unmet biopsychosocial needs in long-term care can include loneliness, boredom, pain, hunger, toileting issues, difficulty communicating needs, medical interventions, changes in routine, interpersonal conflicts, staff issues, and conflicts with other residents.
- Signs of potential BPSD can include restlessness, aggression, agitation, sundowning, wandering, exit seeking, social withdrawal, repetitive behaviors, and increased anxiety.
- Potential signs of psychosis in those with MNCDs can include screaming out, picking at the skin, extreme agitation with personal care, talking to oneself, signs of compulsive behaviors, and the presence of paranoia. The presence of psychosis in MNCD may warrant the use of antipsychotic agents.

References

1. Aigbogun, M. S., Cloutier, M., Gauthier-Loiselle, M., Guerin, A., Ladouceur, M., Baker, R. A., Grundman, M., Duffy, R. A., Hartry, A., Gwin, K., & Fillit, H. (2019). Real-world treatment patterns and characteristics among patients with agitation and dementia in the United States: Findings from a large, observational, retrospective chart review. *Journal of Alzheimer's Disease*, 77 (3), 1181–1194. https://doi.org/10.3233/JAD-200127

Further Reading

Ballard, C., Corbett, A., Orrell, M., Williams, G., Moniz-Cook, E., Romeo, R., Woods, B., Garrod, L., Testad, I., Woodward-Carlton, B., Wenborn, J., Knapp, M., & Fossey, J. (2018). Impact of person-centered care training and person-centered activities on quality of life, agitation, and antipsychotic use in people with dementia living in nursing homes: A cluster-randomized controlled trial. *PLoS Medicine*, 15 (2). https://doi.org/10.1371/journal.pmed.1002500

Carrarini, C., Russo, M., Dono, F., Barbone, F., Rispoli, M. G., Ferri, L., Di Pietro, M., Digiovanni, A., Ajdinaj, P., Speranza, R., Granzotto, A., Frazzini, V., Thomas, A., Pilotto, A., Padovani, A., Onofrj, M., Sensi, S. L., & Bonanni, L. (2021). Agitation and dementia: Prevention and treatment strategies in acute and chronic conditions. *Frontiers in Neurology*, 12, 644317.

Published 2021 Apr 16. doi:10.3389/fneur.2021.644317

Grossberg, G. T., Kohegyi, E., Mergel, V., Josiassen, M. K., Meulien, D., Hobart, M., Slomkowski, M., Baker, R. A., McQuade, R. D., & Cummings, J. L. (2020). Efficacy and safety of brexpiprazole for the treatment of agitation in Alzheimer's dementia: Two 12-week, randomized, double-blind, placebo-controlled trials. *The American Journal of Geriatric Psychiatry*, 28 (4), 383–400. https://doi.org/10.1016/j.jagp.2019.09.009

Ijaopo, E. O. (2017). Dementia-related agitation: A review of non-pharmacological interventions and analysis of risks and benefits of pharmacotherapy. *Translational Psychiatry*, 7 (10), e1250. https://doi.org/10.1038/tp.2017.199

Marcinkowska, M., Śniecikowska, J., Fajkis, N., Paśko, P., Franczyk, W., & Kołaczkowski, M. (2020). Management of dementia-related psychosis, agitation and aggression: A review of the pharmacology and clinical effects of potential drug candidates. *CNS drugs*, 34 (3), 243–268. https://doi.org/10.1007/s40263–020-00707-7

Watt, J. A., Goodarzi, Z., Veroniki, A. A., Nincic, V., Khan, P. A., Ghassemi, M., Lai, Y., Treister, V., Thompson, Y., Schneider, R., Tricco, A. C., & Straus, S. E. (2020). Comparative efficacy of interventions for reducing symptoms of depression in people with dementia: Systematic review and network meta-analysis. *The BMJ*, 372. https://doi.org/10.1136/bmj.n532

Case

"I Saw the Heavenly Gates"
10 End-of-Life Care in MNCD

Mr. U, a 78-year-old male in the late stages of MNCD due to Alzheimer's disease, had developed acute bleeding from the rectum and his wife was not sure if she should admit him to the hospital or opt for hospice care. The long-term care provider involved in Mr. U's treatment helped Mrs. U understand the futility of hospitalization and that Mr. U would have wanted only comfort care at that point. Mrs. U agreed that her husband would have wanted comfort care only, but she wanted to be sure that she was not "giving up" on him. The couple's daughter and son felt sure that their father would want comfort care only. After their children's input, Mrs. U decided to forgo hospitalization and opted for hospice care. Her dilemma was understandable because just three months before, Mr. U was walking, seemed to enjoy his wife's company, and could feed himself with assistance although he could not recognize family members (including his wife) by name. He had developed pneumonia and Mrs. U had opted for hospitalization and treatment at that time. Although the pneumonia was treated successfully, Mr. U developed severe agitation and delirium in the hospital and needed antipsychotic medication to control agitation. When he returned to the nursing home, he used a wheelchair, had lost the ability to feed himself, had severe speech problems (was extremely difficult to understand), and was able to articulate only some words but not full sentences.

After Mr. U was enrolled in a hospice, the family and staff were surprised to learn that two staff members on different occasions had heard Mr. U clearly state, "I saw the heavenly gates" and "I was told to come back later." Mrs. U asked their pastor to come for spiritual support and to help her understand Mr. U's statements. The pastor suggested that maybe Mr. U was waiting for his wife to say goodbye and say that it was okay for him to go. Mrs. U followed the pastor's advice, and three days later Mr. U died peacefully with his wife holding his hand and their children present at the bedside.

Teaching Points

Even in the terminal stages of MNCD, an individual may be able to say complete sentences on rare occasions. Spiritual needs are more important than ever in the care of a resident during this time. The help of chaplains, members of the clergy, and fellow members of the resident's faith community is crucial for the well-being of many residents and their families. Families may also need guidance to say "goodbye" and understand that allowing nature to take its course (and thus allowing a natural dying process) is not "giving up" but "letting go."

Primary healthcare providers and mental health professionals are likely to be engaged with family or care staff with questions regarding end-of-life care issues in those in the terminal stages of MNCDs. Those who provide care in the long-term care setting should be familiar with issues regarding end-of-life care in MNCD. Medical mental health providers and primary providers should also be comfortable initiating conversations with family members of those with progressing MNCDs. Important issues to discuss with families of those with terminal MNCD are listed in Box 10.1.

Family members may be relatively uninformed when it comes to the true diagnosis of a declining loved one with MNCD. Systems of care are often fragmented at the end of life, without the long-term support of a single primary care physician. This fragmentation of care often leaves families with a suboptimal understanding of diagnoses and anticipated progression of illness.

Goals of care conversations are often difficult and time-consuming for providers. This can result in families that may be underprepared for end-of-life issues when they arise. A suggested template for goals of care conversations is presented in Box 10.2.

Physicians and advanced practice providers (APPs) working with older adults may receive less training in issues of palliative care and hospice care in those with MNCD than is ideal. Palliative care is an approach to medical care that focuses on providing relief from pain, other symptoms, and the physical, emotional, and psychosocial stress that individuals with serious illnesses may experience. The primary goal of palliative care is to improve the quality of life for patients and their families, particularly when dealing with complex, chronic, or terminal medical conditions. Palliative care is usually provided with the oversight of a physician or APP with additional training in the management of

---

Box 10.1   Important topics to cover with families of those with late-stage MNCD

1. Diagnosis.
2. Prognosis.
3. Goals of care.
4. Palliative care versus hospice care.
5. Eligibility for hospice care for those with MNCD.
6. Code status.
7. Receiving appropriate legal counsel regarding end-of-life financial/legal matters.
8. Issues involving nutrition and hydration.

Box 10.2   Important topics to discuss when addressing goals of care with patients and families

1. Assess the level to which patients or surrogates have previously discussed goals of care.
2. Gauge the level of understanding of patients/families of diagnosis and likely disease progression.
3. Discuss the patient's previously expressed end-of-life wishes or documentation thereof.
4. Discuss remaining treatment options or lack thereof for the life-limiting illness.
5. Discuss what an acceptable quality of life would be for a patient.

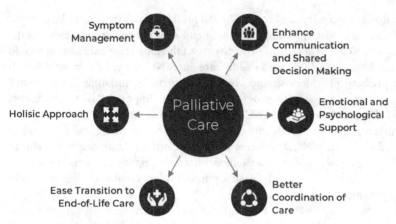

Figure 10.1 Goals of palliative care.

progressive conditions that impact length and quality of life. A good palliative care program is meant to improve symptom management, enhance end-of-life education and shared decision-making, provide additional emotional and psychological support for patients and families, better coordinate care, provide a holistic approach, and ease the transition to end-of-life care when appropriate. See Figure 10.1.

Hospice care is appropriate for patients that are entering the terminal stage of illness and is provided through a licensed hospice agency. The hospice care model focuses on improving comfort and quality of life. It is a holistic approach that encompasses physical, emotional, social, and spiritual support. Hospice care can be provided in almost any care setting including long-term care, assisted living, or private homes. Hospices provide the essential supplies and equipment that are necessary for end-of-life care such as hospital beds, specialty mattresses, Hoyer lifts, wheelchairs, and wound care supplies, among many others. It provides regular nursing assessments and care by nurses specifically trained in end-of-life care. Services through hospice are covered through a patient's Medicare or Medicaid benefits or through a private insurance plan. Some hospice agencies provide free care for those who have no funding source.

Hospice services are not appropriate for all patients and they must have one or more hospice-eligible diagnoses (see Box 10.3). Hospice patients and their families should also be "hospice minded". This refers to a mindset or perspective that aligns with the principles and values of hospice care, with patient-centered care focusing on comfort and symptom management above likely futile disease-focused management. A useful decision tree for determining hospice eligibility is presented in Figure 10.2.

Discussions of code status are delicate but important to have with patients and their surrogate decision-makers. Code status refers to a patient's wishes to undergo "heroic measures" such as CPR, intubation with mechanical ventilation, and advanced life support in the event of cardiopulmonary collapse. Patients and caregivers should be informed that such heroic measures are much less likely to be successful in cases of terminal illness and may be contrary to efforts to comfort the dying and ease the transition from life to death. These conversations may be ongoing with patients and families and can be seen as continuing opportunities to educate them on the dying process.

Determining Hospice Eligibility

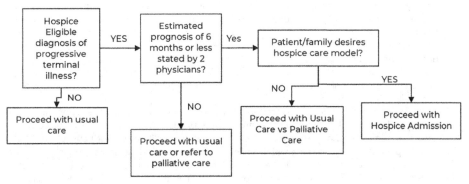

Figure 10.2 Determining hospice eligibility.

Box 10.3   Hospice-eligible conditions

1. Advanced cancer.
2. End-stage heart disease. Congestive heart failure, valvular heart disease, coronary heart disease, and so on.
3. End-stage pulmonary diseases such as chronic obstructive pulmonary disease (COPD), pulmonary fibrosis, cystic fibrosis, and so on.
4. Progressive brain diseases such as Alzheimer's disease, cerebrovascular disease, amyotrophic lateral sclerosis, late effects of cerebrovascular accident, and Parkinson's disease.
5. End-stage renal disease. Dialysis eligible or dependent.
6. Advanced HIV/AIDS.
7. Multiple organ failure.
8. Other progressive terminal illnesses that warrant a predicted prognosis of six months or less.

The interventions of artificial hydration and nutrition in those with late-stage MNCDs can be important to discuss with patients and their families. Primary caregivers are often concerned with their loved one uncomfortably "starving to death" at the end of life. In reality, these conversations can be opportunities to educate families that artificial nutrition and hydration are not in fact adding comfort to the patient in the last days or weeks of life. The absence of food and fluid intake results in ketosis and a release of opioids in the brain, which may produce a sense of comfort or even euphoria [1]. Additionally, the physiologic stress of processing nutrition will eventually be more than the multiple failing organs can handle during the dying process, thereby hastening the end result.

In summary, physicians and other healthcare providers involved in direct patient care of older adults should have a baseline knowledge of end-of-life care topics. Alternatively, many hospice and palliative care physicians and APPs are easily available for consultation and guidance on these topics. Providers should strive to provide excellent care to patients during both life and the dying process.

Take-Home Points

- Primary healthcare providers and mental health professionals are likely to be engaged with family or care staff with questions regarding end-of-life care issues in those in the terminal stages of MNCD. Those who provide care in the long-term care setting should be familiar with the issues regarding end-of-life care in MNCD.
- Hospice care is appropriate for patients who are entering the terminal stage of illness and is provided through a licensed hospice agency. The hospice care model focuses on improving comfort and quality of life. It is a holistic approach that encompasses physical, emotional, social, and spiritual support. Hospice care can be provided in almost any care setting.
- Palliative care is an approach to medical care that focuses on relieving pain, other symptoms, and the physical, emotional, and psychosocial stress that individuals with serious illnesses may experience. The primary goal of palliative care is to improve the quality of life for patients and their families, particularly when dealing with complex, chronic, or terminal medical conditions.
- Discussions of code status are delicate but important to have with patients and the surrogate decision-makers. Patients and caregivers should be informed that heroic measures are much less likely to be successful in cases of terminal illness and may be contrary to efforts to comfort the dying and ease the transition from life to death.

References

1. Schwartz, D. B., Posthauer, M. E., & O'Sullivan, M. J. (2021). Advancing nutrition and dietetics practice: Dealing with ethical issues of nutrition and hydration. *Journal of the Academy of Nutrition and Dietetics*, 121 (5), 823–831. DOI: 10.1016/j.jand.2020.07.028. PMID: 32988795; PMCID: PMC7518202.

Further Reading

Aldridge, M. D., Hunt, L., Husain, M., Li, L., & Kelley, A. (2022). Impact of comorbid dementia on patterns of hospice use. *Journal of Palliative Medicine*, 25 (3), 396–404. https://doi.org/10.1089/jpm.2021.0055

Bartley, M. M., Manggaard, J. M., Fischer, K. M., Holland, D. E., & Takahashi, P. Y. (2023). Dementia care in the last year of life: Experiences in a community practice and in skilled nursing facilities. *Journal of Palliative Care*, 38 (2), 135–142. https://doi.org/10.1177/08258597221125607

Dressler, G., Garrett, S. B., Hunt, L. J., Thompson, N., Mahoney, K., Sudore, R. L., Ritchie, C. S., & Harrison, K. L. (2021). "It's case by case, and it's a struggle": A qualitative study of hospice practices, perspectives, and ethical dilemmas when caring for hospice enrollees with full-code status or intensive treatment preferences. *Journal of Palliative Medicine*, 24 (4), 496–504. https://doi.org/10.1089/jpm.2020.0215

Gilissen, J., Hunt, L., Tahir, P., & Ritchie, C. (2020). Protocol: Earlier initiation of palliative care in the disease trajectory of people living with dementia: A scoping review protocol. *BMJ Open*, 11 (6). https://doi.org/10.1136/bmjopen-2020-044502

Hui, D., Heung, Y., & Bruera, E. (2022). Timely palliative care: Personalizing the process of referral. *Cancers*, 14 (4) https://doi.org/10.3390/cancers14041047

Lassell, K. F., Moreines, L. T., Luebke, M. R., Bhatti, K. S., Pain, K. J., Brody, A. A., & Luth, E. A. (2022). Hospice interventions for persons living with dementia, family members and clinicians: A systematic review. *Journal of the American Geriatrics Society*, 70 (7), 2134. https://doi.org/10.1111/jgs.17802

Miranda, R., Bunn, F., Lynch, J., & Goodman, C. (2019). Palliative care for people with dementia living at home: A systematic review of interventions. *Palliative Medicine*, 33 (7), 726–742. https://doi.org/10.1177/0269216319847092

Mo, L., Geng, Y., Chang, Y. K., Philip, J., Collins, A., & Hui, D. (2021). Referral criteria to specialist palliative care for patients with dementia: A systematic review. *Journal of the American Geriatrics Society*, 69 (6), 1659. https://doi.org/10.1111/jgs.17070

Parast, L., Tolpadi, A. A., Teno, J., Elliott, M. N., & Price, R. A. (2022). Variation in hospice experiences by care setting for patients with dementia. *Journal of the American Medical Directors Association*, 23 (9), 1480. https://doi.org/10.1016/j.jamda.2022.03.010

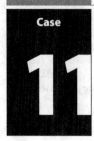

"Leave Me Alone"
Pain Control in MNCD

Mrs. L was an 82-year-old married woman living in a nursing home who had chronic pain, MNCD-mixed-vascular and Alzheimer's type, and chronic major depressive disorder. She had been doing well taking antidepressants (mirtazapine 15 mg at bedtime and duloxetine 60 mg daily) and using a fentanyl pain patch (25 mcg/hour every three days) for more than six months but started showing drowsiness and unsteadiness over the course of two days.

Staff reported that Mrs. L had been shouting at various staff members, "Leave me alone. I don't feel like getting up." The staff called her provider to request as-needed lorazepam to calm her or to reduce her "psych medications" due to drowsiness. The provider recommended an urgent same-day assessment as this behavior was new, of sudden onset, and uncharacteristic. Mrs. L was calm and pleasant during the visit and the provider asked Mr. L if he was aware of Mrs. L's drowsiness and aggressive behavior. Mr. L replied that he had figured out why Mrs. L's condition had changed. He had checked Mrs. L's pain patch and found that the staff had forgotten to remove the previous one when they put on a new patch two days before.

Teaching Points

Although psychiatric medications may sometimes be responsible for sedation and unsteady gait, we recommend a thorough assessment to identify various other potential causes of an acute change in behavior. The healthcare provider should always keep the possibility of medication error in the differential diagnosis, especially if the patient has been stable for some time. Additionally, an informed and astute caregiver (the husband in this case) can often help identify the cause of an acute change in behavior quickly.

The proper assessment and treatment of acute and chronic pain in those with MNCD has a strong influence on mental health. One study found the prevalence of pain from osteoarthritis alone in those over 85 years old to be 72% [1]. Another study estimated that between 40% and 80% of people living with dementia in long-term care homes experience significant acute or chronic pain [2].

Common sources of pain in older adults in the long-term care setting include osteoarthritis/degenerative joint disease, peripheral neuropathy, peripheral vascular disease, osteoporosis with compression fractures, cancer, and pressure wounds. Older adults may present additional challenges to the medical provider when evaluating chronic pain. Some patients may tend toward stoicism and be hesitant to discuss pain issues with their providers. Others may fear the treatment for chronic pain. Some patients are very afraid of addiction, even in the absence of any personal history of substance use or dependence.

The implications of unrecognized pain in those with MNCD are far-reaching. Untreated pain can lead to the destabilization of psychiatric conditions such as anxiety, depression, and agitation. Those with cognitive impairments are more likely to have longer waits for the evaluation of pain and receive weaker analgesia [3]. In 2015, a meta-analysis revealed that individuals residing in nursing homes with MNCD were administered fewer pain-relieving medications compared to those without MNCD, even though they experienced similar occurrences of painful conditions [4]. Undertreated pain can lead to declines in ADL independence and thereby increase the burden on caregivers [5].

The identification of pain in the setting of MNCD can be particularly challenging. Older adults with cognitive impairment have a more difficult time communicating pain and discomfort. Individuals may struggle to remember or accurately describe their pain, leading to inconsistent or unreliable information about their discomfort. Major neuro-cognitive disorders can alter the way pain signals are processed in the brain and can lead to unusual pain responses. The gradually declining ability to communicate can force providers and caregivers to be more observant of behavioral changes that can indicate pain. Behavioral changes such as agitation can be from pain but may also result from frustration, thirst, hunger, and fatigue.

Evaluating pain in those with MNCD is more challenging than in those without dementia. Observational assessments that focus on nonverbal cues of pain include obser-vations of facial expressions, body movements, and vocalizations. Behavior scales such as the PAINAD scale [6] and the Abbey Pain Scale [7] evaluate behaviors associated with pain and provide a numerical score that can be used to assess pain relief interventions. Caregiver input is important as they can offer insights into changes in behavior, mood, and activities that may be associated with pain. Some patients with dementia may still be able to self-report pain to some extent using simple words, gestures, or visual aids. Response to pain medications can also provide clues to the presence of pain. Box 11.1 summarizes the strategies that can assist in pain management in those with MNCD.

Individualized care plans should be developed once pain is recognized and assessed. These care plans should consider the pain source, pain severity, cognitive status of the patient, family preferences, potential side effects, and caregiver abilities. Those condi-tions likely to produce chronic pain should be treated with round-the-clock analgesia. Cognitively intact patients may still be able to express pain and request pain medications for intermittent pain. Pain medications given as needed may be adequate for these patients. Potential side effects should be anticipated such as constipation, sedation, and

---

Box 11.1 Strategies to improve pain evaluation in those with MNCD

1. Observational assessments. These can include observations of facial expressions, body movements, and vocalizations that may indicate pain.
2. Behavioral scales such as PAINAD and the Abbey Pain Scale. These scales can help evaluate and quantify behaviors associated with pain [6,7].
3. Caregiver input. Input from caregivers, family, and nursing staff can provide useful insights into the presence of pain.
4. Self-reporting. Some patients with MNCD are still able to express themselves adequately enough to indicate the presence and nature of pain.
5. Trial of pain medication. A brief trial of pain medication can provide clues to the presence or absence of chronic pain.

worsening cognition. Constipation can be avoided by utilizing prophylactic bowel regimens. Stimulant laxatives (senna or bisacodyl) or osmotic laxatives (polyethylene glycol) are preferred for opioid-induced constipation [8].

As-needed pain medications given to those with MNCD in the long-term care setting may depend too heavily on the judgment of those inadequately trained to assess pain. A long-term care facility often relies heavily on medication aides to pass medications. A registered nurse or licensed practical nurse may be required to assess pain in a long-term care setting and staffing issues often preclude timely assessments or assessments that happen with the frequency needed for adequate pain control. For this reason, regularly scheduled pain medications may be a more appropriate option.

There are usually several options for pain management for any given patient's pain treatment plan. Options can be classified into opiate and non-opiate. Table 11.1 describes the pros and cons of various pain medication classes often used to treat pain in the long-term care setting.

Nonpharmacologic interventions can provide good pain relief in selected individuals. Physical therapy can improve biomechanical issues that may be contributing to musculoskeletal pain. Occupational therapy can provide optimization of day-to-day activities to reduce strain on muscles and joints. Stretching and strength training as directed by a physical trainer or physical therapist can improve day-to-day pain control when part of a comprehensive pain management plan. Heat and cold therapy are low-risk interventions that can provide quick, albeit short-lived pain relief. Transcutaneous electrical nerve stimulation (TENS) devices deliver low-level electrical currents to nerve pathways, potentially providing relief from certain types of musculoskeletal pain [10].

Regular reassessments are required to ensure continuing adequacy of pain management strategies. Pain-causing pathologies are often chronic and progressive and warrant periodic adjustments in pain medication dosing. The assistance offered by a well-trained palliative care provider can be a welcome addition to the care team.

Ethical dilemmas are commonly encountered by those who treat chronic pain in long-term care patients. Balancing pain relief with the potential risks and benefits of medication use in individuals with cognitive impairment involves ethical considerations. This includes understanding the principle of beneficence and ensuring the individual's dignity and quality of life.

Table 11.1 Options for pharmacologic pain management in long-term care settings [9,10].

Drug class	Pros	Cons
Acetaminophen	Generally safe and well tolerated. A good option for mild pain. Few drug–drug interactions and no respiratory depression or sedation issues.	Generally less effective for moderate-to-severe pain. Some patients may have no improvement.
Nonsteroidal anti-inflammatory drugs (NSAIDS)	Can provide pain relief for mild-to-moderate pain. Minimal risk of respiratory depression and sedation. Can decrease inflammation involved in many pain syndromes.	Many drug–drug interactions with medications commonly used in older adults. Should not be given with blood thinners due to increased bleeding risk.

Table 11.1 (cont.)

Drug class	Pros	Cons
		Older adults are at increased risk of GI side effects/bleeding from NSAID. Older adults may be at higher risk of renal side effects due to comorbidities and other medications. Potential increased risk of cardiac complications in those with pre-existing cardiac conditions. May cause blood pressure to increase in those with high blood pressure.
Opiates and opiate derivatives	More effective for moderate-to-severe pain. Doses can be easily titrated to effect.	The risk of sedation, respiratory depression, and worsening cognition is dose-dependent. Chronic use may lead to tolerance and dependence. Potential increase in fall risk due to sedation and dizziness. May be less effective for neuropathic pain.
Antidepressants SNRIs Tricyclics	No risk of respiratory depression. May help treat comorbid mood disorders that often accompany chronic pain. May be used as adjunct agents in chronic pain.	Likely not adequate as monotherapy for moderate or severe chronic pain.
Anticonvulsants Gabapentin Carbamazepine Oxcarbazepine Valproic acid	Preferentially effective for neuropathic pain.	May increase the risk of falls. Cognitive side effects.
Topical agents NSAIDS (diclofenac) Lidocaine patches Menthol	Generally, little if any systemic side effects.	Limited pain relief for some.

Take-Home Points

- The implications of unrecognized pain in those with MNCD are far-reaching. Untreated pain can lead to the destabilization of psychiatric conditions such as anxiety, depression, and agitation. Those with cognitive impairments are more likely to have longer waits for the evaluation of pain and receive less than adequate analgesia.
- Always keep the possibility of medication error in the differential diagnosis for apparent changes in mental status.

- Those with MNCD with inadequately controlled pain may present with atypical symptoms when compared to those without MNCD.
- As-needed pain medications given to those with MNCD in the long-term care setting may depend too heavily on the judgment of those inadequately trained to assess pain. Regularly scheduled pain medication may be a more appropriate option.
- Consider both pharmacologic and nonpharmacologic interventions when formulating a treatment plan for chronic pain in older adults. Opiates may have the best benefit/risk ratio for the treatment of chronic pain in some older adults.

References

1. Duncan, R., Francis, R. M., Collerton, J., Davies, K., Jagger, C., Kingston, A., & Birrell, F. (2011). Prevalence of arthritis and joint pain in the oldest old: Findings from the Newcastle 85+ study. *Age and aging*, 40 (6), 752–755.

2. van Kooten, J., Smalbrugge, M., van der Wouden, J. C., Stek, M. L., & Hertogh, C. M. (2017). Prevalence of pain in nursing home residents: The role of dementia stage and dementia subtypes. *Journal of the American Medical Directors Association*, 18 (6), 522–527.

3. McDermott, J. H., Nichols, D. R., & Lovell, M. E. (2014). A case-control study examining inconsistencies in pain management following fractured neck of femur: An inferior analgesia for the cognitively impaired. *Emergency medicine journal*, 31 (e1), e2–e8.

4. Tan, E. C., Jokanovic, N., Koponen, M. P., Thomas, D., Hilmer, S. N., & Bell, J. S. (2015). Prevalence of analgesic use and pain in people with and without dementia or cognitive impairment in aged care facilities: A systematic review and meta-analysis. *Current clinical pharmacology*, 10 (3), 194–203.

5. van Dalen-Kok, A. H., Pieper, M. J. C., de Waal, M. W. M., van der Steen, J. T., Scherder, E. J. A., & Achterberg, W. P. (2021). The impact of pain on the course of ADL functioning in patients with dementia. *Age Ageing*, 50 (3), 906–913.

doi: 10.1093/aging/afaa247. PMID: 33300044.

6. Paulson, C. M., Monroe, T., & Mion, L. C. (2014). Pain assessment in hospitalized older adults with dementia and delirium. *Journal of Gerontological Nursing*, 40 (6), 10. https://doi.org/10.3928/00989134-20140428-02

7. Tegenborg, S., Fransson, P., & Martinsson, L. (2022). Physicians' and nurses' experience of using the Abbey Pain Scale (APS) in people with advanced cancer: A qualitative content analysis. *BMC Nursing*, 22. www.ncbi.nlm.nih.gov/pmc/articles/PMC10071650/

8. Giorgio, R. D., Zucco, F. M., Chiarioni, G., Mercadante, S., Corazziari, E. S., Caraceni, A., Odetti, P., Giusti, R., Marinangeli, F., & Pinto, C. (2020). Management of opioid-induced constipation and bowel dysfunction: Expert opinion of an Italian multidisciplinary panel. *Advances in Therapy*, 38 (7), 3589–3621. www.ncbi.nlm.nih.gov/pmc/articles/PMC8279968/

9. Wongrakpanich, S., Wongrakpanich, A., Melhado, K., & Rangaswami, J. (2018). A comprehensive review of non-steroidal anti-inflammatory drug use in the elderly. *Aging and Disease*, 9 (1), 143–150. https://doi.org/10.14336/AD.2017.0306

10. Schwan, J., Sclafani, J., & Tawfik, V. L. (2019). Chronic pain management in the elderly. *Anesthesiology Clinics*, 37 (3), 547. https://doi.org/10.1016/j.anclin.2019.04.012

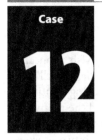

"I Am in Hell and I Will Die in Hell"
Treatment-Resistant Depression and Electroconvulsive Therapy

Mr. S. was an 80-year-old white male with a history of atrial fibrillation, hypertension, Type 2 diabetes, and major depressive disorder (MDD). He was originally admitted to long-term care as he lived alone and was no longer able to look after himself. The consultation with geriatric psychiatry was initially requested as Mr. S had been recently noted to be calling his daughter and making statements of fear regarding his feelings that someone was out to harm him or that people were intentionally ignoring him. He reported to the consulting psychiatrist that he was having intermittent feelings of sadness and was feeling guilty with regard to choices he had made in his younger days. He denied any suicidal or homicidal thoughts, paranoia/delusions, or hallucinations on the day of initial psychiatric evaluation. At the time of the initial evaluation he was on escitalopram 5 mg daily, which was increased to 10 mg daily with thoughts that the patient's MDD was only in partial remission and would respond to a higher dose of SSRI. As time went on Mr. S mentioned several times that he was lonely and felt little ability to connect with others. His one living family member was his daughter, who lived six or more hours away and was only able to see Mr. S once a month or so.

As time went on the increase in SSRI dose, along with weekly psychotherapy, helped the patient's mood symptoms improve. He began to participate in more social activities and started to foster some friendships. After about eight months psychiatry was asked to reevaluate Mr. S as he was again having increasing symptoms of depression. In recent months he had been switched by his primary provider from escitalopram 10 mg daily to sertraline 50 mg daily and mirtazapine 15 mg qhs.

His depression was exacerbated by an abrupt worsening of vision in his right eye. He was already blind in his left eye and was found to have a retinal bleed that made him legally blind. He felt more isolated as his blindness left him much less able to participate in social or recreational activities in the facility. He was also less able to participate in his own care and had become almost totally dependent on caregivers.

Anxiety had become more prominent. His sertraline was increased to 100 mg daily, mirtazapine continued, and buspirone was titrated up to 10 mg tid. Despite medication adjustment, Mr. S continued to become more despondent and was noted to perseverate on his loss of sight and increasing dependence on others. He began making regular passive suicidal statements. His sertraline was stepped up further to 200 mg daily.

During a follow-up visit it was discovered that the patient had a love of classical music. The clinician and patient would spend 30 minutes during visits listening to and discussing their favorite classical music pieces. These interactions seemed to open the patient up to further brief motivational interviewing with a focus on adapting to his new disabilities in positive ways to help his mood and overall outlook. On the next couple of follow-up visits he seemed somewhat improved, and no medication adjustments were made. After two months, Mr. S began again to make passive suicidal statements such as looking forward to the possibility of dying in his sleep. He became continually frustrated and irritable with care staff and increasingly anxious. At a follow-up visit soon after, Mr. S stated to the psychiatry team that "I am in hell, and I will die in hell". His depression was clearly no better and somewhat worse, and he was having continuing difficulty adjusting to his blindness. He was lonely and bored but lacked the motivation to leave his room to participate in activities or be around others. Aripiprazole was started at a dose of 2.5 mg qhs with plans to increase the dose to 5 mg in one to two weeks.

After four weeks Mr. S was found to be no better with regards to his mood symptoms. He had little interest in food and his weight had declined about 10 lbs over six weeks. Mr. S continued to have persistent feelings of guilt and worthlessness and continued to feel that his current life was punishment for misdeeds in his younger years. He was found by nursing staff to be in bed 75% of the day and night and did little else but sit in his room quietly. He declined any efforts by facility staff to include him in facility activities.

The physician discussed the situation with the patient and his daughter. It was pointed out that Mr. S had failed to improve with multiple different medication strategies for his depression. The option of ECT was discussed with the patient and his daughter in great detail. After weighing the risks and benefits of the procedure they decided to proceed with ECT and arrangements were made to transport Mr. S to a local hospital for the treatment. The prescribed course was three treatments weekly for four weeks.

Mr. S tolerated ECT well with only some mild increase in fatigue on days of treatment. After the third treatment, Mr. S admitted to less rumination about past perceived misdeeds and he was noted by facility nursing staff to be eating 50–75% of his meals (up from bites and sips only). After the final treatment, Mr. S was reevaluated and found to be in generally better spirits. He was coming out of his room and participating in facility activities. He was also eating normal portions of meals and was open to participating in individualized psychosocial activities.

Teaching Points

This is a complex case for several reasons. It was felt that the patient never fully adjusted to his move from his home in the community to the nursing home. His limited family/ social support was his daughter, who lived hours away. Mr. S was still cognitively intact and being surrounded by others he saw as cognitively worse off than himself was a source of stress. Despite being in a facility full of friendly residents and staff he had difficulty mixing into the community. The unfortunate development of near-total blindness from a retinal bleed further exacerbated the patient's depression and isolation.

Several appropriate medication interventions were trialed over the course of months with Mr. S. He was started on escitalopram and the dose was increased to the maximum dose recommended in geriatric patients (10 mg). When this proved ineffective, he was switched by his primary team to sertraline. The sertraline was increased to the maximum dose and augmentation was later started with buspirone and then later aripiprazole. This was a clinically sound progression of medication management of MDD with anxiety in a geriatric patient. Consideration was then given to ECT.

A relatively large number of older patients will be resistant to multiple medications and pharmacologic combination strategies. Only 60–70% of patients respond to an adequate trial of two different antidepressants [1]. Treatment-resistant depression (TRD) may require consideration of nonpharmacologic options (see Box 12.1). In cases of TRD, ECT may be a solid choice for treatment in older adults. The efficacy of ECT is high. Studies show response rates of 80–90% for those with severe, especially psychotic depression and response rates of 40–50% for those with TRD [1].

Electroconvulsive therapy is the use of electrical current to induce tonic-clonic seizure activity to produce a therapeutic effect. The technique was first utilized in the 1930s and has had varying popularity over the decades. Despite a negative stigma by the lay public, ECT is considered by many experts to be an underutilized treatment in older adults. Indications for ECT include severe depression, depression with psychotic symptoms, TRD, severe mania, and catatonia (see Box 12.2). It can be particularly useful in

---

Box 12.1 Nonpharmacologic treatment options for those with TRD

1. Transcranial magnetic stimulation (TMS). Expensive. Limited availability [5].
2. Vagal nerve stimulator. Invasive. Very costly. Not covered fully by insurance [4].
3. Psychotherapy. Often helpful but may have limited utility in those with moderate to severe cognitive impairment.
4. Deep brain stimulation. Still considered experimental and trials are available only at limited tertiary centers. Invasive. Risk of infection, intracerebral bleeding, and neurological complications [2].
5. Electroconvulsive therapy. Response rates of 40–50% for those with TRD. Generally well tolerated. Response to treatment is often brisk.

Box 12.2 Major indications for ECT

1. Major depressive disorder with features of:

   a. Suicidality.
   b. Malnutrition.
   c. Psychosis.
   d. Intolerance to effective medications (e.g. severe hyponatremia with SSRIs/SNRIs).
   e. Previous positive response to ECT.

2. Bipolar disorder with features of:

   a. Severe mania with psychosis.
   b. Severe depression with suicidality, inability to care for self, psychosis.

3. Schizophrenia with:

   a. Severe psychosis resistant to antipsychotics.
   b. Severe mood symptoms or severe agitation resistant to medications.
   c. Catatonia.

4. Parkinson's disease with severe depression:

   a. May improve both mood and movement symptoms.

5. Catatonia irrespective of the cause [3].

depression when symptoms are severe and life-threatening, such as in instances of severely reduced nutritional intake, active suicidal ideation, or self-harm. At times like these, there may be more urgency and less time to wait for trials of typical antidepressants that may take weeks for a clinical response.

Side effects of ECT are usually relatively mild and may include transient confusion, headache, retrograde amnesia, nausea, hypertension, and jaw pain. Headache, nausea, and hypertension can be easily treated with medications. Occasionally retrograde amnesia can be significant enough to make future ECT courses less desirable.

The mechanisms by which ECT yields clinical improvement are still not well known. Research has suggested that therapeutic effects are related to neuroinflammation reduction, promotion of new synaptic connections, monoaminergic systems modulation, and the normalization of the activity of the hypothalamus–pituitary–adrenal (HPA) and hypothalamus–pituitary–thyroid (HPT) axes [4].

Despite misunderstandings of the treatment by the lay public, ECT is generally well tolerated and considered one of the most effective treatments for severe MDD. It is safe and rapidly effective in many. Older adults have also been found to have a relatively greater response to ECT than younger adults [1].

Electroconvulsive therapy does pose challenges for patients and caregivers. It can be logistically difficult to arrange the required transportation from a long-term care facility to a facility equipped to provide ECT. The treatments are typically three times weekly for four to six weeks. Electroconvulsive therapy is also not widely available in all smaller community settings. When ECT is indicated and available the results are often likely to be worth the effort.

Transcranial magnetic stimulation is a treatment utilizing an electromechanical medical device to deliver magnetic stimulation using rapidly alternating magnetic fields. The rapidly alternating magnetic fields stimulate the creation of electrical currents within carefully controlled areas of the brain. The first TMS device was FDA approved for the treatment of depression in 2008. A standard course of treatment is five daily treatments per week over the course of four to six weeks. Fewer than one in 1,000 patients will experience a seizure during treatment. Transcranial magnetic stimulation can be done while a patient is receiving antidepressants or other psychotropic medications. Some patients who have benefited from TMS can be continued on less frequent maintenance TMS with good results. Response rates to TMS among those with TRD are reported to be between 45 and 60%. Remission rates are between 30 and 40% [5]. There are challenges to the use of TMS in TRD. It is not widely available in many areas and also involves a commitment from the patient and family to attend daily appointments for four to six weeks. Cost and insurance coverage can also be factors in patient selection for the treatment.

Take-Home Points

- Major depressive disorder is a serious and potentially life-threatening condition common in older adults.
- Only 60–70% of patients respond to an adequate trial of two different antidepressants.
- When patients have TRD a clinician may need to consider nonpharmacologic therapies for depression such as ECT or TMS.

- Reasonable strategies to address TRD in older adults include adding an antidepressant in another class or adding one or more of many available augmentation agents.
- Electroconvulsive therapy is thought by many to be underutilized in those with TRD. Treatment responses to ECT can be brisk and dramatic.

References

1. Dominiak, M., Antosik-Wójcińska, A. Z., Wojnar, M., & Mierzejewski, P. (2021). Electroconvulsive therapy and age: Effectiveness, safety and tolerability in the treatment of major depression among patients under and over 65 years of age. *Pharmaceuticals*, 14 (6) https://doi.org/10.3390/ph14060582

2. Rosenquist, P. B., Miller, B., & Pillai, A. (2014). The antipsychotic effects of ECT: A review of possible mechanisms. *The Journal of ECT*, 30 (2), 125–131.

3. Rojas, M., Ariza, D., Ortega, Á., Riaño-Garzón, M. E., Chávez-Castillo, M., Pérez, J. L., Cudris-Torres, L., Bautista, M. J., Medina-Ortiz, O., Rojas-Quintero, J., & Bermúdez, V. (2022). Electroconvulsive therapy in psychiatric disorders: A narrative review exploring neuroendocrine–immune therapeutic mechanisms and clinical implications. *International Journal of Molecular Sciences*, 23 (13). https://doi.org/10.3390/ijms23136918

4. Kelly, M. S., Oliveira-Maia, A. J., Bernstein, M., Stern, A. P., Press, D. Z., Pascual-Leone, A., & Boes, A. D. (2017). Initial response to transcranial magnetic stimulation treatment for depression predicts subsequent response. *The Journal of Neuropsychiatry and Clinical Neurosciences*, 29 (2), 179. www.ncbi.nlm.nih.gov/pmc/articles/PMC5592731/

5. Mancusi, G., Santovito, M. C., Marrangone, C., Martino, F., Santorelli, M., Miuli, A., Carlo, F. D., Signorelli, M. S., Clerici, M., Pettorruso, M., & Martinotti, G. (2023). Investigating the role of maintenance TMS protocols for major depression: Systematic review and future perspectives for personalized interventions. *Journal of Personalized Medicine*, 13 (4). https://doi.org/10.3390/jpm13040697

Further Reading

Bottomley, J. M., LeReun, C., Diamantopoulos, A., Mitchell, S., & Gaynes, B. N. (2020). Vagus nerve stimulation (VNS) therapy in patients with treatment-resistant depression: A systematic review and meta-analysis. *Comprehensive Psychiatry*, 98, 152156.

Desai, A., & Grossberg, G. (2018). *Psychiatric Consultation in Long-Term Care. A Guide for Healthcare Professionals.* 2nd ed. (Cambridge University Press.) pp. 139–142.

van Rooij, S. J., Riva-Posse, P., & McDonald, W. M. (2020). The efficacy and safety of neuromodulation treatments in late-life depression. *Current Treatment Options in Psychiatry*, 7, 337–348.

"My Mom Looks Like a Zombie!"
Antipsychotic-Related Movement Disorders

Ms. R was a 77-year-old female who had been a resident in long-term care for almost two years. Prior to living in long-term care she lived in a local senior housing building and retained her independence there with the help of her daughter. Her daughter would visit daily and make sure her mother had all her basic needs met and was receiving her medications as prescribed, but was forced to move an hour away because of work. Ms. R had a lifelong history of bipolar disorder. She was diagnosed in her early 30s, at which time she was hospitalized for two to three weeks following her first manic episode. She was on and off her medications frequently and had recurrent hospitalizations related to this throughout her adult life. She became more stable in her 50s when she qualified for federal disability income and her life became less stressful and more routine.

Ms. R had a happy childhood. She had a loving home with two parents and two siblings. Her father was a Methodist minister and her mother stayed at home, taking care of the children and home. She did well in school and went to college for two years where she studied office management. She had been a rather accomplished pianist as well. She married her high school sweetheart and had a happy marriage. She was employed to run a dental office for some years prior to showing signs of extreme stress from both her work and family obligations. She began using over-the-counter weight loss pills to "help me keep up". She then began having difficulty keeping up with her work responsibilities and was eventually hospitalized for a mental breakdown and diagnosed as being "manic depressive".

As Ms. R approached her mid-60s, again she began having more frequent hospitalizations for her bipolar disorder. She was hospitalized on average once every year or two. Her medications were adjusted often as her lithium monotherapy became less and less effective at mood stabilization. She would be stable on a particular combination of medications for an average of two to three years before major medication adjustments would be necessary

At the age of 75, Ms. R moved into a Medicaid-funded bed at a long-term care facility in her small town after one of her psychiatric hospitalizations. This was at the urging of her daughter who was no longer able to provide adequate care oversight in her home due to work obligations. Ms. R settled in surprisingly well at the facility. She was described as sweet and friendly by all the staff at the facility, and she had many friends.

Two years after moving into long-term care, Ms. R started behaving erratically and becoming quite irritable. Her sleep patterns became unusual and she began having conversations with herself, or at times appeared to be speaking to the wall, according to staff. Complicating the situation was the fact that her facility psychiatrist had retired and there were no other psychiatrists that serviced the small town where she lived. She was transferred to the city and was hospitalized for two weeks for an acute manic episode. She was discharged on divalproex 750 mg twice daily and aripiprazole 15 mg qhs, along with prn lorazepam 1 mg q6 hours for anxiety.

Ms. R's daughter came to visit her at the facility and expressed her shock at her mother's appearance. "My mom looks like a zombie!" At the first physician visit post-discharge, she appeared quite different to before her hospitalization. Ms. R was now dependent on a wheelchair for mobility when she had been using a walker before her hospitalization. Her face had a drawn and frozen appearance, her extremities were stiff, and she had a subtle slow tremor noted in her left hand. Ms. R was also much less interactive, and her cognition had slowed. She had a hard time feeding herself and needed help from staff to eat her meals.

The long-term care provider examined Ms. R and reviewed all of her recent hospital documents. She had a head CT with her recent hospitalization that was negative for any acute findings and showed mild age-appropriate changes. Ms. R was checked for a UTI and had her labs checked again, but they did not reveal any acute metabolic issues. Her exam was consistent with Parkinsonism and her long-term care provider thought it likely that these symptoms were induced by the recent addition of aripiprazole as a mood stabilizer during her hospitalization. Her dose of aripiprazole therefore was tapered over two weeks to 5 mg nightly. This improved the Parkinson's features, but Ms. R again began showing signs of impending mania with increased agitation and decreased need for sleep. After consulting with the long-term care provider, Ms. R's daughter requested something be done for the mania short of another hospitalization. The long-term care provider started Ms. R on quetiapine and titrated the dose to 200 mg twice daily. This seemed to avert another manic episode, but Ms. R continued to demonstrate Parkinsonian characteristics. The patient and her daughter were disappointed at the side effects of her medication but were very pleased with the good control of her bipolar disorder.

Teaching Points

Antipsychotic medications are part of the pharmacologic treatment of many psychiatric disorders, including schizophrenia, schizoaffective disorder, bipolar disorder, MDD, and delusional disorder, among others. Much of the management of these conditions is through a mental health specialist such as a psychiatrist or psychiatric nurse practitioner. But many places in the US are underserved by mental health specialists and long-term care providers may be required to provide psychiatric care to their patients.

Some of the more difficult challenges that antipsychotic providers may face are side effects involving drug-induced movement disorders. These are collectively referred to as extrapyramidal side effects (EPS) and are due to the dopamine blocking mechanism of the antipsychotic class of medications.

There are four well-known extrapyramidal symptoms that the provider should be familiar with (see Box 13.1). Three of these presentations can be seen within days and weeks after initiating antipsychotic treatment and include acute dystonia, akathisia, and Parkinsonism. Tardive akathisia and tardive dyskinesia (TD) are considered manifestations of chronic antipsychotic use. Extrapyramidal side effects are more likely to occur with older first-generation antipsychotic medications and are seen less commonly now that the use of second-generation antipsychotics far surpasses older first-generation

Box 13.1 EPS related to antipsychotic use

1. Acute dystonia. Uncontrollable muscle spasms that lead to uncontrollable body movements or postures.
2. Akathisia. A sense of inner restlessness and inability to remain still.
3. Drug-induced Parkinsonism. The presence of Parkinson-like symptoms such as tremors, bradykinesia, rigidity, and difficulty walking.
4. Tardive dyskinesia. Repetitive involuntary movements of the head/neck, trunk, or extremities can develop after long-term use of antipsychotics.
5. Neuroleptic malignant syndrome. An antipsychotic-related acute illness involving severe muscle rigidity, fever, altered mental status, and autonomic instability. Not classically considered to be an EPS but is often discussed with other, more classic extrapyramidal symptoms.

Box 13.2 Potential symptoms of acute dystonia related to antipsychotic use

1. Torticollis. The neck muscles contract involuntarily, causing the head to twist to one side. This is usually uncomfortable or painful.
2. Oculogyric crisis. The eyes involuntarily roll upwards, causing distress and visual disturbances.
3. Opisthotonus. This is extreme arching of the back and can be particularly severe and distressing.
4. Buccolingual crisis. This is the involuntary movement of the tongue or jaw which can be seen as tongue protrusion, lip smacking, and difficulty speaking or swallowing.
5. Retrocollis. Similar to torticollis. The neck arches posteriorly, causing the head to tilt backward.
6. Facial grimacing. This is seen as involuntary puckering of the lips or squinting of the eyes.
7. Laryngospasm. This can potentially lead to difficulty breathing or speaking.
8. Limb and trunk movements. These are less common but can result in unusual, uncontrollable movements of the limbs and unusual body postures.

antipsychotics. The majority of newly-diagnosed EPS are now in patients who are on atypical second-generation antipsychotics.

Acute dystonia is a relatively uncommon occurrence and usually happens early in the treatment with an antipsychotic. Most of the acute dystonic reactions involve the muscles of the face and neck. Box 13.2 lists some common manifestations of acute dystonia related to antipsychotic use.

The treatment of acute dystonic reactions is the swift administration of an antihistamine such as diphenhydramine or benztropine. In the emergency room, these are usually given intramuscularly or intravenously and often produce a swift and dramatic relief of symptoms. Strategies to handle the need for antipsychotics in patients with a history of acute dystonic reactions include prophylactic or ongoing use of an antihistamine medication such as benztropine, using the lowest dose necessary to control the side effects.

Akathisia is a distressing and uncomfortable movement disorder in which patients have a feeling of restlessness and an objective increase in motor activity. People with akathisia often experience an inner sense of restlessness, a strong urge to move, and an inability to sit still. These sensations can be quite distressing and may lead to significant discomfort and agitation. Patients can demonstrate akathisia in several ways. Leg restlessness is common and can be seen as continuous tapping of the feet, pacing, or constantly shifting weight from one leg to the other while standing. It can also be seen when sitting as frequent shifting in the seat or rocking back and forth. Patients with akathisia may also demonstrate an almost complete inability to stand or sit still. Restlessness can also lead to increased anxiety and agitation.

Several interventions can help manage akathisia. Lowering the dose of the antipsychotic can be helpful if this is possible and switching the antipsychotic to an alternative agent may be useful. If these interventions are not successful several medication options may help to lessen the akathisia. These include beta-blockers (propranolol) and benzodiazepines. Beta-blockers such as propranolol may be effective at lower doses and tolerated by older adults. Benzodiazepines may be effective in ameliorating symptoms of akathisia in younger long-term care residents but should be avoided if possible in older adults. Trazodone has shown promise in the treatment of akathisia and is well tolerated in older adults [1]. Low-dose mirtazapine (7.5 mg daily) has also shown promise as a potential treatment for akathisia and is generally well tolerated in older adults.

Parkinsonism related to antipsychotic use clinically looks quite similar to the symptoms of Parkinson's disease with features such as tremors, muscle rigidity, bradykinesia, and postural instability. It can be seen with the use of both first- and second-generation antipsychotics and can develop acutely or gradually. These are relatively common with antipsychotic medications but are much more likely with potent first-generation antipsychotics such as haloperidol. It is estimated that over 50% of patients over 60 on long-term therapy with antipsychotics will experience medication-related Parkinsonism [2]. Drug-induced Parkinsonism is generally treated by stopping the offending antipsychotic medication. If an antipsychotic is required one should be utilized that is known to have less risk of drug-induced Parkinsonism. These agents will have less affinity for dopamine d2 receptors and include quetiapine, clozapine, olanzapine, and brexpiprazole [3]. Parkinsonism usually dissipates within weeks to months after discontinuing the offending agent, but 10–50% of patients may retain Parkinsonian features even after the medication is discontinued. Some of the Parkinsonism seen in older patients on antipsychotics may also suggest a possible unmasking of a previously preclinical Parkinson's disease.

Tardive dyskinesia is considered a late-occurring side effect of antipsychotic medications. It most frequently involves involuntary repetitive movements of the facial muscles but can also affect the neck, hands, limbs, and even walking. It is one of the most feared complications of chronic antipsychotic use as it can dramatically affect a patient's quality of life and lead to social withdrawal and increased depression and anxiety. Older adults have been shown to be at higher risk of TD than younger patients. This is true even when lower doses and shorter courses of antipsychotics are used [4]. Tardive dyskinesia symptoms include grimacing, lip smacking, tongue movements, uncontrolled chewing or teeth grinding, blinking, and arrhythmic head or limb movements. It is hard to treat and often irreversible. Therapeutic strategies to address TD may include changing to another antipsychotic medication less inclined to be associated with TD, adjusting the dose of the implicated medication, or utilizing medications indicated to treat TD. Box 13.3 reiterates strategies to deal with TD.

> **Box 13.3 Strategies to therapeutically address TD**
>
> 1. Regularly monitor antipsychotic medications to ensure that the lowest effective dose is being used to control symptoms.
> 2. Switch medications. Sometimes switching to an antipsychotic less likely to lead to TD can be helpful.
> 3. Reduce or discontinue the antipsychotic medication if possible.
> 4. Use of medications approved to treat TD, including valbenazine, tetrabenazine, and deutetrabenazine.
> 5. Consider referral to a movement disorder neurology specialist for severe or refractory cases.

Valbenazine, tetrabenazine, and deutetrabenazine are FDA-approved agents for the treatment of TD. Chronic antipsychotic use in the long term is thought to upregulate the expression of dopamine receptors in the postsynaptic neuron and also upregulate the release of dopamine into the synaptic cleft by the presynaptic neuron, thereby leading to dysregulation in movement-related brain pathways. Valbenazine, deutetrabenazine, and tetrabenazine inhibit vesicular monoamine transporter 2 (VMAT2) and thereby inhibit the release of dopamine into the synaptic cleft. This reduction in the synaptic concentration of dopamine is postulated to be responsible for the therapeutic reduction in TD movements [5].

Finally, neuroleptic malignant syndrome is a rare but life-threatening emergency related to antipsychotic use. It is more commonly seen with first-generation antipsychotics but can also be seen with atypical antipsychotics. It occurs in 0.04% of the population who receive antipsychotic drugs and can be fatal. Symptoms can develop rapidly and include hyperthermia, severe muscle rigidity, autonomic dysregulation, mental status changes, muscle tremors, difficulty swallowing, and signs of muscle breakdown such as elevated creatine kinase. These patients appear quite ill and are evaluated and treated in emergency and acute care settings. Bromocriptine (a dopamine agonist) and dantrolene (a skeletal muscle relaxant) will likely be the pharmacologic agents used to treat these patients in the acute care setting.

Take-Home Points

- Extrapyramidal symptoms are movement disorders associated with antipsychotics.
- Antipsychotic-related Parkinsonism and akathisia are the most commonly encountered antipsychotic-related movement disorders.
- Extrapyramidal symptoms include acute dystonias, akathisia, Parkinsonism, TD, and neuroleptic malignant syndrome.
- Tardive dyskinesia occurs with long-term antipsychotic use and can be very impactful on quality of life. Treatment options exist for those with TD dependent on antipsychotics.

References

1. Stryjer, R., Rosenzcwaig, S., Bar, F., Ulman, A. M., Weizman, A., & Spivak, B. (2010). Trazodone for the treatment of neuroleptic-induced acute akathisia: A placebo-controlled, double-blind, crossover study. *Clinical Neuropharmacology*, 33, 219–222.

2. Estevez-Fraga, C., Zeun, P., & López-Sendón Moreno, J. L. (2018). Current methods for the treatment and prevention of drug-induced Parkinsonism and tardive dyskinesia in the elderly. *Drugs Aging*, 35, 959–971. doi: 10.1007/s40266-018-0590-y.

3. Shin, W., & Chung, S. J. (2012). Drug-induced Parkinsonism. *Journal of Clinical Neurology (Seoul, Korea)*, 8 (1), 15–21. https://doi.org/10.3988/jcn.2012.8.1.15

4. Solmi, M., Pigato, G., Kane, J. M., & Correll, C. U. (2018). Clinical risk factors for the development of tardive dyskinesia. *Journal of Neurological Sciences*, 389, 21–27.

5. Luo, R., Bozigian, H., Jimenez, R., & Loewen, G. (2017). Single dose and repeat once-daily dose safety, tolerability and pharmacokinetics of valbenazine in healthy male subjects. *Psychopharmacology Bulletin*, 47 (3), 44–52. www.ncbi.nlm.nih.gov/pmc/articles/PMC5546550/

Further Reading

Ali, T., Sisay, M., Tariku, M., Mekuria, A. N., & Desalew, A. (2021). Antipsychotic-induced extrapyramidal side effects: A systematic review and meta-analysis of observational studies. *PLoS ONE*, 16 (9). https://doi.org/10.1371/journal.pone.0257129

Caroff, S. N. (2020). Recent advances in the pharmacology of tardive dyskinesia. *Clinical Psychopharmacology and Neuroscience*, 18 (4), 493–506. https://doi.org/10.9758/cpn.2020.18.4.493

Duma, S. R., & Fung, V. S. (2019). Drug-induced movement disorders. *Australian Prescriber*, 42 (2), 56–61. https://doi.org/10.18773/austprescr.2019.014

Poyurovsky, M., Bergman, J., Pashinian, A., & Weizman, A. (2014). Beneficial effect of low-dose mirtazapine in acute aripiprazole-induced akathisia. *International Clinical Psychopharmacology*, 29, 296–298.

Poyurovsky, M., & Weizman, A. (2018). Very low-dose mirtazapine (7.5 mg) in treatment of acute antipsychotic-associated akathisia. *Journal of Clinical Psychopharmacology*, 38, 609–611.

Ricciardi, L., Pringsheim, T., Barnes, R. E., Martino, D., Gardner, D., Remington, G., Addington, D., Morgante, F., Poole, N., Carson, A., & Edwards, M. (2019). Treatment recommendations for tardive dyskinesia. *Canadian Journal of Psychiatry. Revue Canadienne de Psychiatrie*, 64 (6), 388–399. https://doi.org/10.1177/0706743719828968

Case

"My Soul Is in England"
Treatment of Depression and Anxiety at End of Life

14

Mrs. S was a 91-year-old retired schoolteacher, recovering from recent hospitalization for aspiration pneumonia. She had been lethargic for the first few days after returning from the hospital and then started becoming more anxious, stating, "My soul is in England ... I left it at the airport ... When will it arrive back?" Psychiatric consultation was requested to start antipsychotics as Mrs. S was severely distressed and agitated, yelled off and on for hours, had not slept for two consecutive days, could not be consoled or distracted, and hit staff during personal care.

After a comprehensive assessment, the primary provider diagnosed multifactorial delirium (due to pneumonia and high-dose prednisone [tapered off by the time of the assessment]), as the work-up otherwise was negative. The provider educated the staff and Mrs. S's son that, due to underlying moderate-stage vascular dementia, advanced age, high medical comorbidity, and frailty, Mrs. S was at high risk of adverse effects from antipsychotics, had a limited life expectancy, and was at high risk of recurrent delirium. This was Mrs. S's second aspiration pneumonia and second hospitalization in three months and, per her son, both hospitalizations were a "harrowing experience" for Mrs. S. The primary provider explained to Mrs. S's son and staff that pneumonia in this context could be seen as a friend rather than a foe and discussed the goals of palliative care, as the son shared that this would be in keeping with Mrs. S's values and wishes. The provider prescribed low-dose quetiapine (12.5 mg twice daily) after explaining the risks, including risks of stroke, mortality, dysphagia, and ventricular arrhythmias (as Mrs. S had pre-existing prolonged QTc interval [512 msec] and quetiapine prolongs QTc interval). Her son wanted Mrs. S to be comfortable and not in so much distress. The provider chose quetiapine over haloperidol, risperidone, and olanzapine because Mrs. S had pre-existing mild Parkinsonism due to cerebrovascular disease.

The medical provider also asked the facility chaplain to visit Mrs. S and recommended that the staff and family provide soothing hand massages with lavender lotion and make extra efforts to distract Mrs. S by showing her photos of her grandson and videos of his piano recital. Her son also started visiting more, giving the staff some breaks. Mrs. S's anxiety, agitation, and psychotic symptoms improved with these interventions, and over the subsequent two weeks, quetiapine was decreased and discontinued. The son opted for Do Not Hospitalize intervention and comfort measures only if Mrs. S developed pneumonia again. The pharmacist and primary care team reviewed Mrs. S's medications and discontinued statins, vitamins, aspirin, clopidogrel, and calcium. Staff were educated about the importance of ensuring that Mrs. S regularly wore her glasses and used her dentures to address visual deficits and prevent malnutrition, as both are reversible risk factors for delirium.

Teaching Points

The primary care provider is often the first clinician to recognize the high burden of life-prolonging treatment for a resident who has limited life expectancy and high medical and neurocognitive comorbidity. It is important to explain to residents, their families, and staff about the significant burdens imposed by hospitalization, steroids, and antibiotics on residents who have advanced MNCD. The value of palliative care goals is ensuring that the last weeks and months of life are peaceful, dignified, and without the burden of excessive treatment. The management of delirium also offers an opportunity for the primary provider to provide case-based education that is tailored to the staff's educational needs (in this case, poor recognition of the resident's limited life expectancy, limited understanding of the high burdens of life-prolonging care on many residents, and lack of recognition of the importance of inquiring into Mrs. S's values and wishes regarding palliative care).

There is much crossover in the fields of palliative care and psychiatry. Palliative care refers to specialized medical care provided to individuals with serious illnesses or conditions that are not curable. The goal of palliative care is to improve the quality of life for patients by alleviating symptoms, managing pain, and addressing the physical, emotional, social, and spiritual needs associated with their condition. Common psychiatric syndromes that are encountered in palliative care patients include anxiety with agitation, depression, delirium, insomnia, and others. The approach to psychiatric care in the palliative care setting can be somewhat different as goals of care often focus more on patient comfort than on life-prolonging interventions.

Causes of anxiety in palliative care patients can be categorized as primarily psychiatric, organic, iatrogenic, and existential. Psychiatric causes of anxiety include poorly controlled underlying anxiety or mood disorder or PTSD, for example. Organic causes of anxiety include underlying physical processes such as hypoxia, pain, or sepsis. Examples of iatrogenic causes of increased anxiety would include supratherapeutic doses of thyroid replacement or the use of psychiatric medications that have a potential to be over-stimulating. Existential causes of anxiety include concerns about increasing dependency, disfigurement, the meaning of one's life, leaving one's loved ones, and concerns about what happens after death. Psychosocial stressors can also be contributors to increased anxiety (see Box 14.1).

Clinical depression is also relatively common at the end of life. The prevalence of MDD at the end of life for cancer patients is estimated to be between 5–20% [1]. The contributors to depression at the end of life include: (1) Grief and loss: The awareness of impending death and the experience of significant losses, such as declining health, independence, or the loss of relationships, can trigger feelings of grief and sadness. This grief can manifest as depressive symptoms. (2) Physical discomfort: Pain, fatigue, and other physical symptoms associated with advanced illness can contribute to a decline in overall well-being, affecting mood and potentially leading to depressive symptoms. (3) Social isolation: The end-of-life phase may involve changes in social support networks, as individuals may become more confined to home or require specialized care. Social isolation or a decreased ability to engage in meaningful social interactions can contribute to feelings of loneliness and depression. (4) Existential distress: Reflecting on mortality and the meaning of life can evoke existential questions and concerns. Existential distress, including feelings of hopelessness, regret, or a loss of purpose, can contribute to

Box 14.1 Causes of anxiety at end of life

1. Psychiatric causes include poorly controlled primary psychiatric disorders such as anxiety, depression, PTSD, insomnia, and so on.
2. General medical causes. These are related to physical discomfort from underlying diseases such as dyspnea, pain, nausea, constipation, and so on.
3. Existential causes of anxiety:

   a. concerns about increasing dependency.
   b. concerns of physical disfigurement at end of life.
   c. concerns over leaving loved ones.
   d. concerns over what happens after death.
   e. loss of autonomy.

4. Psychosocial stressors:

   a. dysfunctional family dynamics.
   b. unmet financial needs.
   c. concerns about advancing caregiving needs.
   d. social isolation at the end of life.
   e. legal matters at the end of life.
   f. caregiver burden.

depressive symptoms. (5) Medications and medical treatments: Certain medications or medical interventions used to manage symptoms or prolong life may have side effects that impact mood and contribute to depressive symptoms.

Unfortunately, studies specific to issues regarding the treatment of depression in end-of-life patients are lacking. A common misconception is that depression is an unavoidable and expected response to the dying process. In reality, most terminal cancer patients do not meet the diagnostic criteria for major depression. It can be more difficult to assess for MDD in those at the end of life as many of the vegetative symptoms of depression such as sleep disturbances, alterations in appetite, fatigue, psychomotor retardation, and generalized pain can be attributed to the underlying terminal disease process. For this reason, a high index of suspicion for depression by the healthcare provider is warranted. Thankfully, those that choose to enroll in a hospice at the end of life may have easier access to clinical social workers and spiritual care coordinators that assist them through the psychological and spiritual issues that accompany the dying process.

There are some unique considerations when thinking of treatment options for suspected depressive symptoms at the end of life (Box 14.2).

Box 14.2 Considerations in managing mood symptoms for patients nearing end of life

1. Have a high index of suspicion for depression or anxiety at the end of life.
2. Realize that depression and anxiety are not expected complications of end of life.
3. Early recognition and treatment of depression and anxiety can reduce significant suffering in those at the end of life.
4. Make sure that physical symptoms at the end of life are adequately controlled. Anxiety and depression can be directly related to poorly controlled symptoms such as pain or dyspnea.

Box 14.2 (cont.)

5. Choose psychotropic medications that have a quicker response time when possible. Examples include stimulants for depressive symptoms and benzodiazepines for anxiety. The use of SSRIs, SNRIs, and other more commonly prescribed medications for depression and anxiety may take up to four to six weeks for clinical response.
6. Keep a high index of suspicion for delirium related to the underlying terminal disease process. Modest doses of antipsychotic medications can be effective for treating delirium at the end of life.
7. Hypoactive delirium can be mistaken for depression. Hyperactive delirium can be mistaken for anxiety.
8. Collaboration with other professionals such as clinical social workers, case managers, spiritual care professionals, and psychologists can be essential to providing adequate care to those at the end of life.
9. Side effects of unnecessary treatments can contribute to mood symptoms. Consider the removal of unessential medications that can be of limited benefit and add to morbidity at the end of life. Medications to consider deprescribing might include statins, blood thinners, osteoporosis medications, acetylcholinesterase inhibitors and NMDA receptor blocker medications for MNCD, and any others that do not directly or indirectly contribute to a patient's comfort.
10. Consider the early use of antidepressants that have indications for chronic pain. The use of antidepressants for pain management can address both pain and assist with the relief of mood symptoms. Using SNRIs such as duloxetine and venlafaxine may be particularly helpful for these dual indications.

Take-Home Points

- The primary care provider is often the first clinician to recognize the high burden of life-prolonging treatment for a resident who has limited life expectancy and high medical and neurocognitive comorbidity.
- Clinical depression is relatively common at the end of life. The prevalence of MDD at the end of life for cancer patients is estimated to be up to 20%.
- Palliative care refers to specialized medical care provided to individuals with serious illnesses or conditions that are not curable. The goal of palliative care is to improve the quality of life for patients by alleviating symptoms, managing pain, and addressing the physical, emotional, social, and spiritual needs associated with their condition.
- Choose psychotropic medications that have a quicker response time when possible. Examples include stimulants for depressive symptoms and benzodiazepines for anxiety. The use of SSRIs, SNRIs, and other more commonly prescribed medications for depression and anxiety may take up to four to six weeks for clinical response.

References

1. Rosenstein, D. L. (2011). Depression and end-of-life care for patients with cancer. *Dialogues in Clinical Neuroscience*, 13 (1), 101–108. https://doi.org/10.31887/DCNS.2011.13.1/drosenstein

Further Reading

Almeida, S. S., Zizzi, F. B., Cattaneo, A., Comandini, A., Dato, G. D., Lubrano, E., Pellicano, C., Spallone, V., Tongiani, S., & Torta, R. (2019). Management and treatment of patients with major depressive disorder and chronic diseases: A multidisciplinary approach. *Frontiers in Psychology*, 11. https://doi.org/10.3389/fpsyg.2020.542444

Desai, A., & Grossberg, G. (2017). *Psychiatric Consultation in Long-Term Care (A Guide for Healthcare Professionals)*. (Cambridge University Press.) Kindle Edition. p. 118.

Khouzam, H. R. (2016). Psychopharmacology of chronic pain: A focus on antidepressants and atypical antipsychotics. *Postgraduate Medicine*, 128 (3), 323–330.

Smith, H. R. (2015). Depression in cancer patients: Pathogenesis, implications and treatment. *Oncology letters*, 9 (4), 1509–1514.

Walker, J., Hansen, C. H., Martin, P., Sawhney, A., Thekkumpurath, P., Beale, C., & Sharpe, M. (2013). Prevalence of depression in adults with cancer: A systematic review. *Annals of oncology*, 24 (4), 895–900.

Yang, X., Wu, X., Gao, M., Wang, W., Quan, L., & Zhou, X. (2020). Heterogeneous patterns of posttraumatic stress symptoms and depression in cancer patients. *Journal of Affective Disorders*, 273, 203–209.

"I Feel Terrible"

15 SSRIs and Treatment-Resistant Depression

Mrs. U, a 90-year-old resident in a nursing home who had MNCD due to Alzheimer's disease, had been experiencing severe depressive symptoms for four months. Symptoms included tearfulness, lack of interest in activities, severe anxiety, insomnia, lack of appetite, weight loss, and irritability. A referral to a psychiatrist was made as Mrs. U had not responded to two adequate trials of antidepressants. The psychiatrist found that the patient had been tried on citalopram 20 mg daily for eight weeks and then sertraline 50 mg for eight weeks before the referral. The patient's primary care physician was reluctant to use higher doses of antidepressants because of the patient's advanced age and MNCD.

In the week before evaluation by the psychiatrist, Mrs. U had developed lower abdominal pain and was found to have a UTI so was put on antibiotics. At the time of the interview, the psychiatrist found her to be severely depressed and tearful throughout the interview, expressing statements indicating hopelessness and a wish that she was dead. Mrs. U was also distraught because she had developed mild antibiotic-induced diarrhea. She told the psychiatrist, "I feel terrible." Her SLUMS score was 13. The psychiatrist considered restarting one of the SSRIs but because of the risk of worsening antibiotic-induced diarrhea, decided to avoid them and start mirtazapine instead. Mrs. U was put on 7.5 mg of mirtazapine daily at bedtime and the dose was increased after seven days to 15 mg daily at bedtime. She started sleeping better after two weeks of treatment, the diarrhea resolved when the antibiotic course was over, the UTI resolved, and the abdominal pain improved. However, her tearfulness, daytime agitation, and hopelessness persisted. Hence, the dose of mirtazapine was further increased to 22.5 mg daily at bedtime for seven days. Mrs U. was able to tolerate this dose without sedation or other adverse effects.

An individualized, pleasant activity schedule was created and initiated for Mrs. U, after consultation with the family and staff. The family and staff were counseled to try to walk with her daily as she had been active all her life, and bright light therapy was started (exposure to bright light for one hour every morning while Mrs. U was perusing her favorite magazines). Mrs. U enjoyed hugs from the staff, and staff who were comfortable were encouraged to hug her off and on throughout the day. Mrs. U enjoyed classical and instrumental music, and listening to this music was added to her daily schedule. The family hired a massage therapist to come twice a week. After eight weeks, her mood had improved significantly, her anxiety decreased, her appetite had returned to near normal, and her feelings of hopelessness had resolved.

Teaching Points

This case provides the opportunity to examine some common treatment challenges in depression for older adults. One of the first dilemmas is often which antidepressant to choose as initial treatment for newly-diagnosed MDD. Current guidelines still support the use of an SSRI as the first choice for the treatment of depression in older adults. Although no SSRI has been shown to be more efficacious than other SSRIs, sertraline is the favorite choice of this author due to its safety, tolerability, effectiveness, and ability to titrate the dose. The potential benefits and challenges of individual SSRIs are listed in Table 15.1.

A second question is how to proceed in patients who do not have an initial full and positive remission with a dose of sertraline that has reached a therapeutic dose. A potential treatment algorithm for newly-diagnosed MDD is represented in Box 15.1 [1].

Clinicians should keep in mind the old adage "start low, go slow, but go" with regard to the prescribing of antidepressants in older patients. With older adults, it is a good idea to start at half or quarter of the normal adult starting dose but to increase the dose to well within the therapeutic range for a given antidepressant. This escalation to a therapeutic

Table 15.1 Potential positives and negatives to the available generic SSRIs.

SSRI	Potential positive	Potential negative
Citalopram	Ease of use. Tolerability.	The top dose is now limited to 20 mg daily due to concerns of QTc prolongation in those over 60 years.
Escitalopram	Ease of use. Tolerability.	Dose now limited to 10 mg daily in those over 60 years due to concerns of QtC prolongation.
Paroxetine	Effective and may be ok to continue in those well controlled and who have been on for years.	Should generally be avoided in older adults due to the anticholinergic burden. Has the highest incidence of erectile dysfunction.
Fluoxetine	Long half-life. Active metabolites have a half-life of 4–16 days. Good for those who may miss the occasional dose. Can be self-tapered should there be a need to discontinue.	Tends to be activating and may worsen comorbid anxiety or add to insomnia issues.
Fluvoxamine	Has a low anticholinergic burden.	May impair cognition in older patients.
Sertraline	Wide therapeutic dose range allows for the opportunity for dose increase if necessary. Ease of use. Tolerability. Low potential for drug–drug interactions.	May have a somewhat higher incidence of GI side effects.

Box 15.1 Treatment suggestion for new diagnosis depression in older adults

1. Start with an SSRI such as sertraline at a dose that is a half or quarter of the normal adult starting dose (12.5 or 25 mg daily).
2. Institute patient-specific nonpharmacologic interventions such as psychotherapy, recreation therapy, exercise, pet therapy, massage, increased family involvement, and so on.
3. In two weeks increase the dose of sertraline to 50 mg daily.
4. Reassess every four weeks for response or remission of symptoms. If there is an inadequate response, consider increasing the dose of sertraline by 25–50 mg/day to a max dose of 200 mg daily.
5. Reassess in four weeks. If inadequate response, initiate a trial of aripiprazole 2 mg daily [1].
6. Reassess in four weeks. If inadequate response, increase the dose of aripiprazole to 5 mg daily.
7. If there is an inadequate response, after four weeks the patient can be considered treatment resistant. At this point, a consultation with a psychiatrist may be warranted. If not available, consider proceeding to step 8.
8. Consider adding a third agent from a different antidepressant class such as an SDRI (bupropion) or SNRI (venlafaxine, duloxetine, or desvenlafaxine). Start at half of the normal adult starting dose.
9. Titrate the dose of the SDRI or SNRI to mid to upper therapeutic dose by small steps every two to four weeks.
10. If the patient does not respond adequately to treatments at this point it may be advisable to consult a geriatric psychiatrist.

dose should happen slowly over the course of one to two months. If an older patient does not respond to a typical therapeutic dose the clinician should not feel overly cautious about prescribing a dose at the upper limit of FDA-approved doses.

This case also highlights the nonpharmacologic interventions important in the treatment of depression. Pharmacologic treatments have a higher likelihood of failing in the absence of nonpharmacologic interventions.

Loneliness is an epidemic in the lives of older adults and can contribute greatly to the development and persistence of mood and anxiety disorders. Loneliness can be due to both inadequate quantity and quality of social relationships [2,3]. Insufficient quantity and poor-quality relationships can be problematic even in a long-term care setting with a relatively large number of residents and staff. Boredom can also significantly impact mental health. The more successful long-term care facilities have active social, spiritual, and recreational activity programs to enhance connections and give more meaning to the life of seniors.

The healing effect of human touch is also highlighted in this case study. Studies have shown that psychosocial interventions can be as effective or more effective than pharmacological therapies for the treatment of depression [4]. Animal therapy, cognitive stimulation, massage therapy, and reminiscence therapy should be considered as options for supportive interventions in those with depression in long-term care [5]. There can be time, financial, and access issues to these services in long-term care facilities that may make utilization of these interventions problematic.

Bright light therapy, also referred to as phototherapy, is a non-invasive approach used to alleviate symptoms of depression by exposing individuals to specific wavelengths of intense light. It is particularly successful in addressing seasonal affective disorder (SAD), a form of depression typically experienced during the darker months of fall and winter. The fundamental concept behind bright light therapy is based on the notion that light exposure can regulate both circadian rhythms and neurotransmitter function, ultimately leading to improved mood and a reduction in depressive symptoms. The therapy usually involves sitting near a specialized lightbox, which emits bright light at intensities of 10,000 lux or higher. The duration of exposure is typically prescribed and can range from 30 minutes to several hours per day. Numerous studies have substantiated the efficacy of bright light therapy in the treatment of depression, including SAD. This therapy has been found to have positive effects on mood, increasing energy levels, and diminishing feelings of fatigue and lethargy associated with depression. Furthermore, it has the potential to regulate sleep–wake cycles and enhance overall well-being [6].

It is also interesting to note that the patient in this case had a Montreal Cognitive Assessment (MoCA) score of 13 in the setting of MDD. Abnormal cognitive testing (MoCA, SLUMS, neuropsychiatric testing) may not reflect a patient's true cognitive baseline. Major depressive disorder is well known to cause impairments in cognitive domains such as processing speed, attention, and executive function. These deficits will likely be reflected in formal cognitive testing [7,8]. The term "pseudodementia" used to be used frequently for this phenomenon of apparent cognitive impairment in a patient with MDD. Preferable terms are now "depression-related cognitive impairment" or "the dementia syndrome of depression". In the case presented here it is possible that the patient may score higher on her SLUMS exam after her MDD has responded or remitted with appropriate treatment.

As a final note, depression is prevalent in older adults in long-term care with estimated prevalence from 11% to 45%. Depression is associated with poor overall health outcomes and poor quality of life. Interventions are often effective if these patients are identified but treatment can be challenging and require multiple adjustments in medications or treatment strategies. There can be little more gratifying to a healthcare provider than seeing a patient emerge from a state of depression to a state of enjoying life again and contributing to the community where they live.

Take-Home Points

- Depression is prevalent in older adults in long-term care with an estimated prevalence of 11–45%. Depression is associated with poor overall health outcomes and poor quality of life. Interventions are often effective if these patients are identified, but treatment can be challenging and require multiple adjustments in medications or treatment strategies.
- Current guidelines still support the use of an SSRI as the first choice for the treatment of depression in older adults.
- Clinicians should keep in mind the old adage "start low, go slow, but go" with regard to the prescribing of antidepressants in older patients. With older adults, it is a good idea to start at half or quarter of the normal adult starting dose but to increase the dose to well within the therapeutic range for a given antidepressant.
- Clinical depression is relatively common at the end of life. The prevalence of MDD at the end of life for cancer patients is estimated to be up to 20%.

References

1. Lenze, E. J., Mulsant, B. H., Roose, S. P., Lavretsky, H., Reynolds III, C. F., Blumberger, D. M., & Karp, J. F. (2023). Antidepressant augmentation versus switch in treatment-resistant geriatric depression. *New England Journal of Medicine*, 388 (12), 1067–1079.

2. Lee, S. L., Pearce, E., Ajnakina, O., Johnson, S., Lewis, G., Mann, F., Pitman, A., Solmi, F., Sommerlad, A., Steptoe, A., Tymoszuk, U., & Lewis, G. (2021). The association between loneliness and depressive symptoms among adults aged 50 years and older: A 12-year population-based cohort study. *Lancet Psychiatry*, 8 (1), 48–57. doi: 10.1016/S2215-0366(20)30383-7. Epub 2020 Nov 9. PMID: 33181096; PMCID: PMC8009277.

3. National Academies of Sciences, Engineering, and Medicine. (2020). *Social Isolation and Loneliness in Older Adults: Opportunities for the Health Care System*. National Academies Press.

4. Watt, J. A., Goodarzi, Z., Veroniki, A. A., Nincic, V., Khan, P. A., Ghassemi, M., Lai, Y., Treister, V., Thompson, Y., Schneider, R., Tricco, A. C., & Straus, S. E. (2020). Comparative efficacy of interventions for reducing symptoms of depression in people with dementia: Systematic review and network meta-analysis. *The BMJ*, 372. https://doi.org/10.1136/bmj.n532

5. Macleod, F., Storey, L., Rushe, T., & McLaughlin, K. (2021). Towards an increased understanding of reminiscence therapy for people with dementia: A narrative analysis. *Dementia (London, England)*, 20 (4), 1375–1407. https://doi.org/10.1177/1471301220941275

6. Al-Karawi, D., & Jubair, L. (2016). Bright light therapy for nonseasonal depression: Meta-analysis of clinical trials. *Journal of Affective Disorders*, 198, 64–71.

7. Riddle, M., Potter, G. G., McQuoid, D. R., Steffens, D. C., Beyer, J. L., & Taylor, W. D. (2017). Longitudinal cognitive outcomes of clinical phenotypes of late-life depression. *The American Journal of Geriatric Psychiatry*, 25 (10), 1123–1134.

8. Zaremba, D., Kalthoff, I. S., Förster, K., Redlich, R., Grotegerd, D., Leehr, E. J., & Dannlowski, U. (2019). The effects of processing speed on memory impairment in patients with major depressive disorder. *Progress in Neuro-Psychopharmacology and Biological Psychiatry*, 92, 494–500.

Further Reading

Conroy, R., Golden, J., Jeffares, I., O'Neill, D., & Mcgee, H. (2010). Boredom-proneness, loneliness, social engagement and depression and their association with cognitive function in older people: A population study. *Psychology, Health & Medicine*. 15, 463–473. 10.1080/13548506.2010.487103.

Domènech-Abella, J., Mundó, J., Haro, J. M., & Rubio-Valera, M. (2019). Anxiety, depression, loneliness and social network in the elderly: Longitudinal associations from The Irish Longitudinal Study on Ageing (TILDA). *Journal of Affective Disorders*, 246, 82–88.

Furukawa, Y., Hamza, T., Cipriani, A., Furukawa, T., Salanti, G., & Ostinelli, E. (2022). Optimal dose of aripiprazole for augmentation therapy of antidepressant-refractory depression: Preliminary findings based on a systematic review and dose-effect meta-analysis. *The British Journal of Psychiatry*, 221 (2), 440–447. doi:10.1192/bjp.2021.165

"I Don't Care"

16 SSRIs/SNRIs and Bleeding Risk

Mr. B was an 82-year-old retired accountant living in a long-term care facility. He had been experiencing a lack of interest in activities, decreased appetite, decreased energy, and agitation during personal care. He had been expressing statements such as "I don't care" for three months. The symptoms started a few weeks after he was moved from an AL home to a skilled nursing home due to advancing MNCD and recurrent falls. He also had a recent history of GI bleeding due to peptic ulcer disease.

On clinical exam, the long-term care provider noted that Mr. B had a depressed mood and poor eye contact. Major neurocognitive disorder due to Alzheimer's disease with MDD was diagnosed. The primary provider considered prescribing SSRIs but did not due to Mr. B's recent history of GI bleeding and the potential for an SSRI to increase the risk of bleeding. Mirtazapine was considered but not prescribed because of its propensity to cause weight gain and Mr. B had morbid obesity with related mobility impairment. Bupropion was started at 75 mg daily in the morning and after seven days increased to 75 mg in the morning and at 5 pm. An individualized, pleasant activity schedule was created for Mr. B after a discussion with him, his family, and staff. The family was encouraged to bring grandchildren to visit Mr. B as they always cheered him up, and it was recommended that staff bring Mr. B's former roommate to visit as they had become close friends over the two years that they lived together in the AL home.

Over the next four weeks, Mr. B gradually started talking more and eating more. The bupropion was changed to bupropion sustained-release preparation, given as 150 mg once daily in the morning. After eight weeks Mr. B was attending activities and eating better and the agitation during personal care had reduced dramatically.

Teaching Points

Major depressive disorder is a prevalent cause of disability worldwide and can cause significant and enduring impairment in older adults. According to the Diagnostic and Statistical Manual of Mental Disorders–5–TR (DSM–5–TR), MDD is characterized by a duration of at least two weeks during which a patient experiences five or more of the following symptoms nearly every day: depressed mood, lack of interest or pleasure (anhedonia), changes in weight or appetite, sleep disturbances (insomnia or hypersomnia), psychomotor retardation, fatigue or loss of energy, feelings of worthlessness or excessive guilt, difficulty concentrating or making decisions, and recurrent thoughts of death, suicide, or a suicide attempt. The most prominent theory regarding the underlying mechanisms of MDD is the monoamine deficiency hypothesis, which proposes that depression arises from the depletion of serotonin, norepinephrine, or dopamine in key areas of the CNS. Among these neurotransmitters, serotonin has received considerable attention in the study of depression's pathophysiology. Research has shown that reduced synthesis and effective concentrations of serotonin at the neural synapses in key areas of the brain contributes to depressive symptoms in individuals vulnerable to depression.

Antidepressants, when used appropriately and in combination with an individual-ized psychosocial approach, can dramatically improve depressive symptoms and the quality of life of residents who have MDD. The selection of antidepressants needs to consider the patient's medical problems as well as what side effects one wants or wants to avoid for a particular patient. There is no compelling evidence that one antidepressant works better than any other for the treatment of MDD in long-term care populations. Selective serotonin reuptake inhibitors are probably the most commonly selected first-line medications for the treatment of MDD in long-term care residents. They function by impeding the reuptake of serotonin, thereby increas-ing its availability in synapses. This mechanism of action within the CNS explains the efficacy of SSRIs for depression but the effects are not limited to the CNS [1]. Serotonin transporters are present in tissues throughout the body. This fact helps to explain why up to 80% of patients taking SSRIs will experience at least one side effect. Some of the potential side effects include sexual dysfunction, anxiety, dizziness, weight gain, GI problems, and headaches. Other adverse effects include prolongation of the QT interval, coagulopathy, the potential for serotonin syndrome, and SSRI discontinuation syndrome [2].

Increased bleeding risk associated with SSRI use has been reported, notably in the upper GI tract. The existing literature on this subject reveals mixed findings: Some studies indicate no elevation bleeding risk with SSRIs, others demonstrate an increased risk of bleeding in the perioperative period when SSRIs are combined with NSAIDs [3]. The proof of risk of intracranial bleeding associated with SSRIs is lacking. The study by Isokuortti et al. indicated no increased risk or intracranial bleeding in those on SSRIs who sustained head trauma [4]. The study by Jensen et al. demonstrated insufficient data to recommend restricting the use of SSRIs because of concern for increased risk of intracranial bleeding complications [5]. The consensus currently seems to be that SSRIs cause a true increase in GI bleeding complications but that these effects can be lessened with certain precautions.

Serotonin–norepinephrine reuptake inhibitors have also been associated with a potentially increased risk of bleeding, although the risk appears to be lower compared to SSRIs. The potential for bleeding when using SNRIs is generally regarded as modest, and most individuals still experience a favorable balance between the risks and benefits of these medications [6].

The mechanism behind the impact of SSRIs on increased bleeding complications is multifactorial. Inhibition of serotonin reuptake can influence platelet aggregation as platelets also express the serotonin transporter. Selective serotonin reuptake inhibitors can lead to reduced storage of serotonin in platelet-dense granules, potentially impacting bleeding tendencies. Moreover, increased serotonin levels can stimulate gastric acid secretion, thereby raising the risk of ulcers. When SSRIs are combined with NSAIDs or antiplatelet agents, the risk of upper GI bleeding is significantly augmented. Examples of commonly used antiplatelet agents include aspirin, clopidogrel, prasugrel, ticagrelor, persantine, and cilostazol.

Despite the increased risk of bleeding with SSRIs and antiplatelet agents, there are times when a patient may require an antiplatelet agent and it is thought that an SSRI may still be the best antidepressant option. In these cases, the use of a proton pump inhibitor (PPI) should be considered. Proton pump inhibitors have been shown to reduce the risk of GI bleeding in those that have increased risk such as in those patients who require NSAIDs or antiplatelet agents and SSRIs [2].

Some studies have shown an estimated 30–70% increased risk of bleeding when the vitamin K antagonist warfarin is used along with SSRIs in hospitalized patients [7]. It is hard to know if these findings can be generalized to a non-hospitalized patient population as well. The utilization of PPIs may also be beneficial in these cases to help mitigate the risk of combining this blood thinner with SSRIs.

Since 2010 the use of direct oral anticoagulants (DOACs) has increased. Examples of these medications include apixaban (Eliquis), dabigatran (Pradaxa), and rivaroxaban (Xarelto). Their safety and efficacy make them more popular choices for those who need anticoagulation. Before the arrival of DOACs, warfarin was the only choice for oral anticoagulation. Studies have shown an increase in bleeding risk when DOACs are combined with SSRIs and for this reason patients requiring this treatment should be considered for concomitant PPI use [8].

There are strategies to mitigate the increased bleeding risk that can be associated with SSRIs and SNRIs (Box 16.1).

It should be mentioned that the pathophysiology of depression is still in active research with alternative therapeutic targets having been identified in recent years. Ketamine and esketamine have multiple pharmacodynamic targets but the major target is the NMDA receptor, for which they act as an antagonist. By doing so, ketamine modulates the release and function of various neurotransmitters, including glutamate, in several brain regions. This modulation of glutamate transmission is thought to play a crucial role in the antidepressant effects of ketamine. Another important downstream effect of ketamine and esketamine is the rapid and transient increase in the release of brain-derived neurotrophic factor (BDNF), a protein that promotes the growth, survival, and function of neurons. Its deficiency has been associated with depression. The increase in BDNF levels is believed to promote synaptic plasticity and the formation of new connections between brain cells, which may contribute to the antidepressant effects of ketamine. The roles of ketamine and esketamine are still being elucidated for the management of TRD [9,10].

Box 16.1 Strategies to mitigate the increased risk of bleeding seen with SSRIs and SNRIs

1. Antiplatelet agents and NSAIDs strongly increase the risk of upper GI bleeding with SSRIs and SNRIs. Consider if a patient truly needs to be on an antiplatelet agent.
2. If a patient needs to be on an antiplatelet agent or NSAID and an SSRI or SNRI, consider adding a PPI. This can help to decrease the risk of upper GI bleeding with SSRIs.
3. Consider an alternative antidepressant to an SSRI if the antiplatelet agent is necessary and the patient has an increased risk of upper GI bleeding. Alternative agents to be considered include bupropion, trazodone, and mirtazapine.

Take-Home Points

- Antidepressants, when used appropriately and in combination with an individualized psychosocial approach, can dramatically improve depressive symptoms and the quality of life of residents who have MDD.
- The selection of antidepressants needs to consider the patient's medical problems as well as what side effects one wants or wants to avoid for a particular patient.
- SNRIs have also been associated with a potentially increased risk of bleeding, although the risk appears to be lower compared to SSRIs.
- There is no compelling evidence that one antidepressant works any better than any other for the treatment of MDD in long-term care populations. SSRIs are probably the most commonly selected first-line medications for the treatment of MDD in long-term care residents.
- Consider an alternative antidepressant to an SSRI if the antiplatelet agent is necessary and the patient has an increased risk of upper GI bleeding. Alternative agents to be considered include bupropion, trazodone, and mirtazapine.

References

1. Joshi, A. (2018). Selective serotonin re-uptake inhibitors: An overview. *Psychiatria Danubina*, 30 (Suppl 7), 605–609. PMID: 30439857.

2. Edinoff, A. N., Akuly, H. A., Hanna, T. A., Ochoa, C. O., Patti, S. J., Ghaffar, Y. A., Kaye, A. D., Viswanath, O., Urits, I., Boyer, A. G., Cornett, E. M., & Kaye, A. M. (2021). Selective serotonin reuptake inhibitors and adverse effects: A narrative review. *Neurology International*, 13 (3), 387–401. https://doi.org/10.3390/neurolint13030038

3. Edinoff, A. N., Raveendran, K., Colon, M. A., Thomas, B. H., Trettin, K. A., Hunt, G. W., Kaye, A. M., Cornett, E. M., & Kaye, A. D. (2021). Selective serotonin reuptake inhibitors and associated bleeding risks: A narrative and clinical review. *Health Psychology Research*, 10 (4). https://doi.org/10.52965/001c.39580

4. Anglin, R., Yuan, Y., Moayyedi, P., Tse, F., Armstrong, D., & Leontiadis, G. I. (2014). Risk of upper gastrointestinal bleeding with selective serotonin reuptake inhibitors with or without concurrent nonsteroidal anti-inflammatory use: A systematic review and meta-analysis. *Official journal of the American College of Gastroenterology| ACG*, 109 (6), 811–819.

5. Isokuortti, H., Iverson, G. L., Posti, J. P., Ruuskanen, J. O., Brander, A., Kataja, A., Nikula, M., Öhman, J., & Luoto, T. M. (2021) Serotonergic antidepressants and risk for traumatic intracranial bleeding. *Frontiers in Neurology*, 12, 758707. Doi: 10.3389/fneur.2021.758707. PMID: 34777229; PMCID: PMC8581291.

6. Jensen, M. P., Ziff, O. J., Banerjee, G., Ambler, G., & Werring, D. J. (2019) The impact of selective serotonin reuptake inhibitors on the risk of intracranial hemorrhage: A systematic review and meta-analysis. *European Stroke Journal*, 4 (2), 144–152.

7. Cheng, Y. L., Hu, H. Y., Lin, X. H., Luo, J. C., Peng, Y. L., Hou, M. C., Lin, H. C., & Lee, F. Y. (2015). Use of SSRI, but not SNRI, increased upper and lower gastrointestinal bleeding: A nationwide population-based cohort study in Taiwan. *Medicine (Baltimore)*, 94 (46), e2022. doi:10.1097/MD.0000000000002022

8. McIntyre, R. S., Rosenblat, J. D., Nemeroff, C. B., Sanacora, G., Murrough, J. W., Berk, M., Brietzke, E., Dodd, S., Gorwood, P., Ho, R., Iosifescu, D. V., Jaramillo, C. L., Kasper, S., Kratiuk, K., Lee, J. G., Lee, Y., Lui, M. W., Mansur, R. B., Papakostas, G. I., & Stahl, S. (2021). Synthesizing the evidence for ketamine and esketamine in treatment-resistant depression: An international expert opinion on the available evidence and

implementation. *The American Journal of Psychiatry*, 178 (5), 383. https://doi.org/10.1176/appi.ajp.2020.20081251

9. Edinoff, A. N., Akuly, H. A., Hanna, T. A., Ochoa, C. O., Patti, S. J., Ghaffar, Y. A., Kaye, A. D., Viswanath, O., Urits, I., Boyer, A. G., Cornett, E. M., & Kaye, A. M. (2021). Selective serotonin reuptake inhibitors and adverse effects: A narrative review. *Neurology International*, 13 (3), 387–401. https://doi.org/10.3390/neurolint13030038

10. Andrade, C., & Sharma, E. (2016). Serotonin reuptake inhibitors and risk of abnormal bleeding. *Psychiatric Clinics*, 39 (3), 413–426.

Further Reading

Andrade, C., & Sharma, E. (2016). Serotonin reuptake inhibitors and risk of abnormal bleeding. *Psychiatric Clinics of North America*, 39 (3), 413–426. doi: 10.1016/j.psc.2016.04.010. Epub 2016 Jun 28. PMID: 27514297.

Auerbach, A. D., Vittinghoff, E., Maselli, J., Pekow, P. S., Young, J. Q., & Lindenauer, P. K. (2013). Perioperative use of selective serotonin reuptake inhibitors and risks for adverse outcomes of surgery. *JAMA Internal Medicine*, 173 (12), 1075–1081. doi: 10.1001/jamainternmed.2013.714. PMID: 23699725; PMCID: PMC3867199.

Jensen, M. P., Ziff, O. J., Banerjee, G., Ambler, G., & Werring, D. J. (2019). The impact of selective serotonin reuptake inhibitors on the risk of intracranial hemorrhage: A systematic review and meta-analysis. *European Stroke Journal*, 4 (2), 144–152.

Laporte, S., Chapelle, C., Caillet, P., Beyens, M. N., Bellet, F., Delavenne, X., & Bertoletti, L. (2017). Bleeding risk under selective serotonin reuptake inhibitor (SSRI) antidepressants: A meta-analysis of observational studies. *Pharmacological Research*, 118, 19–32.

Lee, T., Park, Y., Kim, S., You, H., Kang, J., & Jung, Y. (2020). Concomitant use of NSAIDs or SSRIs with NOACs requires monitoring for bleeding. *Yonsei Medical Journal*, 61 (9), 741–749. https://doi.org/10.3349/ymj.2020.61.9.741

McIntyre, R. S., Carvalho, I. P., Lui, L. M., Majeed, A., Masand, P. S., Gill, H., & Rosenblat, J. D. (2020). The effect of intravenous, intranasal, and oral ketamine in mood disorders: A meta-analysis. *Journal of Affective Disorders*, 276, 576–584.

Quinn, G. R., Hellkamp, A. S., Hankey, G. J., Becker, R. C., Berkowitz, S. D., Breithardt, G., & Singer, D. E. (2018). Selective serotonin reuptake inhibitors and bleeding risk in anticoagulated patients with atrial fibrillation: An analysis from the ROCKET AF trial. *Journal of the American Heart Association*, 7 (15), e008755.

"I Feel Very Lonely"

Depression/Psychogenomic Testing

Mr. G was a 79-year-old resident who had suffered from a stroke causing left hemiparesis. Staff requested that his long-term care provider evaluate Mr. G because of frequent episodes of irritation, yelling at staff, making sexually inappropriate comments, and attempting to touch staff inappropriately during personal care. These symptoms were present for three months. Mr. G's wife (and legal surrogate decision-maker) had refused antidepressant treatment for Mr. G in the past because he had become "wild" after initiation of an antidepressant (paroxetine) five years earlier after his first stroke.

Following a mental status exam, Mr. G showed evidence of executive dysfunction and depressed mood. He enjoyed socialization and conversation with his provider and seemed to crave social interaction and personal attention. Mr. G told the provider, "Yes, I feel very lonely." A diagnosis of poststroke depression and impulse control disorder due to frontal lobe dysfunction was made. He admitted to feeling sad and hopeless at times. He also expressed that he felt irritable.

The primary provider reviewed previous records, which indicated that Mr. G was treated with 20 mg of paroxetine for depression five years earlier. The provider reviewed the possible adverse effects of antidepressants with Mrs. G and the potential benefits of a second trial with an antidepressant at a low dose. The nursing staff at the long-term care facility encouraged Mrs. G to inquire about the use of pharmacogenetic testing "to see which antidepressant is best". The healthcare provider spoke with Mrs. G and encouraged her to proceed with a trial of one more antidepressant that was likely to be better tolerated in older patients. The provider assured Mrs. G that Mr. G would be started on a very low dose of medication, closely monitored for any adverse effects, and that the antidepressant would promptly be discontinued if the adverse effect was moderate to severe. Mrs. G agreed to this plan.

A decision was made to start Mr. G on sertraline 12.5 mg daily each morning, to be increased to 25 mg daily in the morning after seven days. Mr. G developed transient mild nausea and anxiety for three days, which resolved spontaneously. After treatment for four weeks, the staff noticed that Mr. G was less irritable, although sexually inappropriate behaviors and occasional episodes of yelling out (at least once a week) continued. After four weeks, his dose of sertraline was increased to 37.5 mg daily for seven days and then 50 mg daily in the morning. Mr. G, once again, developed transient mild nausea and anxiety, which cleared up spontaneously over one week.

After six more weeks of treatment, staff reported that sexually inappropriate behavior had decreased considerably and episodes of yelling out now occurred only once a month. Mr. G seemed to be getting along better with other residents and was enjoying day-to-day activities more. His wife was also pleased to report that Mr. G was acting much more like himself with the new medication.

Teaching Points

The selection of initial antidepressants in those requiring treatment has several potential implications for the outcomes. The STAR*D trial showed that the rate of response to initial antidepressant treatment is only 49.6% [1]. Another review indicated that those who failed to respond to the first antidepressant had a 15% likelihood of suicide ideation compared to 6% of patients with treatment-responsive depression and 1% in the general population [2]. The financial costs of treatment for those with depression who do not respond to the first course of antidepressants are also higher. The costs of treatment are estimated to be $10,000/year more than for those that do respond to the initial antidepressant choice. Patients also vary widely in developing side effects to common psychotropic medications. A moderate or severe side effect to an initial choice of antidepressant can negatively impact a patient's or family's likelihood of pursuing further treatment and can place a newly-formed therapeutic relationship on shaky grounds. A study in 2014 by Hampton et al. stated that 25,000 patients in the US go to emergency departments each year due to antidepressant-induced adverse events [3].

A major influence on positive or negative therapeutic responses to a medication is the drug's metabolism in a given individual, which can be hard to predict. Those familiar with the care of older adults know that the metabolism of pharmaceuticals is influenced by age-related factors. The liver plays a crucial role in drug metabolism and undergoes structural and functional changes with age, including reduced blood flow and decreased overall liver mass. These changes can lead to decreased metabolic capacity and slower drug metabolism. Drugs are often metabolized by the cytochrome P450 microsomal enzymes in the liver. The activity of these enzymes may decline with age, which will prolong the rate at which some drugs are broken down. Kidney function also generally declines with advancing age, which overall tends to lead to higher concentrations of medications and their metabolites in older adults. Polypharmacy is also more common in older adults and can up- or down-regulate the metabolism of pharmaceuticals and thereby influence therapeutic effects.

How is a provider to know the likely response of a patient to a given medication when there are so many variables? The therapeutic effects of medications are most predictable at particular therapeutic serum concentrations, which are established during the development and testing of a pharmacologic agent. The efficacy of neuropsychiatric medications must also consider the relationship of serum to CSF levels of drugs, which are very dependent on the permeability of the blood–brain barrier to a given medication.

A possible, but not always reasonable, option to assess therapeutic response (or lack thereof) in a given patient is to measure serum drug levels. The cost of these lab tests can be prohibitive. For example, the estimated cost for a fluoxetine serum level is estimated at $50–200. The cost of an olanzapine serum level is estimated at $100–300 or more. This is more than the cost of a year's supply of this medication and insurance may or may not cover the cost of these tests. Additionally, serum levels of fluoxetine or olanzapine are not reliable and do not directly correlate with clinical efficacy or toxicity. Despite this, it is still important to obtain serum drug levels to manage certain psychiatric conditions and is a standard of care. It is also important to obtain lithium, valproic acid, and carbamazepine levels periodically when these drugs are used in the management of bipolar disorder and some other psychiatric and neurologic conditions. Some clinicians also utilize clozapine levels in the management of treatment-resistant schizophrenia.

Pharmacogenetic testing theoretically has the potential to increase the success rates of initial medication selection in the treatment of depression and other psychiatric disorders. The cost of this testing is significant and needs to be considered, with current estimates around $200–1000. The costs have come down considerably in recent years and the reports generated by these tests will list many commonly prescribed medications from a variety of drug classes. They will estimate a patient's likelihood to be a normal, under, or hyper-metabolizer of a medication. Please see reference [4] for a sample report.

There are several factors to consider before widely implementing psychopharmacogenetic testing in the care of psychiatric patients (Box 17.1), and several benefits may influence a clinician's decision to order psychiatric pharmacogenetic testing (Box 17.2)

Selective serotonin reuptake inhibitors (such as sertraline) are still considered good first-choice antidepressants for people who have vascular disease (cardiovascular and cerebrovascular disease) because of negligible cardiac toxicity and anticholinergic properties. Paroxetine carries a small but significant anticholinergic effect and thus is not the SSRI of first choice for long-term care residents. Fluoxetine and fluvoxamine are long-acting SSRIs with a significant risk of drug–drug interaction and hence are also not

---

Box 17.1 Limitations of psychopharmacogenetic testing

1. The metabolism and serum concentrations of medications do not always correlate well with clinical response.
2. The metabolism and serum concentrations of medications and their metabolites do not always correlate well with side effects.
3. The selection of and side effect profile of medication is often influenced by non-measurable factors such as patient familiarity with a particular pharmaceutical, experiences with a pharmaceutical by friends or family, and advertising.
4. The effect of a medication can be highly influenced by the relationship a patient has with a provider.
5. Psychiatric pharmacogenetic testing and its influence on therapeutic drug choice does not take into account such variables as patient medical comorbidities, which can be highly important when choosing a psychotropic medication.
6. Studies examining the efficacy of utilizing pharmacogenetic testing guided therapy in depression have been done. At this time pharmacogenetic information used to guide antidepressant therapy does not consistently show improved outcomes. Some studies show improved outcomes, and some show no difference in outcomes.

Box 17.2 Potential benefits of psychopharmacogenetic testing

1. Testing may be useful for choosing medications when a patient has a history of multiple drug intolerances or side effects.
2. Testing may be useful when a patient has a history of non-response or poor response to psychiatric medications in the past.
3. Consider ordering when a patient or surrogate specifically requests the testing.

first-line SSRIs for long-term care populations. Selective serotonin reuptake inhibitors are also good first-choice antidepressants for people who have depression coexisting with sexually inappropriate behavior, as serotonin dysfunction is associated with impulse control disorders. Education of the family and staff in the management of adverse effects is also key to a successful outcome.

Take-Home Points

- A major influence on positive or negative therapeutic responses to a medication is the drug's metabolism in a given individual. The metabolism of pharmaceuticals is influenced by age-related factors.
- The metabolism and serum concentrations of medications do not always correlate well with clinical response. Pharmacogenetic information used to guide antidepressant therapy does not consistently show improved outcomes. Some studies show improved outcomes, and some show no difference in outcomes.
- It is still important to obtain lithium, valproic acid, and carbamazepine levels periodically when these drugs are used in the management of bipolar disorder and some other psychiatric and neurologic conditions.
- SSRIs such as sertraline are still considered good first-choice antidepressants for people who have vascular disease (cardiovascular and cerebrovascular disease) because of negligible cardiac toxicity and anticholinergic properties.

References

1. Rush, A. J., Trivedi, M. H., Wisniewski, S. R., Nierenberg, A. A., Stewart, J. W., Warden, D., & Fava, M. (2006). Acute and longer-term outcomes in depressed outpatients requiring one or several treatment steps: A STAR*D report. *American Journal of Psychiatry*, 163 (11), 1905–1917.

2. Mrazek, D. A., Hornberger, J. C., Altar, C. A., & Degtiar, I. (2014). A review of the clinical, economic, and societal burden of treatment-resistant depression: 1996–2013. *Psychiatric services*, 65 (8), 977–987.

3. Hampton, L. M., Daubresse, M., Chang, H. Y., Alexander, G. C., & Budnitz, D. S. (2014). Emergency department visits by adults for psychiatric medication adverse events. *JAMA Psychiatry*, 71 (9), 1006–1014.

4. Genesight. (2021). Pyschotropic Report. https://genesight.com/wp-content/uploads/2021/05/GeneSight.Psychotropic.Report.pdf

Further Reading

Bousman, C., Al Maruf, A., & Müller, D. J. (2019). Towards the integration of pharmacogenetics in psychiatry: A minimum, evidence-based genetic testing panel. *Current Opinion in Psychiatry*, 32 (1), 7–15.

Bradley, P., Shiekh, M., Mehra, V., Vrbicky, K., Layle, S., Olson, M. C., & Lukowiak, A. A. (2018). Improved efficacy with targeted pharmacogenetic-guided treatment of patients with depression and anxiety: A randomized clinical trial demonstrating clinical utility. *Journal of Psychiatric Research*, 96, 100–107.

Corponi, F., Fabbri, C., & Serretti, A. (2018). Pharmacogenetics in psychiatry. *Advances in Pharmacology*, 83, 297–331.

Florio, V., Porcelli, S., Saria, A., Serretti, A., & Conca, A. (2017). Escitalopram plasma levels and antidepressant response. *European Neuropsychopharmacology*, 27 (9), 940–944.

Hicks, J. K., Sangkuhl, K., Swen, J. J., Ellingrod, V. L., Müller, D. J., Shimoda, K., & Stingl, J. C.

(2017). Clinical pharmacogenetics implementation consortium guideline (CPIC®) for CYP2D6 and CYP2C19 genotypes and dosing of tricyclic antidepressants: 2016 update. *Clinical Pharmacology and Therapeutics*, 102 (1), 37.

Maciel, A., Cullors, A., Lukowiak, A. A., & Garces, J. (2018). Estimating cost savings of pharmacogenetic testing for depression in real-world clinical settings. *Neuropsychiatric Disease and Treatment*, 14, 225–230.

"I Don't Feel Right"

18 Bipolar Disorder

Mrs. F, an 85-year-old resident, was admitted to a nursing home for rehabilitation after hip fracture surgery. She had a long history of bipolar disorder type I with multiple suicide attempts and hospitalizations but was stable for 10 years, taking olanzapine 5 mg at bedtime and divalproex extended-release 500 mg twice daily. The olanzapine was discontinued due to her experiencing "lethargy" and not participating in physical therapy. Her daughter strongly opposed this intervention, and after Mrs. F started showing a recurrence of bipolar depression symptoms (frequent tearfulness, loss of appetite), her daughter insisted that olanzapine be restarted. The staff decided to seek input from the consulting psychiatrist.

The psychiatrist obtained input from Mrs. F's daughter, who was her primary caregiver and had helped her through previous bouts of exacerbation of bipolar illness. The psychiatrist felt the daughter was knowledgeable about bipolar disorder and her mother's treatment history. The daughter was concerned about the discontinuation of olanzapine due to her history of severe depression and serious suicide attempts. Mrs. F's valproate levels were 45. During the interview, Mrs. F told the psychiatrist, "I don't feel right." Upon reviewing Mrs. F's medications, the psychiatrist noted that she was prescribed oxycodone (5 mg) as needed for pain and it was being used three to four times daily. Laboratory tests indicated mild dehydration (BUN/creatinine ratio 30 [20 and above suggests dehydration]).

The psychiatrist recommended trying up to 3 grams/day of scheduled acetaminophen, encouraging intake of at least 1000 cc fluids daily, restarting olanzapine 5 mg at bedtime, and using low-dose (2.5 mg) oxycodone as needed for breakthrough pain. Over the next four weeks, as the use of oxycodone decreased to once a day and dehydration resolved, the patient's "lethargy" cleared up, her depressed mood lifted, her appetite and sleep improved, and she started actively taking part in physical therapy.

Teaching Points

Bipolar disorder is a condition that is commonly encountered in the older adult population and estimates are that up to 4.5% of adults in the US are affected. The estimates for older adults are between 0.5 and 1%. Bipolar disorder usually presents early in life with the most common diagnosis age being late adolescence or early adulthood.

There is good evidence to support bipolar disorder as being strongly influenced by genetic factors. Monozygotic twins show a 40–70% concordance rate compared to 5–20% in dizygotic twins. Other studies have estimated the heritability of bipolar disorder to be around 60–80%. Despite the strong influence of genetic factors on the

Box 18.1   Primary symptoms of mania

1. Elevated or irritable mood. An elevated mood or irritable mood should be seen for at least one week.
2. Increased energy or activity. Patients may feel restless, agitated, or excessively energetic.
3. Decreased need for sleep. The patient may function on very little or no sleep for days.
4. Racing thoughts. This can be described as a decreased ability to concentrate or stay on topic.
5. Grandiosity. Patients may show an inflated sense of self-esteem or exaggeration of abilities.
6. Irritability. Patients who are manic may be easily irritated, resulting in more conflicts with others.

development of bipolar disorders, environmental factors and gene–environmental interactions are also known to contribute to the development of the disorder.

The treatment of bipolar disorders can be thought of in terms of acute and maintenance phase treatment. The acute phase of bipolar disorder can present as mania or hypomania or as acute depression. The symptoms of mania are shown in Box 18.1 [1].

The role of the healthcare provider in the long-term care setting is usually most concerned with supervising the maintenance therapy of the disease as the diagnosis has most likely been made many years prior. The treatments for acute and maintenance phase bipolar disorder are mood stabilizers and antipsychotics. Some agents have unique features that require specific monitoring (Box 18.2).

It is important to note that many patients with bipolar disorder may come to the attention of their healthcare provider with signs and symptoms of depression. In these cases, symptoms of mania or hypomania may become evident only after years of treatment for suspected unipolar depression. Those with bipolar disorder in general spend more time in the negative or depressed pole of the condition. Symptoms of depression in bipolar disorder are indistinguishable from the symptoms of depression in those with unipolar depression.

Starting a mood stabilizer or second-generation antipsychotic is a good first choice for those who are depressed with a known personal history of bipolar disorder and who are not already on one. Adding a second-generation antipsychotic approved for bipolar depression is a reasonable step for those already on a traditional mood stabilizer such as lithium, divalproex, or lamotrigine. A third option for those already on a mood stabilizer is adding an antidepressant such as an SSRI, SNRI, or bupropion. Extra caution and monitoring should be used when adding an antidepressant in those with bipolar disorder, even when on a mood stabilizer. There is a small chance of flipping a patient from the depressed pole to a manic episode with the addition of an antidepressant.

Special consideration should be given to those patients who may have symptoms of both depression and mania, giving a so-called mixed episode. These patients can show signs of depression such as depressed mood, decreased appetite, guilt, and suicidal ideation, but may also show signs of mania such as irritability, excessive energy, and racing thoughts. After ruling out new medical comorbidity, long-term care providers should focus first on dose optimization of mood stabilizer medication followed by initiation and titration of second-generation antipsychotic medication. These patients

Box 18.2 Commonly prescribed agents for maintenance of bipolar disorder and monitoring issues

Mood Stabilizers:

1. Lamotrigine. The dose should be titrated slowly due to the potential for serious skin reactions. May have antidepressant effects. Preferred by some as the first line in older adults.
2. Divalproex. Monitor serum levels periodically. Monitor CBC periodically as divalproex can cause thrombocytopenia or leukopenia. Monitor liver function periodically.
3. Lithium. Monitor lithium levels periodically and during acute illness. Monitor thyroid levels and renal function periodically. A minority of patients can experience diabetes insipidus. Generally not favored therapy in older adults due to increased risk of side effects but may be continued if well tolerated and the patient is stable.

Second-generation antipsychotics approved for bipolar mania. Effective but be aware of metabolic side effects. Can produce EPS side effects.

1. Olanzapine
2. Quetiapine
3. Risperidone
4. Ziprasidone

Third-generation antipsychotics approved for bipolar mania. Less likely to produce metabolic side effects. Less likely to produce EPS side effects.

1. Aripiprazole
2. Asenapine
3. Cariprazine

can also be more complicated and may benefit from the input of a geriatric psychiatrist if available.

Special consideration should also be given to those with bipolar mania or depression with psychotic symptoms. These patients are at particularly high risk of further behavioral destabilization and poor outcomes and generally require the assessment and treatment coordinated by a psychiatrist for the best chance of stabilization and recovery. Electroconvulsive therapy has been shown to be particularly helpful in these cases with improvements in symptoms as soon as one or two treatment sessions.

It is also important for healthcare providers in long-term care settings to recognize early signs of psychiatric destabilization in those with bipolar disorder. Signs of destabilization in older adults can be a decreased need for sleep, increased irritability, a general increase in activity, or even the development of psychosis (delusions or hallucinations). The decompensation that can be seen in bipolar patients can happen acutely or subacutely. The clinician should inquire about possible triggers for psychiatric destabilization in bipolar patients. Possible triggers might include changes in medication adherence, recent stressful life events such as the death of a loved one or changes in health conditions, new sleep disturbances, hormonal changes (thyroid), acute medical illness, and disruptions to the day-to-day routine. All of these factors can be implicated in triggering worsening control of symptoms in those with bipolar disorder. Family members can be valuable resources when evaluating changes in behavior. They have often had many years of experience in recognizing early signs of bipolar mania or depression in a loved one.

A basic medical workup is important in ruling out a potential medical trigger such as hypo- or hyperthyroidism, electrolyte imbalances, or infection. A good basic workup can usually be done safely without emergency room evaluation and should include checks of CBC, CMP, thyroid stimulating hormone (TSH), b12 level, mood stabilizer level when indicated, urinalysis, and any other imaging or lab workup suggested by a physical exam. Emergency room evaluation is preferred when new neurologic findings accompany behavioral changes, any suspicion of head injury, or in those with homicidal or suicidal behaviors.

Once underlying medical triggers for the destabilization of bipolar disorder and true medical emergency are ruled out, the long-term care provider should quickly intervene to prevent further worsening of bipolar symptoms and thereby prevent potential hospitalization. Most patients with bipolar disorder will already have mood stabilizers in place, but the provider should assess the appropriateness of dosing. Valproic acid and lithium levels are helpful in these instances. Therapeutic valproic acid levels are in the range of 50–100 mcg/ml. Therapeutic levels of lithium are generally considered to be 0.6–1.2 mEq/L but lower levels may be a better target for those older than 60 years of age. Goal therapeutic levels for lithium in older adults are more appropriately 0.4–0.8 mEq/L. Doses of lithium and divalproex can be safely directed by the long-term care provider. Lamotrigine is another commonly used mood stabilizer. Doses effective for bipolar disorder maintenance are typically 200 mg per day in older adults. Serum levels of lamotrigine are not commonly done or considered useful.

A commonly encountered clinical challenge is what to do if a patient on appropriate doses of mood stabilizer and no obvious underlying medical trigger has a manic or hypomanic episode. In these cases, a second agent may be necessary. Second-generation antipsychotics are the most commonly used add-on options for those with mania uncontrolled by mood stabilizers alone. Common choices include aripiprazole, olanzapine, quetiapine, risperidone, and ziprasidone. As with other medications in older adults, a smaller starting dose with frequent re-evaluation is preferred over starting at a dose that is too high.

The treatment of bipolar disorder in older adults would not be complete without the mention of nonpharmacologic interventions that can improve outcomes in those with the condition. Psychotherapy can assist patients with bipolar disorder to self-identify signs of mania, avoid triggers, and help patients with interpersonal conflicts that can sometimes exacerbate or trigger symptoms of bipolar mania or depression. Lifestyle interventions such as avoidance of stimulants like caffeine, regular physical activity, maintaining and supporting relationships with loved ones, and regular sleep schedules can be key to helping manage those at risk of mania or depression.

Take-Home Points

- Bipolar disorder is a condition that is commonly encountered in the older adult population. Estimates are that up to 4.5% of adults in the US are affected by bipolar disorder. The estimates for older adults are between 0.5 and 1%.
- It is important for healthcare providers in long-term care settings to recognize early signs of psychiatric destabilization in those with bipolar disorder. Signs of destabilization in older adults can be a decreased need for sleep, increased irritability, a general increase in activity, or even the development of psychosis (delusions or hallucinations).

- Starting a mood stabilizer or second-generation antipsychotic is a good first choice for those who are depressed with a known personal history of bipolar disorder and who are not already on one.
- Once underlying medical triggers for the destabilization of bipolar disorder and true medical emergency are ruled out, the long-term care provider should quickly intervene to prevent further worsening of bipolar symptoms and thereby prevent potential hospitalization.

References

1. Desai, A., & Grossberg, G. (2017). *Psychiatric Consultation in Long-Term Care (A Guide for Healthcare Professionals).* (Cambridge University Press.) p. 125.

Further Reading

Chakrabarti, S., & Singh, N. (2022). Psychotic symptoms in bipolar disorder and their impact on the illness: A systematic review. *World Journal of Psychiatry*, 12 (9), 1204–1232. https://doi.org/10.5498/wjp.v12.i9.1204

Harrison, P. J., Cipriani, A., Harmer, C. J., Nobre, A. C., Saunders, K., Goodwin, G. M., & Geddes, J. R. (2016). Innovative approaches to bipolar disorder and its treatment. *Annals of the New York Academy of Sciences*, 1366 (1), 76–89. https://doi.org/10.1111/nyas.13048

Huang, H., Nissen, N., Lim, C. T., Gören, J. L., Spottswood, M., & Huang, H. (2021). Treating bipolar disorder in primary care: Diagnosis, pharmacology, and management. *International Journal of General Medicine*, 15, 8299–8314. https://doi.org/10.2147/IJGM.S386875

McIntyre, R. S., Alda, M., Baldessarini, R. J., Bauer, M., Berk, M., Correll, C. U., Fagiolini, A., Fountoulakis, K., Frye, M. A., Grunze, H., Kessing, L. V., Miklowitz, D. J., Parker, G., Post, R. M., Swann, A. C., Suppes, T., Vieta, E., Young, A., & Maj, M. (2022). The clinical characterization of the adult patient with bipolar disorder aimed at personalization of management. *World Psychiatry*, 21 (3), 364–387. https://doi.org/10.1002/wps.20997

Nolen, W. A., Licht, R. W., Young, A. H., Malhi, G. S., Tohen, M., Vieta, E., Kupka, R. W., Zarate, C., Nielsen, R. E.,

Baldessarini, R. J., & Severus, E. (2019). What is the optimal serum level for lithium in the maintenance treatment of bipolar disorder? A systematic review and recommendations from the ISBD/IGSLI Task Force on treatment with lithium. *Bipolar Disorders*, 21 (5), 394–409. https://doi.org/10.1111/bdi.12805

Novick, D. M., & Swartz, H. A. (2019). Evidence-based psychotherapies for bipolar disorder. *Focus: Journal of Life-Long Learning in Psychiatry*, 17 (3), 238–248. https://doi.org/10.1176/appi.focus.20190004

Poon, S. H., Sim, K., & Baldessarini, R. J. (2015). Pharmacological approaches for treatment-resistant bipolar disorder. *Current Neuropharmacology*, 13 (5), 592–604. https://doi.org/10.2174/1570159X13666150630171954

Rhee, T. G., Olfson, M., Nierenberg, A. A., & Wilkinson, S. T. (2020). 20-year trends in the pharmacologic treatment of bipolar disorder by psychiatrists in outpatient care settings. *The American Journal of Psychiatry*, 177 (8), 706. https://doi.org/10.1176/appi.ajp.2020.19091000

Sajatovic, M., Strejilevich, S. A., Gildengers, A. G., Dols, A., Al Jurdi, R. K., Forester, B. P., Kessing, L. V., Beyer, J., Manes, F., Rej, S., Rosa, A. R., Schouws, S. N., Tsai, Y., Young, R. C., & Shulman, K. I. (2015). A report on older-age bipolar disorder from the International Society for Bipolar Disorders Task Force. *Bipolar Disorders*, 17 (7), 689. https://doi.org/10.1111/bdi.12331

Yatham, L. N., Kennedy, S. H., Parikh, S. V., Yatham, L. N., Kennedy, S. H., Parikh, S. V., Schaffer, A., Bond, D. J., Frey, B. N., Sharma, V., Goldstein, B. I., Rej, S., Beaulieu, S., Alda, M., MacQueen, G., Milev, R. V., Ravindran, A., O'Donovan, C., McIntosh, D., Lam, R. W., Vazquez, G.,

Kapczinski, F., McIntyre, R. S., Kozicky, J., Kanba, S., Lafer, B., Suppes, T., Calabrese, J. R., Vieta, E., Malhi, G., Post, R. M., & Berk, M. (2018). Canadian Network for Mood and Anxiety Treatments (CANMAT) and International Society for Bipolar Disorders (ISBD) 2018 guidelines for the management of patients with bipolar disorder. *Bipolar Disorders*, 20 (2), 97–170. doi:10.1111/bdi.12609

"I Am Feeling Great"
Secondary Mania

19

Mr. L was a 62-year-old male who was recently transferred back to his long-term care facility after being treated for severe pneumonia in hospital. While hospitalized, he was diagnosed with bipolar disorder and was treated with haloperidol and lorazepam for aggressive behaviors. Once transferred back to the long-term care facility, Mr. L was experiencing falls and was described as being belligerent with the staff. The staff believed he was having mood swings and exhibiting progressively worse aggressive verbal and physical behaviors over the one to two months since being hospitalized for pneumonia. He was also frequently irritable.

For some years before being admitted to the long-term care facility, Mr. L had a history of making rude comments during social situations and becoming verbally abusive toward the people he was working with. He became increasingly difficult to live with and, as a result, his wife of 32 years filed for divorce. Mr. L's family described an episode where he had assaulted a friend at a friend's house and then decided to walk two miles home in the bitter cold. Consequently, he developed pneumonia and had to be hospitalized.

He had also become nonadherent with treatment for his diabetes, congestive heart failure, and multiple other medical conditions. As a result, he required two partial foot amputations and needed assistance with multiple ADLs and medication management. This led his family to pursue placement in long-term care.

Up until about ten years ago, Mr. L was described as congenial and easy-going throughout his adult life. Before his 50s, he had no history of psychiatric problems. His brother was diagnosed with FTD at age 58.

During the mental status exam, Mr. L reported feeling great. He had recently physically assaulted an acquaintance at the long-term care facility after they declined to invest money in a real estate scheme proposed by Mr. L. When asked about his actions, Mr. L stated that his friend deserved to be hit because he had declined Mr. L's offer to "make money." Mr. L's SLUMS score was 25. On the neurological exam, he exhibited mild extrapyramidal symptoms, including tremors, stiffness, and bradykinesia.

Mr. L agreed to undergo neuropsychological testing and was found to have significant executive dysfunction. An MRI of the brain revealed moderate to severe asymmetric atrophy of both the frontal lobes and insula. The healthcare provider diagnosed him with FTD with secondary mania.

Treatment for Mr. L was initiated with divalproex and quetiapine, while haloperidol was discontinued. Lorazepam was switched from scheduled dosing to as-needed dosing. Over the next four weeks, Mr. L's aggression significantly decreased, and his behavior became more manageable for the staff. The haloperidol-induced extrapyramidal symptoms completely resolved.

Teaching Points

Mania is most commonly thought of as a phase of bipolar disorder and, for this reason, it can be easily misdiagnosed as such when a secondary cause of mania may truly be the culprit. Primary mania results from bipolar disorder. Secondary mania is a distinct form of mania that arises due to an underlying cause or condition. The symptoms of secondary mania can be indistinguishable from mania associated with bipolar disorder and can include an abnormally elevated or irritable mood accompanied by increased energy, racing thoughts, decreased need for sleep, impulsivity, or other manic features. Mania can occur secondary to metabolic disturbances, infection, neoplasm, epilepsy, and medications. When mania is a symptom of an underlying medical problem it is best considered secondary mania.

Although bipolar disorder can be seen with onset in persons over the age of 55 without a previous psychiatric history, new onset mania in older adults is more commonly secondary to another condition. Mania in older adults can be more debilitating than in younger patients. It is also known to be associated with more cognitive impairment in older adults.

Mania secondary to an underlying medical condition can result from various causes. Conditions to keep in mind include primary neurological disorders, endocrine abnormalities, medications, illicit substances, infectious disease, metabolic abnormalities, autoimmune disorders, and primary brain lesions (Box 19.1).

The workup of suspected secondary mania should first include a good history and physical. The history should focus on current medical symptoms, recent infections, use of medication or abuse of drugs, and any personal or family history of psychiatric conditions. If any neurological findings are demonstrated on a physical exam, a neurological consultation may be helpful. Lab evaluation should include blood counts, basic chemistries, vitamin B12, folate, and TSH levels. Imaging may include a CT of the head or MRI depending on the clinical scenario and acuity of the situation.

The treatment of secondary mania primarily focuses on correcting or optimizing the treatment of the underlying medical condition. There are several good options for treating the manic symptoms themselves. Divalproex is well tolerated in most older adults and is prescribed preferentially over valproic acid as it has much less likelihood of GI side effects. Second-generation antipsychotics, including olanzapine, risperidone, or quetiapine, are also good options and can be titrated easily to achieve the desired

---

Box 19.1   Potential causes of secondary mania in older adults

1. Medication side effects, that is corticosteroids, stimulants, antibiotics (including antitubercular agents, macrolide, and quinolones most commonly), levodopa, and benzodiazepines.
2. Illicit substances such as amphetamines, cocaine, and hallucinogens.
3. Neurologic conditions: Multiple sclerosis, stroke, brain tumors, TBI, seizure disorder, MNCD.
4. Endocrine disorders: Hyperthyroidism, Cushing's syndrome, hyperparathyroidism.
5. Infectious diseases: HIV/AIDS, viral encephalitis, Lyme disease.
6. Metabolic disturbances such as hyponatremia, hyper or hypoglycemia, and uremia.
7. Autoimmune disorders involving the CNS such as lupus and vasculitis.
8. Brain lesions such as tumors and arterial–venous malformations.

> **Box 19.2 Steps in the treatment of secondary mania in the long-term care setting**
>
> 1. Assess the appropriate treatment setting. Consider inpatient treatment if the patient is a potential harm to self or others or has acute medical comorbidities.
> 2. Optimize treatment of the underlying medical disorder.
> 3. Discontinue caffeine and all alcohol if applicable.
> 4. Discontinue antidepressants.
> 5. Initiate a first-line agent such as divalproex or an atypical antipsychotic. Titrate the dose to a therapeutic dose.
> 6. If not responding adequately to a first-line agent consider adding another agent. Add divalproex if already on an atypical antipsychotic or add an atypical antipsychotic if the patient is already on divalproex.
> 7. If symptoms are still not well controlled consider referral to a psychiatrist or geriatric psychiatrist.

response. Some patients require a combination of divalproex together with a second-generation antipsychotic. Clinicians should do their best to avoid benzodiazepines in older adults, but there are cases where a short course of as-needed benzodiazepine may be necessary to control symptoms (Box 19.2).

The case presented here is interesting on several fronts. This patient likely had long-standing hypomania as a result of his underlying FTD, which had probably been present for years prior to diagnosis. The acute exacerbation of his mania could have been triggered by his recent pneumonia with illness-related delirium and potentially even the antibiotics used to treat his pneumonia. The choice of haloperidol and lorazepam as initiated in the hospital was not the best choice for the treatment of his aggressive behaviors. Haloperidol, as a potent first-generation antipsychotic, can produce troubling side effects in older adults, such as Parkinsonism, akathisia, and increased falls. A potentially better therapeutic option would be a mood stabilizer such as divalproex with or without an atypical antipsychotic, such as quetiapine.

This case also demonstrates the importance of obtaining a psychosocial context when evaluating neuropsychiatric symptoms. The patient's history of functioning well before age 50 and then demonstrating progressively erratic behavior, troubled relationships, poor judgment, and irritability out of proportion with the patient's cognitive impairment gave clues to an underlying progressive neuropsychiatric condition. The patient's positive family history of FTD gave additional clues that should have led to further workup along these lines.

> **Take-Home Points**
>
> – Mania is most commonly thought of as a phase of bipolar disorder and, for this reason, it can be easily misdiagnosed as such when a secondary cause of mania may truly be the culprit.
> – The workup of suspected secondary mania should first include a good history and physical. The history should focus on current medical symptoms, recent infections, use of medication or abuse of drugs, and any personal or family history of psychiatric conditions.
> – Mania secondary to an underlying medical condition can result from various causes. Conditions to keep in mind include primary neurological disorders, endocrine abnormalities, medications, illicit substances, infectious disease, metabolic abnormalities, autoimmune disorders, and primary brain lesions.
> – The treatment of secondary mania primarily focuses on correcting or optimizing the treatment of the underlying medical condition. There are several good options for treating the manic symptoms themselves. Divalproex is well tolerated in most older adults.

Further Reading

Cuartas, C. F., & Davis, M. (2022). Valproic acid in the management of delirium. *American Journal of Hospice Palliative Medicine*, 39 (5), 562–569. doi: 10.1177/10499091211038371. Epub 2021 Aug 19. PMID: 34409869.

Devenney, E. M, Ahmed, R. M, & Hodges, J. R. (2019). Frontotemporal dementia. *Handbook of Clinical Neurology*, 167, 279–299. doi: 10.1016/B978-0-12-804766-8.00015-7. PMID: 31753137.

Jasani, R., Deacon, J. W., & Sertich, A. (2021). Corticosteroid-induced mania after previous tolerance of higher doses. *Cureus*, 13 (9), e17719. doi: 10.7759/cureus.17719. PMID: 34650893; PMCID: PMC8489796.

Jochim, J., Rifkin-Zybutz, R. P., Geddes, J., & Cipriani, A. (2019). Valproate for acute mania. *Cochrane Database of Systematic Reviews*, 10 (10), CD004052. doi: 10.1002/14651858.CD004052.pub2. PMID: 31621892; PMCID: PMC6953329.

Kendler, K. S. (2017). The clinical features of mania and their representation in modern diagnostic criteria. *Psychological Medicine*, 47 (6), 1013–1029. doi: 10.1017/S0033291716003238. Epub 2016 Dec 19. PMID: 27989245.

Khoury, R., Liu, Y., Sheheryar, Q., & Grossberg, G. T. (2021). Pharmacotherapy for frontotemporal dementia. *CNS Drugs*, 35 (4), 425–438. doi: 10.1007/s40263-021-00813-0. Epub 2021 Apr 11. PMID: 33840052.

Lekurwale, V., Acharya, S., Shukla, S., & Kumar, S. (2023). Neuropsychiatric manifestations of thyroid diseases. *Cureus*, 15 (1), e33987. doi: 10.7759/cureus.33987. PMID: 36811059; PMCID: PMC9938951.

Sloan, S., & Dosumu-Johnson, R. T. (2020). A new onset of mania in a 49-year-old man: An interesting case of Wilson Disease. *Journal of Psychiatric Practice*, 26 (6), 510–517. doi: 10.1097/PRA.0000000000000505. PMID: 33275388; PMCID: PMC10170309.

Younes, K., & Miller, B. L. (2020). Frontotemporal dementia: Neuropathology, genetics, neuroimaging, and treatments. *Psychiatric Clinics of North America*, 43 (2), 331–344. Doi: 10.1016/j.psc.2020.02.006. Epub 2020 Apr 8. PMID: 32439025.

"I Am Staying Here Illegally"
Major Depressive Disorder with Psychosis

Mr. T, a 78-year-old divorced male, had been reporting fears of being put in jail because he had been living "illegally" in the nursing home. He was also experiencing sleep impairment and lack of appetite with a 15-pound weight loss over three months (from 189 pounds to 174, height was 5' 8") and had been refusing to shave, change clothes, or bathe for three weeks. He was referred to the psychiatrist because for a week he had been saying that he would be better off dead. The psychiatrist noted that Mr. T had a history of a "mini-stroke" six months previously and had recently developed severe abdominal pain requiring gall bladder surgery. Mr. T was admitted to the nursing home for rehabilitation. After completing rehabilitation, he was transferred to the long-term care wing for a continued stay as there was no one to take care of him at home. He also had a history of recurrent falls, cognitive impairment, and refusal to take medication, and required close monitoring of unstable diabetes.

His family reported that Mr. T had been disappointed when he was told he could not return home. He had since become withdrawn, stopped smiling, and even stopped watching sports on TV (one of his favorite activities in the past). During the interview, Mr. T reported feeling nervous and explained that his reason for not shaving or bathing was fear that his skin would somehow "infect" his roommate. He felt that he could not ask for a room change because "I am staying here illegally." Mr. T further explained that he had no money to pay the high cost of the nursing home (he had apparently seen the monthly charge of his stay, which was approximately $6,000). Mr. T had a history of severe depression 15 years previously when he had retired but his daughters did not know the details and Mr. T could not give details except to confirm that he was given "nerve pills." There was no obvious history of previous manic or hypomanic episodes and Mr. T had a family history of depression (sister) and suicide (brother). Medication review did not identify any medication that could cause or exacerbate psychiatric symptoms, and laboratory tests (including thyroid tests and vitamin levels) were unremarkable.

On a mental status exam, Mr. T exhibited a depressed mood and affect, delusions of persecution, and passive suicidal ideas (felt life was not worth living) but denied any specific suicidal intention or plan. His recall was one out of three, his SLUMS score was 16, and his geriatric depression scale (GDS30) score was 20/30 (severe depression). Mr. T was diagnosed with recurrent MDD with psychotic features and probable vascular MNCD. The psychiatrist recommended hospitalization and ECT, but Mr. T declined both. There were insufficient grounds for involuntary commitment, as he agreed to treatment at the nursing home. Mr. T was started on sertraline 25 mg daily, and the dose was gradually increased every four days by 25 mg to 100 mg daily. He was also started on risperidone 0.25 mg at bedtime, which was increased to 0.5 mg at bedtime after one week. Behavioral activation with an individualized pleasant activity schedule (IPAS) was initiated.

After four weeks, family and staff reported that Mr. T's appetite and sleep had improved but he was still refusing to shave and come out of his room. His participation in exercise and other activities was intermittent and brief. During the interview, Mr. T continued to express delusional thinking and depressed affect. Over the next two weeks, risperidone was further increased to 0.25 mg daily in the morning and 0.5 mg at bedtime for seven days and then 0.5 mg daily in the morning and 0.5 mg daily at bedtime.

After four more weeks, Mr. T reported for the first time that he was feeling better and started showing interest in watching sports on TV and allowed staff to shave him and help him bathe. His participation in exercise and other pleasant activities also increased considerably. After four more weeks, he was shaving and bathing regularly and did not express any fears he had before. Mr. T still expressed sadness at not being able to go home and hoped the psychiatrist would help him return. Mr. T's repeat GDS30 score was 8/30 and his repeat SLUMS score was 21.

Teaching Points

Most clinicians treating geriatric patients are comfortable with the diagnosis of MDD. The symptoms of major depression are listed in Box 20.1. Those with depression with psychosis meet the criteria for diagnosis of depression but also experience psychotic symptoms. When individuals with MDD experience delusions, hallucinations, or catatonic symptoms, it is referred to as MDD with psychotic psychosis, also known as psychotic depression. These individuals often display inflexible thinking, more severe depression, and delusions that typically align with their mood. These delusions may involve guilt regarding past events, poverty, somatic illness (such as an obsessive fear of having a terminal illness like cancer), or paranoia. Hallucinations, although less common than delusions in these cases, are more likely to be auditory rather than visual or somatic.

Residents diagnosed with psychotic depression often exhibit agitation, characterized by classic behaviors like pacing and wringing hands. They also experience more pronounced cognitive disturbances and have a higher likelihood of having a family history of MDD or bipolar disorder. If a resident with depression has a history of delusions during a depressive episode or shows profound anxiety, it strongly indicates the possibility of psychotic depression.

The lifetime prevalence of psychotic depression has been estimated between 0.35–1% [1]. In contrast to schizophrenia and schizoaffective disorder, the psychotic symptoms in psychotic depression remit as the depression improves. Psychosis in bipolar disorder is more likely to emerge during a manic episode. The severity of depression is often greater in those with psychotic depression when compared to patients with depression without psychosis.

The nature of psychosis in those with depression is usually mood-congruent somatic, pessimistic, or guilt-related delusions. An example of a mood-congruent somatic delusion might be a patient's fixed belief that they are dying of a malignancy when there is no evidence to support that belief. Delusions of spousal infidelity are also commonly seen.

Healthcare providers must diagnose psychotic depression early due to its high risk of suicide and poor response to antidepressant treatment alone [2]. Additional

Box 20.1 Symptoms of MDD in long-term care populations

Core symptoms

1. Lack of interest in daily activities.
2. Depressed mood/affect.

Additional symptoms

1. Lack of appetite or weight loss; increased appetite or weight gain.
2. Insomnia or hypersomnia.
3. Recurrent thoughts of suicide, wish to die, or suicide attempt.
4. Decreased energy or fatigue.
5. Hopelessness.
6. Helplessness.
7. Worthlessness.
8. Inappropriate or excessive guilt.
9. Loss of self-confidence.
10. Staying in bed excessively.
11. Multiple somatic complaints.
12. Chronic pain not responding to pain medication.
13. Hypochondriasis (excessive fear that one may have or will develop a serious illness).
14. Marked symptoms of anxiety.
15. Agitation (especially by residents who have advanced MNCD).
16. Verbal aggression or verbally abusive behavior (especially by residents who have advanced MNCD).
17. Physical aggression (especially by a resident who has advanced MNCD).
18. Decreased spontaneous speech.
19. Psychomotor retardation or agitation.
20. Refusing medication.
21. Resisting care.
22. Refusing to participate in therapy (physical, occupational, speech).
23. Sudden decline in cognition.
24. Subjective memory complaint.

Borrowed with permission from:

Desai, A., & Grossberg, G. Psychiatric Consultation in Long-Term Care (A Guide for Healthcare Professionals) Cambridge University Press. p. 125.

antipsychotic medication is typically necessary in addition to the antidepressant for an effective response. In severe cases, hospitalization and early consideration of ECT are recommended, particularly in situations where psychotic depression poses a life-threatening risk, such as severe malnourishment or catatonia. Electroconvulsive therapy can be safely used with this population and may be lifesaving in severe cases of psychotic depression.

Electroconvulsive therapy is a highly effective treatment option for those with severe unipolar depression and has been used since the 1920s but declined in popularity due to negative perceptions and the development of new therapeutic agents such as antipsychotics. In recent decades it has again been gaining popularity as a first-line treatment approach. Electroconvulsive therapy is more effective than traditional pharmacotherapies and is more commonly used in those with severe depression with suicidality, catatonia, and those with psychotic depression. Studies have shown a response rate of 70–90% with ECT in those with severe depression. The safety of the procedure has improved due to improvements in ECT and anesthesia techniques. Side effects can be a temporary disorientation that may be accompanied by an anterograde or retrograde amnesia. The amnesia usually recovers over time.

Common indications for ECT include severe depression, psychotic depression, treatment-resistant depression, catatonia, mania, and acute suicidality. Older adults may have an even greater response to ECT than younger patients.

Regarding the case presented here, an important consideration is whether or not the patient can be safely treated in a long-term care setting versus an inpatient setting. Potential reasons for inpatient psychiatric care include, but are not limited to, acute suicidality, catatonia, severe behavioral disturbances, and refusal of oral medications. The clinician recommended that Mr. T be treated in an inpatient setting with ECT but the patient declined this recommendation. His psychotic depression warranted closer follow-up. It should be noted that response to antidepressant/antipsychotic medications can take up to 12 weeks. The improvement in the SLUMS score with treatment of depression underscores the fact that depression is often a reversible factor in the treatment of cognitive impairment in people who have MNCD.

Take-Home Points

- Those with depression with psychosis meet the criteria for diagnosis of depression but also experience psychotic symptoms. When individuals with MDD experience delusions, hallucinations, or catatonic symptoms, it is referred to as MDD with psychotic features, also known as psychotic depression.
- It is crucial for healthcare providers to diagnose psychotic depression early due to its high risk of suicide and poor response to antidepressant treatment alone. Additional antipsychotic medication is typically necessary in addition to the antidepressant for an effective response.
- The nature of psychosis in those with depression is usually mood-congruent somatic, pessimistic, or guilt-related delusions.
- Electroconvulsive therapy is more commonly used in those with severe depression with suicidality, catatonia, and those with psychotic depression. Studies have shown a response rate of 70–90% with ECT in those with severe depression.

References

1. Jääskeläinen, E., Juola, T., Korpela, H., Lehtiniemi, H., Nietola, M., Korkeila, J., & Miettunen, J. (2018). Epidemiology of psychotic depression: Systematic review and meta-analysis. *Psychological Medicine*, 48 (6), 905–918.

2. Zalpuri, I., & Rothschild, A. J. (2016). Does psychosis increase the risk of suicide in patients with major depression?

A systematic review. *Journal of Affective Disorders*, 198, 23–31.

Further Reading

Desai, A., & Grossberg, G. (2017). *Psychiatric Consultation in Long-Term Care (A Guide for Healthcare Professionals)* (Cambridge University Press.) p. 125.

Goegan, S. A., Hasey, G. M., King, J. P., Losier, B. J., Bieling, P. J., McKinnon, M. C., & McNeely, H. E. (2022). Naturalistic study on the effects of electroconvulsive therapy (ECT) on depressive symptoms. *Canadian Journal of Psychiatry. Revue Canadienne de Psychiatrie*, 67 (5), 351–360. https://doi.org/10.1177/07067437211064020

Lloyd, J. R., Silverman, E. R., Kugler, J. L., & Cooper, J. J. (2019). Electroconvulsive therapy for patients with catatonia: Current perspectives. *Neuropsychiatric Disease and Treatment*, 16, 2191–2208. https://doi.org/10.2147/NDT.S231573

Neufeld, N. H., Kaczkurkin, A. N., Sotiras, A., Mulsant, B. H., Dickie, E. W., Flint, A. J., Meyers, B. S., Alexopoulos, G. S., Rothschild, A. J., Whyte, E. M., Mah, L., Nierenberg, J., Hoptman, M. J., Davatzikos, C., Satterthwaite, T. D., & Voineskos, A. N. (2020). Structural brain networks in remitted psychotic depression. *Neuropsychopharmacology*, 45 (7), 1223–1231. https://pubmed.ncbi.nlm.nih.gov/32109935/

Wu, Z., Su, G., Lu, W., Liu, L., Zhou, Z., & Xie, B. (2021). Clinical symptoms and their relationship with cognitive impairment in elderly patients with depressive disorder. *Frontiers in Psychiatry*, 13. https://doi.org/10.3389/fpsyt.2022.1009653

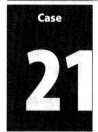

"That Priest Is a Gossip"
Schizophrenia and Long-Acting Injectable Antipsychotics

Ms. S was a 77-year-old resident with a known schizoaffective disorder. She was transferred to long-term care from a local group home as she had become nonadherent with medications and had not been eating well. She had been maintained on aripiprazole for some time, but she decided to stop the medication as she felt it was "mind-altering" and caused her to feel not like herself. She also stated that she felt her visual hallucinations were becoming more frequent and that they were caused by and not helped by the aripiprazole. Her most frequent hallucination was that of a man sitting in her room silently watching her, who would usually disappear once she began speaking. She also had feelings that others were causing her harm without even speaking or interacting with her in any way through a sort of telepathic ability.

The patient's aripiprazole was discontinued due to her feelings that it was causing her harm. She was started on risperidone 0.5 mg every evening but it seemed to have little effect on her hallucinations so it was increased to 1 mg qhs. She had no prominent mood symptoms and was not on any antidepressant medications or medications for anxiety. She felt the higher dose of risperidone caused her GI distress. She then developed worsening delusions, thinking that staff were trying to poison her and that the cleaning products used in the facility were causing her to be essentially paralyzed from the waist down. She rarely left her room and stayed mostly in her bed.

She was sent to the emergency room for making a vague suicidal statement that she later did not recall and continued to feel that her risperidone and the cleaning products used in the facility were causing her lower extremity weakness. She was started on sertraline 25 mg daily for depression which was gradually increased to 100 mg daily, and had continued paranoid delusions. For example, she thought that her priest was telling other residents at the facility about private conversations they had had.

Over the following year, she seemed to settle in at the long-term care facility. Her routine was mostly solitary, leaving her room only for meals and writing mostly unintelligible prose in a tattered notebook. She again began to decline all medications, including her psychotropics. Despite her nonadherence to medications, she did not develop any disruptive behaviors or worsening mood symptoms. It was decided not to push the issue of medication nonadherence with the patient as she was functioning fairly well. Her routine was unfaltering. She left her room only for meals and preferred to be alone and not participate in group activities. She remained content to write in her notebooks and had brief but friendly interactions with a few staff members she had learned to trust. She remained relatively suspicious of most others.

Teaching Points

Ms. S's case presented several challenges over the two to three years she was cared for by her geriatric psychiatrist. Her paranoia regarding medications and staff made it nearly impossible at times to treat her. This is a not an uncommon scenario when providing mental health for those with thought disorders and prominent paranoia. Over the next one to two years the patient settled down into her new community. Facility staff began to get to know her and became less troubled by the occasional odd statements she made. Although long-acting injectable medications (LAIM) were considered it was decided that a more conservative watch-and-wait approach was acceptable as the patient's delusions and hallucinations were generally not troubling to her nor did they lead to behaviors that were disruptive to staff or other residents. It is possible over time that Ms. S learned to be very guarded when discussing her mental health and learned to minimize her symptoms as a way of avoiding unwanted treatments. Regardless of the reason she continued to do well in this environment with periodic brief encounters with her mental health providers to assess behavioral and mood stability.

It is well known that, despite the availability of effective oral antipsychotics for the treatment of schizophrenia, adherence can be low, with 40–50% of patients on antipsychotics for schizophrenia nonadherent to treatment. Nonadherence to treatment can lead to increased relapse rates of serious symptoms and an overall decline in function. Strategies discussed to increase adherence to antipsychotic treatment often involve long-acting injectable antipsychotics (LAIs).

Some benefits of LAIs include improved adherence, reduced relapse rates, reduced hospitalization rates, improved quality of life, and improved therapeutic outcomes. They are typically administered once every four weeks, which eliminates the need for daily medication adherence. A newer formulation of paliperidone can be administered intramuscularly once every three months. This can be especially beneficial for individuals who struggle with adhering to a daily medication regimen. Studies have shown that LAIs are associated with lower rates of relapse compared to oral medications. This may be due to the consistent blood levels of the medication provided by LAIs, which can help to maintain therapeutic levels and prevent symptoms from returning. Long-acting injectable antipsychotics have been shown to reduce the need for hospitalization due to relapse. This can help individuals to maintain their daily lives and avoid disruptions in their routines. Long-acting injectable antipsychotics can provide individuals with a greater sense of control over their illness, as they do not have to worry about missing doses or experiencing medication-related side effects as frequently. They can provide more consistent therapeutic outcomes over time, as the medication is released slowly into the bloodstream over weeks. This can lead to more stable symptom control and a better overall treatment response.

Take-Home Points

- Medication adherence is a major challenge when treating psychiatric conditions, especially conditions that can involve impaired insight and judgment.
- Long-acting injectable antipsychotics are best started by those with experience in their use but continuing therapy may be managed by primary providers in areas underserved by mental health specialists.

- Conditions requiring strict adherence to antipsychotics may be helped by the use of LAIs. Some available LAIs include aripiprazole, paliperidone, olanzapine, and risperidone.
- Benefits of LAIs include better adherence when compared to oral therapies, the bypassing of potentially unpredictable GI pharmacokinetics, and improved steady-state blood levels of medication.

Further Reading

Brissos, S., Veguilla, M. R., Taylor, D., & Balanzá-Martinez, V. (2014) The role of long-acting injectable antipsychotics in schizophrenia: A critical appraisal. *Therapeutic Advances in Psychopharmacology*, 4 (5), 198–219. doi: 10.1177/2045125314540297. PMID: 25360245; PMCID: PMC4212490.

Desai, A., & Grossberg, G. (2017). *Psychiatric Consultation in Long-Term Care. A Guide for Healthcare Professionals.* 2nd ed. (Cambridge University Press.) pp. 165–204.

Schneider-Thoma, J., Chalkou, K., Dörries, C., Bighelli, I., Ceraso, A., Huhn, M., Siafis, S., Davis, J. M., Cipriani, A., Furukawa, T. A., Salanti, G., & Leucht, S. (2022). Comparative efficacy and tolerability of 32 oral and long-acting injectable antipsychotics for the maintenance treatment of adults with schizophrenia: A systematic review and network meta-analysis. *The Lancet*, 399 (10327), 824–836. https://pubmed.ncbi.nlm.nih.gov/35219395/

Tampi, R. R., Young, J., Hoq, R., Resnick, K., & Tampi, D. J. (2019). Psychotic disorders in late life: A narrative review. *Therapeutic Advances in Psychopharmacology*, 9, 2045125319882798.

"He Just Won't Get Up"

Catatonia

22

Mr. S was a 68-year-old male with a history of congestive heart failure, diabetes, morbid obesity, frequent UTIs, bipolar disorder, benign prostatic hypertrophy, urinary retention, remote history of deep vein thrombosis (DVT), and a history of decubitus ulcers. He had lived in long-term care for the past five years as his physical disability from his congestive heart failure (CHF) and obesity progressed. He required a motorized wheelchair for mobility and was dependent on caregivers for nearly all ADLs. He had a supportive family, his wife and two daughters lived close to his care facility and were able to visit often.

Mr. S had been followed by his long-term care psychiatrist for four years. He was doing well on his current regimen of divalproex 500 mg bid and citalopram 20 mg daily. His non-psychiatric medications included tamsulosin 0.4 mg daily, mirabegron 25 mg daily for an overactive bladder, carvedilol 12.5 mg twice daily, fosinopril 10 mg daily, torsemide 20 mg daily, spironolactone 25 mg daily, glipizide 5 mg daily, and aspirin 81 mg daily.

Unfortunately, Mr. S had an injury while being transferred from his bed to his wheelchair and sustained a fracture to his left hip requiring admission to the hospital for an open reduction-internal fixation procedure. He was hospitalized for four days and discharged back to the nursing home. After coming back to the nursing home the patient was noted to be more withdrawn than usual. Facility care staff alerted his psychiatrist that Mr. S was often found in his wheelchair just staring into space and found little interest in the social activities at the facility that he previously enjoyed. His wife also noted that on her most recent visit, Mr. S was inattentive and did not appear to enjoy her visit, which was quite unlike him. Staff also mentioned that Mr. S preferred to stay in his room in the mornings and often skipped breakfast and sometimes lunch.

On examination, the patient was found to be appropriately dressed and he was in his wheelchair as usual. Eye contact was poor, his mood was described as depressed, and his affect was flat. There was no evidence of hallucinations or delusions and Mr. S would generally respond to questions with only brief one-word responses. His psychiatrist diagnosed worsening depression in the setting of bipolar disease and added aripiprazole 2.5 mg, which was later increased to 5 mg daily. At a return visit the following week, the patient had not improved and continued to spend most of the day in bed. He was eating and drinking little and only with much encouragement. It was thought that Mr. S's depression had not had time enough to respond to the addition of aripiprazole. Labs including a urinalysis were recommended but no acute changes to explain his worsening lethargy were found.

One of the members of staff at the facility later reached out to the psychiatrist and said that the patient's status had again worsened, and he was now refusing to get out of bed. He was in bed nearly all of the time with his eyes closed and responding minimally to others. He had no interest in even watching television. He was now eating only bites of nutrition at best in a given day. He was not opening his mouth for medications. An urgent visit by a psychiatrist was requested.

At the follow-up visit Mr. S was found to be in his bed with his eyes closed at 1 pm. His nurse commented, "he just won't get up." His hygiene was poor and he was disheveled. When addressed verbally he would not answer questions and would only briefly open his eyes when shaken. When asked how he felt he would reply with the word "fine", whispered several times. His limbs were described as somewhat stiff. Mr. S's wife was called and permitted the patient to be transferred to a hospital with geriatric psychiatric services for further workup and treatment of presumed catatonia. Mr. S's workup in the emergency department included imaging and labs that did not show any anatomic or metabolic causes for his worsening mental status. An inpatient psychiatric evaluation was obtained and the impression was that of catatonia in the setting of bipolar depression. Psychiatry recommended starting lorazepam at 0.5 mg IV three times daily. Within 24 hours Mr. S became somewhat more alert and responsive, as demonstrated by making eye contact with his family and nursing staff and answering simple yes/no questions appropriately. The dose of lorazepam was increased to 1 mg three times daily. Over the next two days, Mr. S became increasingly alert and began to take in small amounts of food and fluids. Soon he was able to maintain his hydration without IV fluids and was transferred to a geriatric psychiatric unit for further treatment.

Teaching Points

Catatonia is a severe neuropsychiatric condition characterized by a state of immobility, stupor, and unresponsiveness to the environment. In years past the diagnosis of catatonia implied the presence of underlying schizophrenia but now it is known to be associated with a variety of psychiatric, neurological, or medical disorders. It is usually seen in mood disorders but can also be seen in psychotic and various neurological disorders. Estimates vary depending on location, but it is thought to be present in 5–10% of inpatient psychiatric patients.

The symptoms of catatonia are listed in Box 22.1. Signs and symptoms of catatonia can be thought of in terms of motor signs, affective features, and cognitive–behavioral features. Motor signs may include posturing, waxy flexibility, stereotypy, and dyskinesias. Examples

---

Box 22.1 Common symptoms of catatonia

1. Stupor: A state of unresponsiveness and immobility, where the individual appears to be in a trance-like state.
2. Rigidity: A state of muscular rigidity, where the individual may hold their body in awkward or uncomfortable positions.
3. Posturing: A state where the individual may assume fixed, unusual, or bizarre postures.
4. Mutism: A state of silence, where the individual may not speak or respond to questions.
5. Excitement: A state of hyperactivity, where the individual may become agitated, violent, or self-destructive.

Box 22.2 Medical conditions that may be accompanied by catatonia

1. Central nervous system inflammatory conditions such as Lupus, multiple sclerosis, and paraneoplastic autoimmune encephalitis.
2. Psychiatric conditions such as depression, mania, schizophrenia, anxiety disorders, postpartum depression, and autism spectrum disorders.
3. Infectious causes. These can include bacterial meningitis, viral encephalitis, and prion diseases.
4. Endocrine causes. Hyper or hypothyroidism, Addison's disease, hypoparathyroidism.
5. Focal CNS lesions. These can include stroke, TBI, and neoplasms.
6. Medication-related. Catatonia has been seen with a variety of medications including antipsychotics, corticosteroids, certain antibiotics, and other psychiatric medications.
7. Toxin related. Examples include carbon monoxide and inhalants.
8. Medications/drugs. Catatonia can be seen with either the reduction or withdrawal of certain medications including alcohol, benzodiazepines, PCP, ecstasy, and opiates.
9. Metabolic states. Catatonia is sometimes seen in such conditions as diabetic ketoacidosis, advanced renal failure, advanced liver failure, severe hyponatremia, hypercalcemia, and Wilson's disease, among others.
10. Major neurocognitive disorders. Catatonia can sometimes be seen in DLB, Parkinson's disease, and FTD, for example.
11. Acute CNS insults such as TBI, hypoxia, and unrecognized seizure disorder.

of affective features of catatonia can include emotional lability, anxiety, affective latency, impulsivity, and excitement. Cognitive–behavioral features can include such signs as perseveration, echolalia, echopraxia, mutism, and automatic obedience. Rating scales such as the Bush–Francis Catatonia Rating Scale can be used to assist in the evaluation of patients with suspected catatonia [1]. The Bush–Francis rating scale helps clinicians quantify the severity of motor signs, affective signs, and cognitive–behavioral features.

The causes of catatonia can vary and include psychiatric disorders such as schizophrenia, bipolar disorder, and MDD, as well as medical conditions such as encephalitis, brain injury, and metabolic disorders. See Box 22.2 for a partial list of medical conditions which can be accompanied by catatonic features.

The pathophysiology of catatonia is not fully understood, but it is believed to involve dysfunction in the dopamine and gamma-aminobutyric acid (GABA) neurotransmitter systems, as well as abnormalities in the frontal–subcortical circuits and the limbic system.

Some studies suggest that catatonia may be related to changes in the balance of excitatory and inhibitory neurotransmitters in the brain. Specifically, it is thought that decreased GABA activity in the frontal lobes may lead to overstimulation of the basal ganglia and other subcortical regions, resulting in the characteristic motor abnormalities seen in catatonia.

Other studies have implicated abnormalities in the dopamine system, which may contribute to the motor symptoms and cognitive deficits seen in catatonia. For example, dopamine receptor hypersensitivity has been observed in some cases of catatonia, which may explain the hyperactivity and agitation seen in some patients.

In addition to these neurotransmitter abnormalities, catatonia has also been associated with changes in brain structure and function. Some studies have suggested that patients with catatonia may have reduced gray matter volume in certain brain regions including the anterior cingulate cortex and the prefrontal cortex. Other studies have found alterations in functional connectivity between brain regions, particularly in the frontal–subcortical circuits [2].

The pathophysiology of catatonia is complex and likely involves dysfunction in multiple brain regions and neurotransmitter systems. Further research is needed to fully understand the underlying mechanisms of this syndrome and to develop more effective treatments.

The workup of suspected catatonia is in line with the workup of change in mental status and usually includes basic labs including thyroid function, CBC, CMP, urinalysis, and drug screen. Central nervous system imaging is usually helpful in ruling out space-occupying lesions, stroke, and inflammatory CNS findings. An electroencephalogram (EEG) can be necessary to rule out an underlying seizure disorder. After underlying medical conditions have been ruled out, a benzodiazepine challenge test can help diagnose catatonia. First, the examiner evaluates catatonic symptoms using a catatonia rating scale such as the Bush–Francis Catatonia Rating Scale [3]. Then a dose of IV lorazepam is given and the rating scale is repeated. A 50% reduction in the rating scale score is very suggestive of catatonia.

The treatment of catatonia associated with medical illness is primarily the treatment of the underlying disease. In those with catatonia secondary to psychiatric illness, benzodiazepines and ECT are commonly used to treat catatonia. Both are effective in reducing symptoms. Other treatments that have been used with some success include atypical antipsychotics, such as clozapine and olanzapine, and dopamine agonists, such as amantadine.

Benzodiazepines and ECT are the most commonly used treatments for catatonia and both have shown similar efficacy [4]. A benzodiazepine challenge is often a good place to start when initiating treatment for catatonia secondary to underlying psychiatric illness. Lorazepam is the most commonly used benzodiazepine for this indication. In older adults, a common starting dose is 0.5–1 mg IV three times daily, although higher doses may be required. Electroconvulsive therapy can produce the highest success in cases of catatonia [5], but does present some challenges as a treatment option. There may be limited availability of ECT in some settings or delays in accessing it. There are also potential legal issues in obtaining consent for ECT as patients are often not able to consent for themselves.

Overall, the prognosis for individuals with catatonia is generally good, especially when the underlying cause is identified and treated promptly. With appropriate treatment, most individuals with catatonia will recover fully or experience significant improvement in their symptoms.

Take-Home Points

- Catatonia is a severe neuropsychiatric condition characterized by a state of immobility, stupor, and unresponsiveness to the environment.
- Excited catatonia is a less common form in which patients develop prolonged periods of psychomotor agitation.
- Common symptoms of catatonia can include stupor, rigidity, posturing, mutism, or prolonged excitement and agitation.

– Signs and symptoms of catatonia can be thought of in terms of motor signs, affective features, and cognitive–behavioral features.
– Benzodiazepines and ECT are the most commonly used treatments for catatonia. Both treatments have shown similar efficacy.

References

1. Bush, G., Fink, M., Petrides, G., Dowling, F., & Francis, A. (1996). Catatonia. I. Rating scale and standardized examination. *Acta Psychiatrica Scandinavica*, 93 (2), 129–136.

2. Ariza-Salamanca, D. F., Corrales-Hernández, M. G., Pachón-Londoño, M. J., & Hernández-Duarte, I. (2021). Molecular and cellular mechanisms leading to catatonia: An integrative approach from clinical and preclinical evidence. *Frontiers in Molecular Neuroscience*, 15. https://doi.org/10.3389/fnmol.2022.993671

3. Francis A. Catatonia: diagnosis, classification, and treatment. *Curr Psychiatry Rep*. 2010 Jun;12(3):180–185. doi: 10.1007/s11920-010-0113-y. PMID: 20425278.

4. Pelzer, A. C., van der Heijden, F. M., & den Boer, E. (2018). Systematic review of catatonia treatment. *Neuropsychiatric Disease and Treatment*, 14, 317–326.

5. Lloyd, J. R., Silverman, E. R., Kugler, J. L., & Cooper, J. J. (2020). Electroconvulsive therapy for patients with catatonia: Current perspectives. *Neuropsychiatric Disease and Treatment*, 16, 2191–2208. doi: 10.2147/NDT.S231573. eCollection 2020.

Further Reading

Denysenko, L., Sica, N., Penders, T. M., Philbrick, K. L., Walker, A., Shaffer, S., &

Francis, A. (2018). Catatonia in the medically ill: Etiology, diagnosis, and treatment. The Academy of Consultation-Liaison Psychiatry Evidence-Based Medicine Subcommittee Monograph. *Annals of clinical psychiatry: official journal of the American Academy of Clinical Psychiatrists*, 30 (2), 140–155.

Narayanaswamy, J. C., Tibrewal, P., Zutshi, A., Srinivasaraju, R., & Math, S. B. (2012). Clinical predictors of response to treatment in catatonia. *General Hospital Psychiatry*, 34 (3), 312–316.

Rogers, J. P., Oldham, M. A., Fricchione, G., Northoff, G., Wilson, J. E., Mann, S. C., Francis, A., Wieck, A., Wachtel, L. E., Lewis, G., Grover, S., Hirjak, D., Ahuja, N., Zandi, M. S., Young, A. H., Fone, K., Andrews, S., Kessler, D., Saifee, T., & David, A. S. (2023). Evidence-based consensus guidelines for the management of catatonia: Recommendations from the British Association for Psychopharmacology. *Journal of Psychopharmacology (Oxford, England)*, 37 (4), 327–369. https://doi.org/10.1177/02698811231158232

Vaquerizo-Serrano, J., De Pablo, G. S., Singh, J., & Santosh, P. (2022). Catatonia in autism spectrum disorders: A systematic review and meta-analysis. *European Psychiatry*, 65 (1), e4.

"My Body Is Being Taken over by a Fungus!"

23

Delusional Disorder

Mrs. S, an 83-year-old long-term care resident, was referred to psychiatry by the patient's primary care nurse practitioner at the request of the patient's daughters due to persever-ation regarding thoughts that her body was being taken over by a fungal infection. During the first visit, the patient's two daughters were present and assisted with the history. The patient insisted on providing a detailed history of a fungal infection that she claimed started several months earlier as flakiness of her scalp. She was prescribed Nizoral shampoo, which proved to be effective. About a month later, the patient developed a mild candidal rash under her breasts, which also responded well to topical Nystatin cream.

Over the subsequent months, the patient began to perseverate more about her belief that the fungal infection was now "inside me" and "eating me from the inside out!" When asked about the evidence that led her to believe she had a fungal infection, Mrs. S would repeatedly respond, "I just know. I can feel it. It makes me short of breath, I itch, I can't breathe well. It's in my bowels, and I can hear it making noises in there!"

The patient's daughters advised that the patient had seen two different gastroenter-ologists, a dermatologist, and a pulmonologist for these complaints. All of these pro-viders released her from their care after complete workups that were negative for any signs of systemic infection or any other acute pathology, for that matter. Despite these reassurances, Mrs. S would fixate on perceived irregularities in her skin coloration, breathing patterns, and bowel movements, which she was sure proved her systemic fungal infection. These thoughts were intrusive and present every day for many hours.

Mrs. S denied having any visual or auditory hallucinations and her mood seemed somewhat more irritable in recent weeks. Her daughters felt this irritability was second-ary to Mrs. S's frustration about how she felt no one was taking her claims of infection seriously.

Mrs. S denied excessive anger, sleep difficulties, changes in appetite, or major weight changes in the previous months.

Her psychiatric history was significant for being treated for anxiety most of her adult life. Her daughters felt that her anxiety had been very well controlled for years with escitalopram 10 mg daily and trazodone 25 mg at bedtime for sleep. She had never been hospitalized for any mental health reasons. She had never been under the care of a psychiatrist in the past and seemed offended when introduced to a psychiatrist. "I don't need a shrink! My mind is fine. I need someone to tell me what's wrong with my body!"

She had been in long-term care for five to six years after her husband died suddenly. He was instrumental in her care before his death as Mrs. S needed a fair amount of assistance with ADLs secondary to a history of chronic back pain and the effects of multiple back surgeries over the years. She had adjusted quickly and easily to life in long-term care. She enjoyed having the assistance and companionship of care staff and had several close friends in the facility whom she ate meals with regularly. She loved television and could often be found watching old television shows. Her favorites were *Murder She Wrote* and *The Golden Girls*.

On exam, Mrs. S seemed in fairly stable health. She was in a wheelchair and able to answer all questions, and was oriented to her name, birth date, place, and year. She got a 5/5 on her serial 7s and had no deficits in her clock drawing. Her mood could be described as euthymic to mildly anxious when discussing anything related to her perceived fungal infection and had no evidence of any hallucinations. She was somewhat tangential and would often bring any conversation topic back to her "fungal infection".

When asked whether she was bothered by her consistent thoughts of her fungal infections and her physical sensations related to them, she replied, "I'm just pissed that no one believes me or can tell me why this is happening to me!"

At the end of the visit, the provider discreetly asked one of the daughters to help him find his way to the front door of the facility. The patient's daughter expressed exasperation regarding the situation she and her sister found themselves in. "We don't know what to do with Mom … Every doctor has told her that it is in her head, but she is driving us crazy with all this talk of having a fungus in her body." The provider educated the daughter on the condition of delusional disorder and how the disorder can cause those afflicted to be truly convinced of their illness despite multiple medical workups proving otherwise. The patient's daughter was very relieved to hear that medications are often helpful for this form of mental illness and can be well tolerated.

Mrs. S was started on 2 mg of aripiprazole qhs and maintained her low dose of trazodone at night and her daily 10 mg dose of escitalopram, as overall it had been very helpful with the patient's mood and anxiety symptoms in the past. The provider returned for a follow-up visit four weeks later and was pleased to hear that the patient was much less troubled by her perceived illness and was spending much less time speaking of it with her daughters and friends. When the provider sat down to speak to the patient, she shortly began speaking of her ongoing symptoms of her perceived fungal infection. She told the psychiatrist that the symptoms seemed to be getting a little better since the psychiatrist started her on "that new medication" (referring to aripiprazole). The psychiatrist made a small increase in the dose of her aripiprazole to 5 mg qhs. At a second follow-up visit six weeks later, the patient was in a pleasant mood. She felt nearly "cured" of her fungal infection, and it was bothering her very little. She was again a pleasure for her daughters to visit, as she was back to her old self and seemed little troubled by anything, as long as she had plenty of chocolate and *The Golden Girls* to watch on TV.

Teaching Points

Delusional disorder is a mental illness characterized by the presence of one or more delusions for at least one month. Delusional beliefs are based on the misinterpretation of external reality and are not improved by education or persuasion. Major mood symptoms are generally absent. The delusions can result in significant distress or dysfunction and can trouble patients, caregivers, and families alike. Delusions that involve physical symptoms can be particularly burdensome, as the pursuit of these symptoms can lead to unnecessary medical workup and expense.

The American Psychiatric Association estimates the lifetime prevalence of delusional disorder at only 0.2%, which is much lower than other psychotic disorders. This may be somewhat underestimated, as many with delusional disorder do not consider themselves ill and will never seek medical attention [1]. The prevalence of delusional disorder in older adults is thought to be double that seen in younger adults [2]. Older age is a known period of vulnerability for the first occurrence of psychosis or exacerbation of prior psychotic disorders. The occurrence of delusional disorder is more common in later life when compared to other psychotic disorders such as schizophrenia [3], and in older adults is more commonly seen in women than in men [4].

In the past, the pathophysiology of psychotic disorders has been dominated by the dopamine hypothesis, primarily implicating excessive dopamine or high dopamine sensitivity in key neural pathways. Currently, the understanding of the pathophysiology of psychosis has become more complex and also implicates glutamatergic, serotonergic, and GABA neurotransmitters.

A few psychosocial factors have been implicated in the development of susceptibility to delusional disorder. Stressful life events may contribute and those who are socially isolated may be at increased risk of developing delusional disorder. Cultural factors can influence a person's beliefs or perceptions and certain personality types are likely at higher risk of delusional disorder. High levels of suspiciousness and rigidity have been implicated in the increased potential of delusional disorder. Those with a history of trauma, abuse, or neglect may also be more susceptible to distorted beliefs that can act as the precursor to delusional disorder [2].

The diagnosis of delusional disorder relies heavily on the clinical interview, where information about a patient's symptoms, personal history, and current life circumstances are explored. Evaluating potential mood or other more common thought disorders is important. A medical and neurologic examination is conducted to help rule out mimickers of thought disorders, such as structural brain lesions, electrolyte disturbances, or endocrine disturbances, for example. Careful attention should be paid to collateral information provided by family members or friends on the nature of the delusions and their impact on the patient's life. Other more common psychiatric conditions may have prominent delusions, including depression with psychosis.

Once a presumptive diagnosis of delusional disorder is made, attention can be given to the likely subtype. The diagnostic criteria and subtypes of delusional disorder are laid out in the DSM–5–TR and are shown in Box 23.1 [5]. These subtypes are not distinguished by different responses to existing treatment options.

Delusional disorder has been considered a condition more resistant to treatment than some other psychiatric disorders. A review published in 2020 found the overall response to treatment to be 32.3%, and this review showed that first-generation antipsychotics exhibited modest superiority over second-generation antipsychotics. Treatment adherence complicates treatment outcomes, as many with this disorder lack insight into their disease [6].

Most evidence for the effectiveness of antipsychotics in the treatment of delusional disorder has come from studies focusing on the antipsychotic risperidone. Other studies have shown the benefit of olanzapine. A study in 2017 that involved 445 patients with delusional disorder showed no difference in efficacy or tolerability between olanzapine and risperidone [7]. Further review of the research literature shows that multiple other second- and third-generation antipsychotics have been successful in treating delusional

Box 23.1 Diagnostic criteria and subtypes of delusional disorder as described in DSM–5–TR

Diagnostic criteria:

a. The presence of one (or more) delusions with a duration of one month or longer.
b. Criterion A for schizophrenia has never been met. Note: Hallucinations, if present, are not prominent and are related to the delusional theme (e.g., the sensation of being infested with insects associated with delusions of infestation).
c. Apart from the impact of the delusion(s) or its ramifications, functioning is not markedly impaired, and behavior is not obviously bizarre or odd.
d. If manic or major depressive episodes have occurred, these have been brief relative to the duration of the delusional periods.
e. The disturbance is not attributable to the physiological effects of a substance or another medical condition and is not better explained by another mental disorder, such as body dysmorphic disorder or obsessive–compulsive disorder.

Specify whether:

Erotomanic type: This subtype applies when the central theme of the delusion is that another person is in love with the individual.
Grandiose type: This subtype applies when the central theme of the delusion is the conviction of having some great (but unrecognized) talent or insight or having made some important discovery.
Jealous type: This subtype applies when the central theme of the individual's delusion is that his or her spouse or lover is unfaithful.
Persecutory type: This subtype applies when the central theme of the delusion involves the individual's belief that he or she is being conspired against, cheated, spied on, followed, poisoned or drugged, maliciously maligned, harassed, or obstructed in the pursuit of long-term goals.
Somatic type: This subtype applies when the central theme of the delusion involves bodily functions or sensations.
Mixed type: This subtype applies when no one delusional theme predominates.
Unspecified type: This subtype applies when the dominant delusional belief cannot be clearly determined or is not described in the specific types (e.g., referential delusions without a prominent persecutory or grandiose component).

Specify if:

With bizarre content: Delusions are deemed bizarre if they are clearly implausible, not understandable, and not derived from ordinary life experiences (e.g., an individual's belief that a stranger has removed his or her internal organs and replaced them with someone else's organs without leaving any wounds or scars).
Specify if: The following course specifiers are only to be used after a one-year duration of the disorder:
First episode, currently in acute episode: First manifestation of the disorder meeting the defining diagnostic symptom and time criteria. An acute episode is a time period in which the symptom criteria are fulfilled.
First episode, currently in partial remission: Partial remission is a time period during which an improvement after a previous episode is maintained and in which the defining criteria of the disorder are only partially fulfilled.
First episode, currently in full remission: Full remission is a period of time after a previous episode during which no disorder-specific symptoms are present.

Box 23.1 (*cont.*)

Multiple episodes, currently in acute episode
Multiple episodes, currently in partial remission
Multiple episodes, currently in full remission
Continuous: Symptoms fulfilling the diagnostic symptom criteria of the disorder remain for the majority of the illness course, with subthreshold symptom periods being very brief relative to the overall course.

Unspecified

Specify current severity: Severity is rated by a quantitative assessment of the primary symptoms of psychosis, including delusions, hallucinations, disorganized speech, abnormal psychomotor 106 behavior, and negative symptoms. Each of these symptoms may be rated for its current severity (most severe in the last seven days) on a five-point scale ranging from zero (not present) to four (present and severe). (See Clinician-Rated Dimensions of Psychosis Symptom Severity in the chapter "Assessment Measures.")

Note: Diagnosis of delusional disorder can be made without using this severity specifier.

disorder. The choice of antipsychotic should be influenced by medication tolerability and psychiatric comorbidity.

Follow-up visits for delusional disorder may need to be relatively frequent in the initial weeks and months to assess medication tolerability and efficacy. The elimination of delusional thoughts may be difficult or impossible. Improvement in symptoms with related increases in functionality and well-being may be more realistic goals for most patients. Every effort should be made to educate the family on the pointless nature of pursuing symptoms with additional medical workups, as the reassurance provided is usually small and temporary.

This condition can be a particularly difficult one to control. Patients often lack insight, and this can lead to poor adherence to medications. Antipsychotics can also have a higher risk of side effects in the long-term care population. Several antipsychotics may need to be trialed before a medication with an acceptable ratio of benefits to side effects is found. The treatment of secondary anxiety or depression can be successful even in the absence of a response of the delusional disorder to antipsychotics.

Although somewhat uncommon, delusional disorder is a psychiatric diagnosis that will eventually be encountered by long-term care providers. Keys to successful outcomes include good recognition of the disorder, familiarity with antipsychotic medications, patience, and recognizing and treating common psychiatric comorbidities.

Take-Home Points

- Delusional disorder is a mental illness characterized by the presence of one or more delusions for a period of at least one month. Delusional beliefs are based on the misinterpretation of external reality and are not made better with education or persuasion.
- Seven subtypes of delusional disorder are recognized in the DSM–5. These include persecutory type, somatic type, jealous type, grandiose type, erotomanic type, mixed type, and unspecified type.

- The prevalence of delusional disorder in older adults is thought to be double that seen in younger adults. The occurrence of delusional disorder is more common in later life when compared to other psychotic disorders such as schizophrenia.
- Studies have not shown dramatic differences in response rates to different second- or third-generation antipsychotics.
- Choice of antipsychotic depends on clinician familiarity, side effect profile, and comorbidities.

References

1. González-Rodríguez, A., Monreal, J. A., Natividad, M., & Seeman, M. V. (2022). Seventy years of treating delusional disorder with antipsychotics: A historical perspective. *Biomedicines*, 10 (12).

2. González-Rodríguez, A., Seeman, M. V., Izquierdo, E., Natividad, M., Guàrdia, A., Román, E., & Monreal, J. A. (2022). Delusional disorder in old age: A hypothesis-driven review of recent work focusing on epidemiology, clinical aspects, and outcomes. *International Journal of Environmental Research and Public Health*, 19 (13).

3. Gardijan, N., & Szücs, A. (2016). Late-life psychotic disorders: Clinical aspects. *Revue Médicale Suisse*, 12, 1561–1564.

4. Kulkarni, K. R., Arasappa, R., Prasad, M. K., Zutshi, A., Chand, P. K., Murthy, P., & Muralidharan, K. (2017). Gender differences in persistent delusional disorder. *Indian Journal of Psychological Medicine*, 39 (2), 216–217. doi: 10.4103/0253-7176.203123. PMID: 28515568; PMCID: PMC5385760.

5. American Psychiatric Association. (2013). *Diagnostic and Statistical Manual of Mental Disorders*. 5th ed. https://doi.org/10.1176/appi.books.9780890425596

6. Muñoz-Negro, J. E., Gómez-Sierra, F. J., Peralta, V., González-Rodríguez, A., & Cervilla, J. A. (2020). A systematic review of studies with clinician-rated scales on the pharmacological treatment of delusional disorder. *International Clinical Psychopharmacology*, 35, 129–136.

7. Kulkarni, K., Arasappa, R., Prasad, M. K., Zutshi, A., Chand, P. K., Murthy, P., Philip, M., & Muralidharan, K. (2017). Risperidone versus olanzapine in the acute treatment of persistent delusional disorder: A retrospective analysis. *Psychiatry Research*, 253, 270–273.

Further Reading

Tampi, R. R., Young, J., Hoq, R., Resnick, K., & Tampi, D. J. (2019). Psychotic disorders in late life: A narrative review. *Therapeutic Advances in Psychopharmacology*, 9.

Trindade, P., Laginhas, C., Adão, C., Canas-Simião, H., Marques, A. R., & Caetano, R. (2022). Therapeutic challenge in delusional disorder: A case report and literature review. *European Psychiatry*, 65 (Suppl 1), S767. https://doi.org/10.1192/j.eurpsy.2022.1979

"This Is Humiliating"

Clozapine

24

Mr. S was a 58-year-old single male who had chronic paranoid schizophrenia and lived in a community nursing home. He had been moved there several years before from the state hospital ward/unit for chronically mentally ill patients. Mr. S was stable on his antipsychotic drug regimen of clozapine 100 mg qam and 300 mg qhs. He was mostly reclusive but did leave his room to go to the dining room for meals. Mr. S collected pornographic magazines and videotapes, which he would read and watch in the privacy of his room. One day, on returning from breakfast in the dining room, he found his dresser and other belongings in the hallway. He was not told that his room would be recarpeted. His magazines and tapes were also moved into the hallway. He became angry, agitated, and upset – accusing the staff of messing with his personal belongings. "This is humiliating," he stated. His dormant suspiciousness became blatant, and he required hospitalization after a serious suicide attempt.

Teaching Points

Knowing a resident and taking extra precautions to ensure privacy for residents who are managing their own sexual needs appropriately is crucial, not only to support their rights of sexual expression but also to prevent serious trauma and humiliation experienced by residents whose privacy is violated due to lack of mindfulness on the part of staff. The range of sexuality, romance, and sexual identity experiences in later life encompasses various activities and experiences, including self-pleasure, physical intimacy, as well as emotional and intellectual closeness. There is evidence to suggest that sexual expression in later life may have positive psychological and physiological effects, such as enhancing overall quality of life, reducing rates of depressive symptoms, and lowering the risk of certain types of cancers and fatal coronary events [1].

Despite the well-documented benefits of continuing sexual expression in later life, research has shown that the personal perspectives of staff and family members often create limitations for resident sexual expression [2]. Every opportunity should be utilized to educate all staff in long-term care about the rights of residents to privacy and appropriate expression of sexual needs.

This case also mentions the use of clozapine. Clozapine has an important place in the treatment of psychiatric patients. It was developed and introduced to the market in 1972 in Switzerland by the pharmaceutical company Sandoz (now Novartis). However, in the late 1970s and early 1980s, reports emerged linking clozapine to potentially fatal agranulocytosis, which led to the drug being withdrawn from the market in most countries. After extensive research and clinical trials, clozapine was reintroduced to the market in 1990, with additional safety measures in place to monitor for the development of agranulocytosis. Clozapine is now an important medication in the treatment of schizophrenia. It is used primarily in cases of treatment-resistant schizophrenia (TRS) but is also useful in patients with schizophrenia who have had adverse effects to multiple other antipsychotics. Treatment-resistant schizophrenia is defined as a lack of significant improvement in symptoms despite at least two trials of different antipsychotic medications, each given at an adequate dose for an adequate duration of time. Treatment-resistant schizophrenia can also refer to cases in which a person may respond well to an antipsychotic medication initially but then experience a relapse of symptoms later on, despite continuing to take the medication as prescribed [3]. Clozapine has not proven more efficacious than other antipsychotics for the initial choice of treatment of schizophrenia [4].

The use of clozapine has several benefits in addition to improving the control of the symptoms of schizophrenia for those with TRS. Patients who carry the diagnosis of schizophrenia have an elevated mortality compared to the general population, with estimates that it is 2.5 times higher. Those with schizophrenia are also estimated to have a lifespan that is 15–25 years shorter than those without the condition. Clozapine is not only attractive for its benefits for those with TRS but also because it has been shown to reduce overall mortality. It is thought to do this through a reduction in the incidence of suicidality [5]. An additional benefit of clozapine is its documented effects and supporting data on the patterns of illicit substance use in those with schizophrenia [6]. Comorbid illicit substance use in schizophrenia is associated with a poor outcome, including an increased risk of suicide and poor response to treatment. Finally, clozapine is also not known to produce extrapyramidal symptoms that can be more common with other first- and second-generation antipsychotics.

The risks of using clozapine are well known and the most feared side effect is agranulocytosis. Agranulocytosis risk is highest in the first three months of use of the drug but is possible even after years of use [4]. For this reason, most countries have a mandatory system of lab monitoring and reporting to help minimize this complication. Some experts argue that the risk of developing agranulocytosis decreases over time in people who use clozapine, and that ongoing monitoring may not be necessary for those who have been stable on the medication for an extended period. However, others argue that regular monitoring is still necessary to ensure early detection and treatment of agranulocytosis, which can occur even after many years of clozapine use [7]. The current standard of care is for weekly monitoring of blood counts for six months, followed by every other week monitoring for six months, followed by monthly monitoring thereafter. This is the main limitation of clozapine use in older adults.

There are less common but still well-documented side effects of clozapine, which are documented in Box 24.1.

The dosing of clozapine is not complex but warrants discussion. There are recommendations to slowly titrate the dose when initiating therapy in order to minimize side effects. It should be noted that cigarette smoking increases the metabolism of clozapine by up to 50%. Those that suddenly stop smoking, as often happens during hospital admission, can develop the toxic effects of clozapine in as little as several days. Nicotine replacement therapy does not increase the metabolism of clozapine [9].

Box 24.1 Well-documented potential side effects of clozapine

1. Hypersalivation (excessive saliva production): This is a common side effect of clozapine, but it can become more severe in some people and lead to drooling or difficulty speaking.
2. Constipation: Clozapine can slow down the movement of the intestines, which can lead to constipation. This can be particularly problematic in people who already have constipation or bowel problems.
3. Weight gain: Weight gain is a common side effect of many antipsychotic medications, including clozapine. However, some people may experience more significant weight gain with clozapine than with other medications.
4. Seizures: Although rare, seizures can occur in people taking clozapine, particularly at higher doses or in people with a history of seizures.
5. Myocarditis: Clozapine can cause inflammation of the heart muscle (myocarditis) in rare cases. This can lead to symptoms such as chest pain, shortness of breath, and fatigue.
6. Neuroleptic malignant syndrome (NMS): This is a rare but potentially life-threatening side effect of clozapine and other antipsychotic medications. It can cause fever, muscle stiffness, confusion, and other symptoms.
7. Respiratory depression: Clozapine can depress respiratory function, particularly in people with preexisting respiratory problems [8].

There are some off-label uses of clozapine that healthcare providers in long-term care should be aware of. Some studies have suggested that clozapine may be effective in treating TRD and it has been used off-label in the treatment of bipolar disorder, particularly in people who have not responded to other more commonly prescribed medications. Clozapine is sometimes used in Parkinson's disease-related psychosis and some studies have shown that it may also be effective in treating certain symptoms of autism spectrum disorder, such as aggression and irritability [10]. Regardless of the indication, clozapine is probably underappreciated and underutilized in the long-term care population.

Take-Home Points

- Clozapine is an important medication in the treatment of schizophrenia. It is used primarily in cases of TRS but is also useful in patients with schizophrenia who have had adverse effects to multiple other antipsychotics.
- The risks of using clozapine are well known and the most feared side effect is agranulocytosis. Agranulocytosis risk is highest in the first three months of use of the drug but is possible even after years of use.
- The use of clozapine in schizophrenia has several benefits in addition to improving the control of the symptoms of schizophrenia for those with TRS.
- There are some off-label uses of clozapine that healthcare providers in long-term care should be aware of. Some studies have suggested that clozapine may be effective in treating TRD and has been used off-label in the treatment of bipolar disorder, particularly in people who have not responded to other more commonly prescribed medications.

References

1. Syme, M. (2014). The evolving concept of older adult sexual behavior and its benefits. *Generations*, 38 (1), 35–41.

2. Howard, L., Brassolotto, J., & Manduca-Barone, A. (2020). Navigating tensions about resident sexual expression in Alberta's continuing care homes: A qualitative study of leaders' experiences. *Sexuality Research and Social Policy*, 17, 632–642.

3. National Collaborating Centre for Mental Health (UK). (2014). Psychosis and schizophrenia in adults: Treatment and management.

4. Lally, J., & MacCabe, J. H. (2015). Antipsychotic medication in schizophrenia: A review. *British Medical Bulletin*, 114 (1), 169–179.

5. Vermeulen, J. M., van Rooijen, G., van de Kerkhof, M. P., Sutterland, A. L., Correll, C. U., & de Haan, L. (2019). Clozapine and long-term mortality risk in patients with schizophrenia: A systematic review and meta-analysis of studies lasting 1.1–12.5 years. *Schizophrenia Bulletin*, 45 (2), 315–329.

6. Abou-Saleh, M. T. (2004). Psychopharmacology of substance misuse and comorbid psychiatric disorders. *Acta Neuropsychiatrica*, 16 (1), 19–25.

7. Schulte, P. F. (2006). Risk of clozapine-associated agranulocytosis and mandatory white blood cell monitoring. *Annals of Pharmacotherapy*, 40 (4), 683–688.

8. Li, K. J., Gurrera, R. J., & Delisi, L. E. (2018). Potentially fatal outcomes associated with clozapine. *Schizophrenia Research*, 199, 386–389.

9. Haslemo, T., Eikeseth, P. H., Tanum, L., Molden, E., & Refsum, H. (2006). The effect of variable cigarette consumption on the interaction with clozapine and olanzapine. *European Journal of Clinical Pharmacology*, 62, 1049–1053.

10. Newman, W. J., & Newman, B. M. (2016). Rediscovering clozapine: Clinically relevant off-label uses. *Current Psychiatry Reports*, 15, 51–62.

"I Want to Go Home"
Delirium

Mr. A was an 80-year-old male who had hypertension, benign prostatic hypertrophy, hyperlipidemia, and arthritis. In the hospital after hip fracture surgery, Mr. A became disoriented, insisting that he needed to go to work, tried to climb out of bed, and became aggressive when the staff tried to redirect him. He was given haloperidol (2 mg twice daily) and was recommended to continue haloperidol when he was transferred to a nursing home for rehabilitation. Mr. A developed drooling, tremors, and daytime sedation and continued to have periods of agitation. A psychiatric consultation was requested.

The psychiatrist asked Mrs. A about Mr. A's cognitive functioning before surgery. Mrs. A insisted that Mr. A's memory was "quite good" but added, "he is quite old, you know." Mr. A's daughter reported that for the last two years her father had been increasingly forgetful, repeating himself often, and growing irritable. In the last six months he had started making mistakes in bill paying, became lost while driving, started avoiding social gatherings, and refused to wear a hearing aid. During the examination, the psychiatrist found Mr. A somewhat drowsy, with poor attention and concentration. Mr. A stated to the psychiatrist, "I want to go home." He did not recall having been hospitalized and had slurred speech. The psychiatrist reviewed the results of tests done in the hospital. A CT scan of the brain showed diffuse moderate cerebral atrophy, urine analysis was negative for infection, and the results of blood tests, including the chemistry panel, thyroid profile, and folate levels, were within normal limits. Vitamin B12 was at the lower limit of normal (level of 220). The psychiatrist made the diagnosis of MNCD due to probable Alzheimer's disease with postoperative delirium, discontinued haloperidol due to adverse effects caused by it, added vitamin B12 1000 mcg daily, and started donepezil 5 mg daily in the morning to be taken after breakfast. The psychiatrist also met with the family and staff to discuss various psychosocial environmental interventions to be instituted (such as listening to favorite music, aromatherapy with lavender lotion, one-to-one supervision at times, minimizing nighttime noise, and lowering expectations for the resident to remember and follow directions). The psychiatrist then had a lengthy family meeting at which he explained his diagnosis to the family, recommended a support group for the wife and daughter, and discussed the prognosis.

Over the next several days, Mr. A gradually became less agitated and started taking part in physical therapy (although he required constant reassurance, redirection, and encouragement). The drooling was markedly reduced, tremors and slurred speech decreased significantly, and daytime sleepiness resolved completely. After six weeks, Mr. A was found to smile and joke, although he still asked when he could go home.

Teaching Points

The DSM–5–TR of the American Psychiatric Association defines delirium as, "a disturbance in attention (i.e. reduced ability to direct, focus, sustain, and shift attention) accompanied by reduced awareness of the environment" [1]. Unlike dementia, delirium has a rapid onset and fluctuating and reversible symptoms. However, the symptoms are unpredictable and irregular, making delirium under-detected. Delirium is categorized as hyperactive, hypoactive, or mixed based on the predominance of psychomotor symptoms.

Delirium is a frequently encountered syndrome in hospitalized patients, with an estimated occurrence rate of 8–17% in older patients in emergency departments and 29–64% in general medical and older adult inpatients. This syndrome is more commonly observed in patients with risk factors such as pre-existing cognitive impairment, recent surgery, acute infection, or critical illness [2].

The causes of delirium are varied. The most common causes in the long-term care setting are likely to be UTIs, untreated pain, and medication side effects (Box 25.1).

Since the etiology of delirium is multifactorial, there are probably various neurobiological mechanisms that contribute to its pathogenesis, such as neuroinflammation, brain vascular dysfunction, altered brain metabolism, neurotransmitter imbalances, and impaired neuronal network connectivity [3]. While several neurotransmitter systems have been associated with delirium, current literature mostly supports the theory of a relative acetylcholine deficiency and/or dopamine excess.

Several potentially modifiable risk factors for delirium can be addressed and thereby help prevent its development in both the hospital and long-term care settings. Modifiable risk factors for delirium are shown in Box 25.2 [4].

Box 25.1 Potential causes of delirium

1. Medications: Certain medications, especially those with sedative or anticholinergic properties, can contribute to the development of delirium. Examples include benzodiazepines, opioids, antipsychotics, and some over-the-counter medications.
2. Infections: Infections, such as UTIs, pneumonia, sepsis, or other systemic infections, can trigger delirium, particularly in older adults.
3. Metabolic imbalances: Disturbances in electrolyte levels (such as sodium, potassium, or calcium), glucose levels, liver or kidney function, or thyroid abnormalities can lead to delirium.
4. Substance withdrawal or intoxication: Abrupt cessation or excessive use of alcohol, sedatives, opioids, or other substances can result in delirium.
5. Acute medical illnesses: Serious medical conditions, such as heart attacks, strokes, respiratory failure, or severe pain, can contribute to the onset of delirium.
6. Surgical procedures: Delirium can occur as a result of anesthesia, postoperative complications, or the stress of surgery.
7. Traumatic brain injury: Head injuries, concussions, or other forms of brain trauma can lead to delirium, particularly in the acute phase.
8. Sleep deprivation: Prolonged lack of sleep or disturbances in sleep patterns can increase the risk of delirium.
9. Psychological stress: High levels of emotional stress, such as grief, anxiety, or significant life changes, can be contributing factors to delirium.

> **Box 25.2** Potentially modifiable risk factors for delirium in older adults in the long-term care setting
>
> 1. Medication management: Avoiding medications that can cause delirium or adjusting doses to the lowest effective amount.
> 2. Dehydration and malnutrition: Addressing these issues and ensuring adequate hydration and nutrition.
> 3. Infections: Identifying and treating infections promptly.
> 4. Pain: Managing pain effectively to reduce the risk of delirium.
> 5. Sleep deprivation: Encouraging good sleep habits and reducing interruptions to sleep.
> 6. Immobility: Encouraging activity and mobility as much as possible.
> 7. Sensory impairment: Addressing vision and hearing impairment.
> 8. Environmental factors: Reducing noise, providing natural light and orientation cues, and encouraging family involvement and socialization.

The Confusion Assessment Method (CAM) is a validated instrument for delirium detection. The CAM is typically administered within a five to ten-minute timeframe and relies on a concise cognitive assessment. Studies validating its effectiveness have consistently shown high sensitivity (94–100%) and specificity (90–95%) when used by trained clinicians or researchers [5]. The CAM consists of a set of criteria and questions that help evaluate the presence of key features associated with delirium, including acute onset, inattention, disorganized thinking, and altered levels of consciousness. It also incorporates an assessment of the fluctuating nature of symptoms and evidence of an underlying medical cause.

By using the CAM, healthcare providers can systematically evaluate patients for delirium and differentiate it from other conditions that may present with similar symptoms. The tool has been extensively validated and has demonstrated high sensitivity and specificity in detecting delirium when administered by trained clinicians or researchers.

The initial steps recommended in managing delirium involve identifying and addressing underlying medical conditions, reducing environmental triggers, and minimizing exposure to drugs. A range of strategies has been employed, including managing acute medical problems, controlling pain, implementing reorientation techniques, regulating sleep patterns, facilitating safe movement, and investigating potential drug-related causes. Various classes of psychoactive medications, such as antipsychotics, benzodiazepines, opioids, alpha-2 agonists, and cholinesterase inhibitors have been studied for their efficacy in treating delirium in different patient populations. However, the data are inconsistent, and the use of these drugs is largely determined by clinical factors and physician discretion. Due to the uncertainty surrounding the effectiveness of antipsychotics in delirium management, professional organizations recommend limited and cautious use only after nonpharmacological approaches have been attempted and symptoms remain distressing or pose a threat to the patient or healthcare staff [6].

Despite the known risks and lack of evidence showing consistent benefits of antipsychotic use in those hospitalized with delirium, the use of antipsychotics in hospitalized patients is quite high. As demonstrated in the case here, it is not uncommon for a patient to be introduced to long-term care on an antipsychotic drug after being discharged from the hospital. In these cases, obtaining collateral information by examining available hospital records and speaking with knowledgeable family members can be invaluable. Every effort should be made to taper or stop antipsychotics as soon as possible. Their continued use can hinder patient progress in the long-term care setting by causing excessive sedation, movement disorders, and worsening cognition.

When evaluating a patient in the long-term care setting with potential new-onset delirium it is important to consider all possible causes. If symptoms of delirium are severe, transfer to a hospital setting for timely workup and treatment is indicated. If symptoms of delirium are mild a workup in the long-term care setting can usually be justified and would include a urinalysis, basic labs such as a CBC, CMP, TSH, B12, and vitamin D level, and other labs or imaging studies as indicated by history and physical exam findings.

As in the case here, mild Alzheimer's disease often goes unrecognized and undiagnosed. It predisposes the person to develop postoperative delirium. Hence, for any resident who has postoperative delirium, the healthcare provider must inquire about cognitive functioning before surgery. It is also common for delirium to be treated with larger doses of haloperidol in the hospital, and patients are often discharged on haloperidol or another antipsychotic medication. Haloperidol is associated with a high incidence of extrapyramidal adverse effects in older adults who have MNCD, especially at doses larger than 1–2 mg/day (although extrapyramidal symptoms [EPS] can be seen at doses as low as 0.5 mg/day). Hence, in the management of delirium, the healthcare professional must discontinue haloperidol or any other antipsychotic as soon as possible, especially if adverse effects arise.

Finally, besides treatment of the cause, management of delirium primarily involves psychosocial interventions. These can include environmental modifications such as addressing poor lighting, excessive noise, or lack of orientation cues. They should include cognitive stimulation with activities that may include puzzles, games, and other mentally stimulating activities to encourage engagement and interaction with the environment. Family involvement can also help. Family members can provide comfort and support, help with orientation, and monitor the patient for changes in behavior or other symptoms. Music therapy can be an effective nonpharmacological intervention for the treatment of delirium. Listening to music can help promote relaxation and reduce anxiety and agitation. Pet therapy involves the use of animals to provide comfort and support to patients. Studies have shown that pet therapy can be effective in reducing symptoms of delirium in some patients [7].

In summary, delirium can be seen with some frequency in the long-term care setting. Clinicians should be aware of its potential and familiar with the treatment, workup, and prevention.

Take-Home Points

- Delirium is a complex neuropsychiatric syndrome characterized by disturbances in attention, awareness, and cognition that are not explained by a pre-existing neurocognitive disorder.
- The initial steps recommended in managing delirium involve identifying and addressing underlying medical conditions, reducing environmental triggers, and minimizing exposure to drugs.
- Causes of delirium are varied. The most common causes of delirium in the long-term care setting are likely UTIs, untreated pain, and medication side effects.
- Besides treatment of the cause, management of delirium primarily involves psychosocial interventions. These can include environmental modifications such as addressing poor lighting, excessive noise, or lack of orientation cues.

References

1. American Psychiatric Association. (2022). *Diagnostic and Statistical Manual of Mental Disorders.* 5th ed. text rev. (American Psychiatric Association.)

2. Inouye, S. K., Westendorp, R. G., & Saczynski, J. S. (2014). Delirium in elderly people. *The Lancet*, 383 (9920), 911–922.

3. Ormseth, C. H., LaHue, S. C., Oldham, M. A., Josephson, S. A., Whitaker, E., & Douglas, V. C. (2023). Predisposing and precipitating factors associated with delirium: A systematic review. *JAMA Network Open*, 6 (1), e2249950. https://doi.org/10.1001/jamanetworkopen.2022.49950

4. Wilson, J. E., Mart, M. F., Cunningham, C., Shehabi, Y., Girard, T. D., MacLullich, A. M. J., Slooter, A. J. C., & Ely, E. W. (2020). Delirium. *Nature Reviews. Disease primers*, 6 (1), 90. www.nature.com/articles/s41572-020-00223-4

5. Green, J. R., Smith, J., Teale, E., Collinson, M., Avidan, M. S., Schmitt, E. M., Inouye, S. K., & Young, J. (2019). Use of the confusion assessment method in multicentre delirium trials: Training and standardization. *BMC Geriatrics*, 19 (1), 107. doi: 10.1186/s12877-019-1129-8. PMID: 30991945; PMCID: PMC6466721.

6. Burry, L., Mehta, S., Perreault, M. M., Luxenberg, J. S., Siddiqi, N., Hutton, B., Fergusson, D. A., Bell, C., & Rose, L. (2018). Antipsychotics for treatment of delirium in hospitalized non-ICU patients. *Cochrane Database of Systematic Reviews*, 6 (6): CD005594. doi: 10.1002/14651858.CD005594.pub3. PMID: 29920656; PMCID: PMC6513380.

7. Sheikh, A. B., Javed, N., Leyba, K., Khair, A. H., Ijaz, Z., Dar, A. A., Hanif, H., Farooq, A., & Shekhar, R. (2021). Pet-assisted therapy for delirium and agitation in hospitalized patients with neurocognitive impairment: A review of literature. *Geriatrics (Basel)*, 6 (4), 96. doi: 10.3390/geriatrics6040096. PMID: 34698207; PMCID: PMC8544463.

Further Reading

Desai, A., & Grossberg, G. (2017). *Psychiatric Consultation in Long-Term Care. A Guide for Healthcare Professionals.* 2nd ed. (Cambridge University Press.) pp. 102–119.

Fong, T. G., & Inouye, S. K. (2022). The inter-relationship between delirium and dementia: The importance of delirium prevention. *Nature Reviews. Neurology*, 18 (10), 579–596. www.nature.com/articles/s41582-022-00698-7

Gross, A. L., Tommet, D., D'Aquila, M., Schmitt, E., Marcantonio, E. R., Helfand, B., Inouye, S. K., Jones, R. N., & BASIL Study Group (2018). Harmonization of delirium severity instruments: A comparison of the DRS-R-98, MDAS, and CAM-S using item response theory. *BMC Medical Research Methodology*, 18 (1), 92. www.ncbi.nlm.nih.gov/pmc/articles/PMC6131747/

Woodhouse, R., Burton, J. K., Rana, N., Pang, Y. L., Lister, J. E., & Siddiqi, N. (2019). Interventions for preventing delirium in older people in institutional long-term care. *The Cochrane Database of Systematic Reviews*, 4 (4), CD009537. https://doi.org/10.1002/14651858.CD009537.pub3

"I Am a Worrier"

26 Schizoaffective Disorder and Antipsychotics

Ms. S was a 69-year-old single woman who had been living in a long-term care facility for two years due to sequelae of severe arthritis, obesity, CHF, chronic kidney disease, chronic pain, diabetes requiring insulin, poor mobility, and osteoporosis. She had a long history of schizoaffective disorder with multiple hospitalizations for serious suicide attempts, severe psychotic symptoms (paranoid delusions and auditory hallucinations), and severe depressive symptoms, but had been stable for seven years on a medication regimen that included olanzapine 10 mg at bedtime and mirtazapine 30 mg at bedtime. The psychiatrist was consulted for the management of increased agitation, as demonstrated by yelling out instead of using the call light, calling her roommate "the devil", paranoia (accusing staff of stealing her clothes), and insomnia.

Ms. S had relatively intact cognitive function (SLUMS 28) and was able to give a detailed history of her psychiatric illness. She reported that the current medication regimen helped her more than all other medications she had tried since her 20s, and she had avoided hospitalization for the last seven years. Ms. S denied any history suggestive of hypomania or mania and reported a lifelong history of excessive anxiety and added, "I am a worrier." The psychiatrist also noted that Ms. S had a history of recurrent UTIs and was put on antibiotics two days before consultation for another UTI.

On a mental status exam, Ms. S was found to be anxious and eager to please. She denied any suicidal or homicidal ideas or any current auditory or visual hallucinations. She acknowledged that she had called her roommate "the devil" but reported that she was angry with her because she would keep her TV on until late in the night and Ms. S liked to go to sleep by 8 pm. Staff acknowledged to the psychiatrist that this was an ongoing conflict between Ms. S and her roommate. Ms. S denied feeling that the staff were taking her belongings but felt that certain staff were "not nice" to her. The psychiatrist made a provisional diagnosis of schizoaffective disorder–depressed type and generalized anxiety disorder and felt that Ms. S's psychotic symptoms were controlled and hence did not recommend any change in antipsychotic dosage. Trazodone 50 mg q6 hours for anxiety was added as needed. The psychiatrist also recommended that the nursing home social worker address the conflicts between Ms. S and her roommate and requested records from previous psychiatrists. The social worker, over three meetings with Ms. S and her roommate, brokered an agreement that Ms. S's roommate could watch TV in their room until 9 pm and then go to a family room that had a TV if she wanted to continue watching.

After four weeks, staff reported that Ms. S's agitation was much better. She also reported feeling less anxious and irritable. Ms. S was given as-needed trazodone once almost daily for the first week but after that staff were able to manage her anxiety without it. The psychiatrist considered switching olanzapine to another atypical antipsychotic with a lower risk of metabolic complication (e.g. weight gain, hyperglycemia, risk of hyperlipidemia), such as aripiprazole or ziprasidone and discussed this with Ms. S. Psychiatric records indicated that Ms. S had tried taking risperidone, quetiapine, haloperidol, thiothixene, sertraline, fluoxetine, and venlafaxine without adequate response. Records also confirmed the history obtained from Ms. S that she had several serious suicide attempts (primarily by overdose) in the past requiring repeated hospitalization and severe psychotic symptoms that had incapacitated her for several years. Ms. S was nervous about any change in medication and expressed awareness of metabolic risks with olanzapine and mirtazapine. The psychiatrist agreed with Ms. S that the risks of switching (destabilizing the psychiatric illness, relapse of severe depressive and psychotic symptoms, need for hospitalization, and suicide) outweighed the benefits (lower risk of weight gain, better control of diabetes and hyperlipidemia, improved mobility).

Teaching Points

Schizoaffective disorder is a psychiatric disorder in which patients demonstrate a combination of symptoms associated with schizophrenia and a mood disorder such as bipolar disorder or depression. The symptoms of schizophrenia and mood disorder occur concomitantly for a substantial portion of the illness's duration. Schizoaffective disorder can be classified into two subtypes. Schizoaffective disorder–bipolar type involves both manic and depressive episodes alongside psychotic symptoms. Schizoaffective disorder–depressive type is characterized by depressive episodes alongside psychotic symptoms.

Older adults who have a severe persistent mental illness, such as schizoaffective disorder, are as likely as those who do not have such illness to become agitated due to medical issues and/or environmental causes. The healthcare provider should consider these factors before assuming that exacerbation of the underlying psychiatric illness is the cause of increased psychiatric symptoms. Suppose a resident has been stable on a psychiatric drug regimen. In that case, it is advisable to avoid any major change in that regimen because obtaining a similar good therapeutic response from a different drug regimen is not predictable or assured. The provider should decide to switch antipsychotics or antidepressants only after a thorough review of the patient's history and perspectives (and those of the involved family) about changes and a review of previous records. Although drugs like olanzapine and mirtazapine carry substantial metabolic risk (especially for people who are obese and have diabetes), for some people (such as Ms. S) the risk may not outweigh the benefit of stabilization of a serious psychiatric illness.

All antipsychotics have the potential to cause weight gain and increase the risk of obesity and related hyperlipidemia and diabetes. First-generation antipsychotics are used less now than in decades past. Examples of first-generation antipsychotics include haloperidol, fluphenazine, perphenazine, and loxapine. This group of medications is considered relatively low risk for metabolic side effects [1]. The newer atypical antipsychotics are well known to be associated with metabolic syndrome and can be thought of as being high, medium, and low risk for these complications. Medications at high risk for metabolic syndrome include clozapine and olanzapine. Medications at medium risk for causing metabolic syndrome include risperidone, quetiapine, paliperidone,

Table 26.1 Atypical antipsychotics and associated risk of metabolic side effects.

Antipsychotics at low risk for metabolic syndrome	Aripiprazole, ziprasidone, lurasidone, brexpiprazole, cariprazine, lumateperone, pimavanserin
Antipsychotics at medium risk for metabolic syndrome	Quetiapine, risperidone, paliperidone, asenapine, iloperidone
Antipsychotics at high risk for metabolic syndrome	Clozapine, olanzapine

asenapine, and iloperidone. Antipsychotics thought to be low risk for metabolic syndrome include cariprazine, lurasidone, lumateperone, ziprasidone, pimavanserin, aripiprazole, and brexpiprazole [2]. See Table 26.1 for details.

Adults with schizophrenia have three and a half times the mortality risk than the general population, with cardiovascular diseases the most common cause. Antipsychotic medications with a high or medium risk of inducing metabolic abnormalities are associated with almost a three-fold higher risk of major cardiovascular events [1]. Regular monitoring of weight, lipid panel, and screening for diabetes is important for those on long-term antipsychotic treatment.

Take-Home Points

- Schizoaffective disorder is a psychiatric disorder in which patients demonstrate a combination of symptoms associated with schizophrenia and a mood disorder such as bipolar disorder or depression. The symptoms of schizophrenia and mood disorder occur concomitantly for a substantial portion of the illness's duration.
- All antipsychotics have the potential to cause weight gain and increase the risk of obesity and related hyperlipidemia and diabetes. Atypical antipsychotics can be thought of as being high, medium, and low risk for these complications.
- If a resident has been stable on a psychiatric drug regimen, it is advisable to avoid any major change because obtaining a similar good therapeutic response from a different drug regimen is not predictable or assured.
- Antipsychotics thought to be low risk for metabolic syndrome include cariprazine, lurasidone, lumateperone, ziprasidone, pimavanserin, aripiprazole, and brexpiprazole.

References

1. Szmulewicz, A. G., Angriman, F., Pedroso, F. E., Vazquez, C., & Martino, D. J. (2017). Long-term antipsychotic use and major cardiovascular events: A retrospective cohort study. *The Journal of Clinical Psychiatry*, 78 (8), 1161.

2. Stahl, S. M. (2021). *Stahl's Essential Psychopharmacology: Neuroscientific Basis and Practical Applications*. 5th ed. (Cambridge University Press.) Ebook. Kindle Edition. p. 212.

Further Reading

Bernardo, M., Rico-Villademoros, F., García-Rizo, C., Rojo, R., & Gómez-Huelgas, R. (2021). Real-world data on the adverse metabolic effects of second-generation antipsychotics and their potential determinants in adult patients: A systematic review of population-based studies. *Advances in Therapy*, 38 (5), 2491–2512. www.ncbi.nlm.nih.gov/pmc/articles/PMC8107077/

Carli, M., Kolachalam, S., Longoni, B., Pintaudi, A., Baldini, M., Aringhieri, S., & Scarselli, M. (2021). Atypical antipsychotics and metabolic syndrome: From molecular mechanisms to clinical differences. *Pharmaceuticals*, 14 (3), 238.

DeJongh, B. M. (2021). Clinical pearls for the monitoring and treatment of antipsychotic induced metabolic syndrome. *Mental Health Clinician*, 11 (6), 311–319.

Friedrich, M. E., Winkler, D., Konstantinidis, A., Huf, W., Engel, R., Toto, S., Grohmann, R., & Kasper, S. (2020). Cardiovascular adverse reactions during antipsychotic treatment: Results of AMSP, a drug surveillance program between 1993 and 2013. *The International Journal of Neuropsychopharmacology*, 23 (2), 67–75. https://doi.org/10.1093/ijnp/pyz046

Hammoudeh, S., Al Lawati, H., Ghuloum, S., Iram, H., Yehya, A., Becetti, I., & Al-Amin, H. (2020). Risk factors of metabolic syndrome among patients receiving antipsychotics: A retrospective study. *Community Mental Health Journal*, 56, 760–770.

Sneller, M. H., De Boer, N., Everaars, S., Schuurmans, M., Guloksuz, S., Cahn, W., & Luykx, J. J. (2021). Clinical, biochemical and genetic variables associated with metabolic syndrome in patients with schizophrenia spectrum disorders using second-generation antipsychotics: a systematic review. *Frontiers in Psychiatry*, 12, 625935.

Ventriglio, A., Baldessarini, R. J., Vitrani, G., Bonfitto, I., Cecere, A. C., Rinaldi, A., & Bellomo, A. (2019). Metabolic syndrome in psychotic disorder patients treated with oral and long-acting injected antipsychotics. *Frontiers in Psychiatry*, 9, 744.

"Get out of My House"

Medication-Induced Delirium

27

Mr. M, an 82-year-old widowed male who had MNCD due to Alzheimer's disease, was transferred from the hospital to a nursing home for rehabilitation after being treated for syncope due to severe bradycardia with pacemaker implantation and initiation of 200 mg/day of amiodarone. He started developing changes in mental status a week after discharge, including worsening disorientation, agitation, insomnia, aggressive behavior during personal care, and paranoia. Staff at the nursing home requested a psychiatric consult to facilitate hospitalization to an inpatient psychiatric unit, as Mr. M was "violent." The psychiatrist found Mr. M to be agitated and repeatedly yelling, "Get out of my house!" After an emergency assessment, the consulting psychiatrist diagnosed amiodarone-induced delirium. Amiodarone was discontinued (after consultation with the resident's cardiologist) and Mr. M was given risperidone (0.25 mg twice a day, increased the next day to 0.5 mg twice a day) for agitation and aggression. The aggression improved dramatically after two days and resolved completely after seven days. Risperidone was discontinued soon after.

Teaching Points

Delirium is identified when there is an abrupt onset of a condition affecting focus and consciousness, occurring rapidly and differing from the usual state. This condition tends to vary in intensity and is accompanied by cognitive deficits (like memory loss, confusion, language issues, visuospatial problems, or perception abnormalities). Delirium can present with hyperactivity, restlessness, and agitation but can also present as a more hypoactive variant [1]. Those with hypoactive delirium may be more at risk of delayed workup as they have fewer easily-recognized symptoms such as sleepiness and social withdrawal and this variant may be more serious [2] (Figure 27.1).

Older adults are at higher risk of drug-induced (or any other) delirium due to heightened sensitivity to medications, more comorbidities, and less cognitive reserve. Older adults with cognitive impairment have an even higher incidence of delirium and are also more likely to suffer from sensory impairment due to poor vision and hearing. This can increase the risk of drug-induced delirium. They are more likely to be subject to polypharmacy, a well-known risk factor for drug-related mental status changes.

Although drugs can be instigators of delirium, a multifactorial model of delirium is probably more accurate. In this model, even a relatively benign-appearing medication such as a commonly prescribed antibiotic can lead to delirium in those with a baseline high vulnerability to the condition.

Amiodarone (and many other prescription drugs) has the potential to cause significant adverse cognitive effects in older adults, especially those who have MNCD. Several

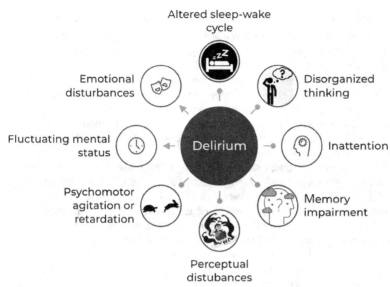

Figure 27.1 Symptoms of delirium.

Box 27.1 Medications commonly associated with delirium

- Anticholinergics (sclopolamine, benztropine, trihexyphenidyl, oxybutynin, tolterodine)
- Anticonvulsants: depakote, carbamazepine, topiramate, levatiracetam
- Antidepressants: especially anticholinergic tricyclics. Less commonly SSRIs
- Antihistamines: especially centrally-acting agents such as diphenhydramine or doxylamine
- Corticosteroids
- Muscle relaxers: cyclobenzaprine, carisoprodol, baclofen
- Sedative/hypnotics: zolpidem, benzodiazepines
- Antibiotics: ertapenem, cefepime, imipenem, ofloxacin, ceftazidime, clarithromycin, cefaclor, levofloxacin, linezolid, moxifloxacin, azithromycin, piperacillin-tazobactam, trimethoprim-sulfamethoxazole, metronidazole, ciprofloxacin, and cefuroxime

---

case reports exist in the literature. The unique pharmacokinetics of amiodarone can also lead to delayed neuropsychiatric symptoms and prolonged symptoms after discontinuation of the medication [3,4].

Medications well known to cause delirium in those with MNCD include anticholinergics, benzodiazepines, antihistamine medications, steroids, and opiate analgesics. Less commonly known to cause acute mental status changes are antiparkinsonian agents, antibiotics, antihypertensives (b blockers), NSAIDs, anticonvulsants, and diuretics (Box 27.1).

A review of medications is warranted with each case of delirium in older adults. A thorough medication review should focus on the considerations detailed in Box 27.2.

Laboratory evaluation of suspected drug-induced delirium can be helpful and is individualized to the suspected offending agent. Labs potentially important in the evaluation of suspected drug-induced delirium are shown in Box 27.3.

Box 27.2 Important considerations in cases of suspected medication-induced delirium

1. Review the patient's current and recent medication list, including prescription, over-the-counter, and herbal supplements. Identify any new medications or changes in dosage that might coincide with the onset of delirium.
2. Timing: Determine the timeline of medication administration in relation to the onset of delirium. Consider whether delirium developed shortly after starting a new medication, adjusting the dose, or discontinuing a medication.
3. Polypharmacy: Assess whether the patient is taking multiple medications that could potentially interact with and contribute to the development of delirium. Drug–drug interactions can amplify the risk of adverse effects.
4. Dose and route of administration: Examine the dosage and route of administration of the medications. High doses, rapid titration, and certain routes of administration (e.g. intravenous) can increase the risk of adverse effects, including delirium.
5. Pharmacokinetics: Understand the pharmacokinetic properties of the medications involved, including metabolism and elimination. Impaired renal or hepatic function can lead to increased drug levels and a higher risk of adverse effects.
6. Pharmacodynamics: Consider the pharmacodynamic effects of the medications on the CNS. Some medications can directly affect neurotransmitter systems and cognitive function.
7. Underlying medical conditions: Evaluate the patient's overall medical condition, including any preexisting cognitive impairment, organ dysfunction, or conditions that might increase susceptibility to medication-induced delirium.
8. Age and sensitivity: Recognize that older adults are generally more susceptible to medication-induced delirium due to age-related changes in metabolism, increased sensitivity to medications, and potential accumulation of drugs.
9. Withdrawal effects: In cases where delirium develops after abrupt discontinuation of medication (especially sedatives, opioids, or benzodiazepines), consider the possibility of withdrawal-induced delirium.
10. Other contributing factors: Rule out other potential causes of delirium, such as infections, metabolic disturbances, electrolyte imbalances, and other medical or neurological conditions.

Box 27.3 Labs that may be helpful in the workup of suspected drug-induced delirium

1. Serum electrolytes. Useful when the patient is on diuretics, lithium, or trimethoprim/sulfa and there is suspicion of drug-induced electrolyte disturbances.
2. Serum liver function tests. Use especially in cases of suspected medication-induced hepatic encephalopathy (acetaminophen, amiodarone).
3. Renal function panel. Acute changes in renal function can lead to a buildup of previously tolerated doses of medication known to cause neuropsychiatric side effects.
4. Thyroid function tests. Hypo or hyperthyroid states triggered by medications such as lithium and amiodarone can lead to mental status changes.
5. Blood glucose levels. Medications like beta blockers can mask the other physical signs of hypoglycemia that would otherwise accompany acute mental status changes. Fluoroquinolone antibiotics are known to increase the risk of hypoglycemia, especially in older adults.
6. Therapeutic drug levels. Older adults, those with impaired kidney function, and those with low body weight are especially vulnerable to digoxin toxicity and lithium toxicity.
7. Vitamin levels. Certain drugs (anticonvulsants, methotrexate, diuretics, and antacids) are well known to influence thiamine, b12, and folate absorption and metabolism.

The treatment of drug-induced delirium depends on the cause and severity. Of course, discontinuation of the offending agent should be of priority. Hospitalization may be required for severe delirium and less severe cases may be evaluated and treated in the long-term care setting with close monitoring. Low-dose antipsychotic medications are often helpful while waiting for the clearing of mental status. The lowest possible dose of antipsychotic medication for the shortest amount of time should be the goal. The resolution of delirium can occur within hours or days or even longer depending on the pharmacodynamics and pharmacokinetics of the medication, comorbidities, and baseline cognitive reserve of the patient.

Take-Home Points

- Delirium is more common in older adults, especially those with MNCDs.
- Medications and infections are the most common causes of delirium in older adults.
- Always do a thorough review of medication when considering any mental status changes in older adults.
- Delirium is a medical emergency and warrants immediate medical evaluation and treatment.

References

1. Woodhouse, R., Burton, J. K., Rana, N., Pang, Y. L., Lister, J. E., & Siddiqi, N. (2018). Interventions for preventing delirium in older people in institutional long-term care. *The Cochrane Database of Systematic Reviews*, 2019 (4). https://doi.org/10.1002/14651858.CD009537.pub3

2. Yang, F. M., Marcantonio, E. R., Inouye, S. K., Kiely, D. K., Rudolph, J. L., Fearing, M. A., & Jones, R. N. (2009). Phenomenological subtypes of delirium in older persons: Patterns, prevalence, and prognosis. *Psychosomatics*, 50 (3), 248–254.

3. Bahr, J., Lackner, T., & Pacala, J. T. (2008). Amiodarone-induced central nervous system toxicity in the frail geriatric patient: A case report and review of the literature. *Annals of Long-Term Care*, 16 (8), 37–40.

4. Sharma, R., Singh, R., & Sharma, M. (2022). Use of haloperidol in amiodarone-induced delirium. *Annals of Indian Psychiatry*, 6 (4), 390–392. | DOI: 10.4103/aip.aip_72_21

Further Reading

Fong, T. G., & Inouye, S. K. (2022). The inter-relationship between delirium and dementia: The importance of delirium prevention. *Nature Reviews. Neurology*, 18 (10), 579–596. www.nature.com/articles/s41582-022-00698-7

Oh-Park, M., Chen, P., Romel-Nichols, V., Hreha, K., Boukrina, O., & Barrett, A. M. (2018). Delirium screening and management in inpatient rehabilitation facilities. *American Journal of Physical Medicine & Rehabilitation*, 97 (10), 754. https://doi.org/10.1097/PHM.0000000000000962

Ormseth, C. H., LaHue, S. C., Oldham, M. A., Josephson, S. A., Whitaker, E., & Douglas, V. C. (2023). Predisposing and precipitating factors associated with delirium: A systematic review. *JAMA Network Open*, 6 (1). https://doi.org/10.1001/jamanetworkopen.2022.49950

Wilson, J. E., Mart, M., Cunningham, C., Shehabi, Y., Girard, T. D., MacLullich, M. J., Slooter, J. C., & Ely, E. W. (2020). Delirium. *Nature Reviews. Disease Primers*, 6 (1), 90. www.nature.com/articles/s41572-020-00223-4

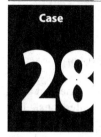

"My Whole Life Is in There!"
Hoarding Disorder

Ms. T was a 77-year-old female who had recently moved into Shady Oaks, a local long-term care facility. Before her move to the facility, she had been living in a trailer home near the outskirts of her small town. She had never married and had no children. Her only living relative was a sister who lived several states away and who had limited contact with Ms. T.

Ms. T had a fall at home about three months before moving to Shady Oaks. She was unable to reach her phone and was only rescued after a concerned neighbor noted Ms. T had not been seen feeding the neighborhood cats for a couple of days, which was her habit. This neighbor was unable to reach Ms. T by phone or get her to answer her door. Local law enforcement were able to see Ms. T on her bathroom floor through the window. Paramedics and firefighters were alerted and successful in gaining entry to the trailer but were nearly unable to reach her due to obstructing debris stacked floor to ceiling.

It took over an hour to clear a path allowing Ms. T to be extracted from her home. She was brought to the hospital where she was diagnosed with a hip fracture, rhabdomyolysis, and renal failure from her prolonged time on the ground after her fall. After surgery for her fracture and a seven-day hospital stay, she was transferred to a unit of the local skilled nursing facility. She recovered somewhat after nearly two weeks of daily therapy and was able to walk with a walker. Her discharge was complicated because her home had been condemned by the local building inspector as being unsafe for habitation. The social worker at the facility accompanied the building inspector for a brief visit to assess the living situation of Ms. T's prior residence and was shocked to find her home at least 90% unusable and crammed full of what could only be described as random discarded items and trash. Ms. T's living area consisted of a small trail extending from a dilapidated recliner to both the bathroom and an extremely cluttered and unhygienic kitchen. Cat feces were found throughout the home and an infestation of roaches was evident.

Carol, the facility social worker, scheduled a meeting with Ms. T to inform her that returning to her home was not possible as it had been condemned by the city as uninhabitable. Ms. T sobbed, "Oh no! What is going to happen to all my things? I have to have my things! My whole life is in there!" Carol assisted Ms. T with finding a local contractor to clean the rented trailer but it was more than she could afford. Arrangements were made for her to stay at Shady Oaks in the long-term care wing of the facility in a Medicaid-funded room with one roommate.

Her transition to her new home was problematic. Ms. T was extremely private and refused to let staff into her side of the room, even to do basic cleaning. Her roommate was unhappy as the room became cluttered with various items collected from throughout the facility that Ms. T thought might later "come in handy for something". She had several meetings with the facility administrator about the situation and was forced to keep her room to an acceptable level of clutter. The facility psychiatrist was asked to evaluate Ms. T for her "behaviors".

The interview with Ms. T was initially difficult. She was reserved and somewhat aloof at first after understanding that the provider was a mental health professional. Her answers to questions were generally short and direct. She started sobbing when asked about her life before coming to the care facility. "I miss my cats. I miss my house. I miss my things. I don't know why I am here. They had no right!"

She expressed sadness and regret over the loss of her home but seemed to have little insight into how it came to be condemned as an unsafe dwelling. "I hate being here. This isn't living. Everything I own is now in this tiny room. I have nothing!" The examiner noted that the patient's small room was already becoming cluttered with items such as bags of empty food containers, stacks of newspapers, and even sacks of empty toilet paper rolls.

She expressed that she was very sad and had little-to-no enjoyment in the day-to-day activities or social interactions at Shady Oaks. She was sleeping poorly, often watching home shopping networks or infomercials into the early hours of the morning and then sleeping through breakfast and sometimes through lunch. She felt tired. When asked about feelings of guilt she admitted that she could not stop thinking about how she had let her life come to this and felt very sad and guilty for all of the neighborhood cats that she had left behind. Her appetite was also poor. When asked about suicidal thoughts she said, "I would never do that, but living like this is pointless." She admitted to the depression symptoms starting soon after finding out she could not return to her home three weeks prior.

Ms. T seemed to have at least average intelligence. She scored a 29/30 on her SLUMS exam and her patient health questionnaire (PHQ-9) score was 22. Her GAD-7 score was 15.

Ms. T was diagnosed with MDD with comorbid hoarding disorder. She was not open to discussing her tendency to "keep things" but was open to the examiner's suggestion that she had clinical depression. She was agreeable to treatment with an antidepressant and was started on sertraline 25 mg daily, which was increased to 50 mg daily in one week. She agreed to speak with the facility psychotherapist for therapy once per week.

At a follow-up appointment four weeks later Ms. T seemed a little less depressed. The nursing staff informed the examiner that she seemed to be adjusting a bit better to the facility routine and could be seen eating with one or two other women at the facility that she seemed to have befriended. She was coming out to the dining room for some of her meals. She told her doctor that she was feeling a little bit better although she would still cry at least daily when she thought of her home and the things that she had lost. She had begrudgingly agreed to limit her collected items to one corner of her room and had started supportive psychotherapy with the on-site licensed clinical social worker. She told the physician that she liked the visits with the therapist and that it was "nice to have someone to talk to about everything."

Teaching Points

Hoarding disorder is now considered one of the obsessive–compulsive (OCD) and related disorders. It is characterized by the urge to save and acquire new items and the difficulty in discarding collected items regardless of value. These urges lead to the progressive accumulation and clutter of living spaces severe enough to lead to consequences such as unsafe living conditions and the development of impairment in social or occupational arenas. The condition is often associated with poor insight or even delusional thinking such as beliefs that worthless items will become indispensable in the future.

The prevalence of hoarding disorder is thought to be about 6% in patients over the age of 70. The symptoms usually begin in young adulthood and increase in severity with age. Seniors with hoarding disorder are at risk of multiple adverse outcomes that are thought to be secondary to the high concurrence of malnutrition, medication mismanagement, falls, food contamination, and eviction from their homes/housing insecurity [1]. Approximately two-thirds of patients with hoarding disorder have comorbid psychiatric diagnoses, most commonly mood or anxiety disorders.

Hoarding disorder is considered to be a chronic and progressive disease and most adults will recall that their hoarding behaviors began before the age of 20. Epidemiological studies seem to show no real differences in the prevalence of the disorder between males and females [2].

Those who suffer from hoarding disorder often form strong emotional attachments to their possessions, making it very difficult for them to throw anything away, even if items are useless or unsanitary. The behaviors can be distressing and difficult to control. The disorder can lead to significant impairment in social, occupational, and family functioning. Patients with this condition may have little-to-no insight into their condition and others may fully realize the magnitude of their pathology. The diagnostic features of hoarding disorder as specified in DSM–5–TR are listed in Box 28.1 [3].

Diagnosing hoarding disorder can be difficult as patients often present late in the stage of their disease, if at all. Typically, poor to absent insight contributes to late presentations. These individuals also experience significant shame and societal stigmatization related to the condition [4].

The causes of hoarding disorder are not fully known. As with many psychiatric conditions, genetic predisposition, environmental/developmental factors, and psychological factors are thought to be at play. Half of those with hoarding disorder will identify a family member who also hoards [5].

Older adults with hoarding disorder commonly suffer from self-neglect and are at risk of food contamination, malnutrition, medication mismanagement, falls, and eviction from their homes. In older adults, 25% with hoarding disorder admit to having an insect infestation in their homes and 58% report that their home is a fire hazard [6]. Comorbid neuropsychiatric illnesses are common, including mood and anxiety disorders, and attention deficit disorder [7].

Treatment options are fairly limited due in part to the fact that the condition has only been officially recognized as a psychiatric condition with clear diagnostic criteria since 2013. The most effective treatment for older adults with hoarding disorder is cognitive rehabilitation and exposure/sorting therapy (CREST). This therapy pairs cognitive training to improve executive functioning with behavioral exposure to the distress of discarding or not acquiring objects [8]. This therapy is challenging for several reasons, including its time-consuming nature, limited availability of trained therapists, and the tendency of some patients to have limited insight into their condition.

Box 28.1 Diagnostic features of hoarding disorder as specified in DSM–5–TR

1. Persistent difficulty discarding or parting with possessions, regardless of their actual value.
2. This difficulty is due to a perceived need to save the items and distress associated with discarding them.
3. The difficulty discarding possessions results in accumulation that congests and clutters active living areas and substantially compromises their intended use. If living areas are uncluttered, it is only because of the interventions of third parties (e.g. family members, cleaners, authorities).
4. The hoarding causes clinically significant distress or impairment in social, occupational, or other important areas of functioning (including maintaining a safe environment for self and others).
5. The hoarding is not attributable to another medical condition (e.g. brain injury, cerebrovascular disease, Prader–Willi syndrome).
6. The hoarding is not better explained by the symptoms of another mental disorder (e.g. obsessions in OCD, decreased energy in MDD, delusions in schizophrenia or another psychotic disorder, cognitive deficits in MNCD, restricted interests in autism spectrum disorder).

Specify if:

With excessive acquisition: If difficulty discarding possessions is accompanied by excessive acquisition of items that are not needed or for which there is no available space.

Specify if:

With good or fair insight: The individual recognizes that hoarding-related beliefs and behaviors (pertaining to difficulty discarding items, clutter, or excessive acquisition) are problematic.
With poor insight: The individual is mostly convinced that hoarding-related beliefs and behaviors (pertaining to difficulty discarding items, clutter, or excessive acquisition) are not problematic despite evidence to the contrary.
With absent insight/delusional beliefs: The individual is completely convinced that hoarding-related beliefs and behaviors (pertaining to difficulty discarding items, clutter, or excessive acquisition) are not problematic despite evidence to the contrary.

Take-Home Points

– Hoarding disorder is now considered one of the obsessive–compulsive and related disorders. It is thought to affect about 6% of those over the age of 70.
– Symptoms of hoarding disorder are thought to begin in young adulthood and increase in severity with age.
– Those with hoarding disorder are likely to be diagnosed late in the course of their disease due to a prominent lack of insight, shame, and social stigma.
– Complications of hoarding disorder include food contamination, malnutrition, medication misman-agement, falls, and eviction from the home.
– The best treatment outcomes have been shown with CREST. This treatment can be limited by the availability of appropriately-trained professionals and the lack of insight by patients.

References

1. Davidson, E. J., Dozier, M. E., Pittman, J. O. E., Mayes, T. L., Blanco, B. H., Gault, J. D., Schwarz, L. J., & Ayers, C. R. (2019). Recent advances in research on hoarding. *Current Psychiatry Reports*, 21 (9), 91. www.ncbi.nlm.nih.gov/pmc/articles/PMC7294597/

2. Cath, D. C., Nizar, K., Boomsma, D., & Mathews, C. A. (2017). Age-specific prevalence of hoarding and obsessive-compulsive disorder: A population-based study. *The American Journal of Geriatric Psychiatry: Official Journal of the American Association for Geriatric Psychiatry*, 25 (3), 245. https://doi.org/10.1016/j.jagp.2016.11.006

3. American Psychiatric Association. (2022). *The Diagnostic and Statistical Manual of Mental Disorders.* 5th ed. text rev. (American Psychiatric Publishing.)

4. Morein-Zamir, S., & Ahluwalia, S. (2023). Hoarding disorder: Evidence and best practice in primary care. *The British Journal of General Practice*, 73 (729), 182–183. https://doi.org/10.3399/bjgp23X732513

5. Ivanov, V. Z., Nordsletten, A., Mataix-Cols, D., Serlachius, E., Lichtenstein, P., Lundström, S., Magnusson, P. K. E., Kuja-Halkola, R., & Rück, C. (2017). Heritability of hoarding symptoms across adolescence and young adulthood: A longitudinal twin study. *PLoS ONE*, 12 (6), e0179541. doi: 10.1371/journal.pone.0179541. PMID: 28658283; PMCID: PMC5489179.

6. Ayers, C. R., & Dozier, M. E. (2015). Predictors of hoarding severity in older adults with hoarding disorder. *International Psychogeriatrics*, 27 (7), 1147–1156. doi: 10.1017/S1041610214001677. Epub 2014 Aug 13. PMID: 25115688; PMCID: PMC5612621.

7. Gleason, A., Perkes, D., & Wand, A. P. (2021). Managing hoarding and squalor. *Australian Prescriber*, 44 (3), 79–84. https://doi.org/10.18773/austprescr.2021.020

8. Ayers, C. R., Dozier, M. E., Twamley, E. W., Saxena, S., Granholm, E., Mayes, T. L., & Wetherell, J. L. (2018). Cognitive rehabilitation and exposure/sorting therapy (CREST) for hoarding disorder in older adults: A randomized clinical trial. *The Journal of Clinical Psychiatry*, 79 (2). https://doi.org/10.4088/JCP.16m11072

Further Reading

Ayers, C. R., Saxena, S., Espejo, E., Twamley, E. W., Granholm, E., & Wetherell, J. L. (2014). Novel treatment for geriatric hoarding disorder: An open trial of cognitive rehabilitation paired with behavior therapy. *The American Journal of Geriatric Psychiatry*, 22 (3), 248–252.

"My Vision Has Been Worsening in the Last Two Weeks"

Generalized Anxiety Disorder

Mrs. U was a 96-year-old widowed woman who was admitted to the nursing home because of frailty, blindness due to macular degeneration, and recurrent falls. She had a sister who was two years younger and in good health, one son, three grandchildren, eight great-grandchildren, and one great-great-grandchild. For eight to nine months Mrs. U had been having increased anxiety and nervousness, had used her call light excessively, was shouting "help, help" for long periods of time, and was grabbing passers-by and asking them to help her.

Mrs. U had been in the long-term care facility for several years and had always been somewhat anxious, but these symptoms were much more severe and triggered by a severe UTI nine months earlier. The staff was initially able to manage her behavior with psychosocial approaches, such as taking her to church service twice a day (Mrs. U was a Methodist and religious but did not mind attending church services of different denominations), hand massage, and soothing music. However, over five months, the symptoms became severe and difficult to manage. Mrs. U usually slept well and, although she had been eating less for a few weeks, had no weight loss.

The family started decreasing their visits because they felt Mrs. U became more agitated when they visited and asked her how she was feeling. The family felt helpless when they could not calm her down and the staff told them that she was having "another bad day."

The primary care physician (PCP) had tried citalopram and mirtazapine with her, but Mrs. U could not tolerate either of these medications. Hence, the PCP referred her to the consulting psychiatrist. The psychiatrist found Mrs. U to be pleasant and talkative, and she anxiously stated, "My vision has been worsening in the last two weeks." She described herself as being a "worrier," and her son confirmed that she had always been extremely nervous and impatient, would be "easily stressed," and thought and feared the worst in any situation. Mrs. U denied any depressive symptoms, and her son confirmed that she had not had any significant depressive symptoms in the past.

Mrs. U's PCP evaluated her for a UTI, constipation, pain, electrolyte imbalance, thyroid dysfunction, and vitamin deficiency and did not find any problems. Mrs. U's vision complaints were not new and were due to macular degeneration, which was being addressed by the ophthalmologist. The pharmacist reviewed Mrs. U's medications and recommended discontinuing cyclobenzaprine (which the PCP subsequently did) but did not find any other medication that could cause anxiety. Mrs. U's SLUMS score was 24 (indicating relatively intact cognitive function, given her age and vision problems), and her Geriatric Depression Scale (GDS) score was 5 (suggesting minimal depression). The psychiatrist diagnosed Mrs. U as having general anxiety disorder (GAD) and mild cognitive impairment and started her on buspirone 5 mg twice daily, increasing to 10 mg twice daily after one week. After another week, the dosage was further increased to 15 mg twice daily.

The psychiatrist also recommended that the family visit as often as possible, have an "active visit" rather than asking questions, and counseled them regarding some of the activities they could do with her. The family would sit with Mrs. U and encourage her to tell stories about her younger days on the farm. They would also take her for a ten-minute walk each time they visited, listen to Mrs. U's favorite music and reminisce, and watch baseball games on TV and keep her informed about the game. The staff was encouraged to avoid telling the family that Mrs. U "was not doing well" but instead to reassure the family that, with time, she should start feeling better with the current care plan. After four more weeks, the family and staff noticed that Mrs. U was better, and her anxiety was less. Over the next three months, she continued to show further improvement, with only one to two episodes of anxiety and yelling per week.

Teaching Points

It is not uncommon for a resident to try multiple medications to manage anxiety disorder before finding a tolerated and effective psychotropic. Although an SSRI or SNRI is usually the first-line agent for pharmacotherapy of GAD, the healthcare professional should also consider prescribing buspirone. The full effects of medication for anxiety disorder may take a few months. Specific guidance and counseling of family and staff regarding psychosocial approaches have a much higher success rate than nonspecific recommendations.

Generalized anxiety disorder is the most commonly encountered anxiety disorder. Other anxiety disorders include panic disorder, agoraphobia, social anxiety disorder, and specific phobias. Symptoms of GAD include chronic and pervasive anxiety and excessive worry. These can be accompanied by various physical symptoms such as increased heart rate, shortness of breath, muscle tension, sweating, GI symptoms, dizziness, sleep disturbances, fatigue, and changes in appetite.

Older adults diagnosed with GAD often have a lifelong history of excessive worry and anxiety, which will usually be corroborated by family members or caregivers. Diagnosing the condition is relatively straightforward. Older adults able to participate in a history may describe feelings of anxiety, worry, irritability, difficulty sleeping, and a variety of physical symptoms that are difficult to attribute to other specific medical conditions. Concern for anxiety is often brought up by caregivers when patients demonstrate disruptive behaviors related to anxiety, such as yelling out, resisting care, becoming frightened with personal care, and repetitive behaviors such as pushing a call light many times a day, pacing, or restlessness.

Those with GAD may have frequent exacerbations of their condition that can be triggered by changes in routine, loneliness, boredom, new staff, changes in medical conditions, and pain. Those older adults with more severe GAD may be triggered by the smallest inconveniences or irritants.

Diagnosing GAD is possible with a good history, mental status exam, review of medications, and review of pertinent labs. Cognitively intact patients will often readily and eagerly describe their anxiety and may describe an inability to enjoy day-to-day activities due to excessive worry. Perseveration may be prominent. The family may tell

Box 29.1 Anxious behaviors in those with advanced MNCD

1. Pacing.
2. Wringing hands.
3. Inability to sit still.
4. Difficult time winding down and going to bed at night.
5. Being excessively irritable with caregivers or other residents.
6. Repeated exit-seeking behaviors.
7. Decreased appetite.
8. Repeated verbalizations such as "help me, help me".
9. Shadowing. Shadowing is when one with severe cognitive impairment needs to keep their caregiver in sight at all times.
10. Constant looking for or calling out for a loved one.

providers that their loved one will call excessively or be excessively focused on physical symptoms and their potentially dire implications. The mental status exam is usually positive for an anxious mood. The workup should include pertinent labs such as thyroid status, electrolyte status, b12, and vitamin D levels. A brief neurological exam focusing on the presence or absence of focal neurologic signs, tremors, and gait is helpful.

Recognizing and diagnosing anxiety in an older adult with advanced MNCD can be more challenging. These patients often cannot express themselves sufficiently to tell the clinician or caregiver their feelings. The provider can then look for outward signs of anxiety or ask for detailed behavior descriptions from caregivers. Those with advanced MNCD may show signs of restlessness, which can be seen as pacing, wringing of hands, or fidgeting. Anxious behaviors can also be seen to include frequent nonsensical verbalizations or vocalizations. Patients who are anxious are often easily irritated, may lash out verbally or physically at times, and may have a hard time getting to sleep at night. Some other signs of anxious behavior in those with severe cognitive impairment are shown in Box 29.1.

The differential diagnosis for general and persistent anxiety symptoms can include endocrine causes such as overreplacement of thyroid hormone and functioning thyroid nodules. Very rarely catecholamine-producing neuroendocrine tumors can lead to anxiety symptoms, tachycardia, and episodic hypertension. Symptoms of hyper or hypoglycemia can be mistaken for anxiety. Cardiac causes such as uncontrolled atrial fibrillation can lead to tachycardia and shortness of breath that may be mistaken for anxiety symptoms. Those with chronic pulmonary disease often deal with anxiety secondary to chronic shortness of breath, hypoxia, and hypercapnia.

Once the diagnosis of GAD is made treatment options can be considered. First-line agents for the treatment of GAD are SSRIs. Of the six SSRIs commonly prescribed sertraline and fluoxetine may be preferred due to lack of dosing restrictions from a cardiac standpoint and lack of anticholinergic effects. Serotonin–norepinephrine reuptake inhibitors are also a good choice and include duloxetine and venlafaxine. In those who may have a contraindication or intolerance to SSRIs or SNRIs, there are several good alternatives. Buspirone is generally well tolerated in older adults and doses should quickly be titrated up to 30 or 60 mg daily. It may then take weeks to have a full clinical response. Mirtazapine is a similarly well-tolerated second-line medication. A summary of some commonly used pharmaceuticals used in anxiety is listed in Box 29.2.

Implementing psychosocial–spiritual interventions can also be quite helpful and should always be considered along with pharmacologic interventions. Some psychosocial–spiritual interventions are listed in Box 29.3.

Generalized anxiety disorder is common enough in the older adult population that almost any provider will encounter patients that are particularly difficult to treat. These patients may not respond to first-line agents or may only have a partial response. There are several options to consider in these cases. Box 29.4 gives several suggestions for those who respond poorly or inadequately to first-line agents for GAD.

Box 29.2   Therapeutic options for GAD

First-line agents

1. SSRIs. Sertraline and fluoxetine are good choices but may need higher doses than effective for depressive disorders. Some others (citalopram/escitalopram) have dose limitations due to risk of prolonged QTc interval.
2. SNRIs. (duloxetine/venlafaxine). May be a good first choice for patients with comorbid chronic pain.

Second-line agents

1. Buspirone. The dose should be titrated to 30 or 60 mg daily. May take weeks for clinical response.
2. Mirtazapine. May take weeks for clinical response. Good if increased appetite is desired.
3. Propranolol. Even low doses of propranolol are unlikely to have a cardiovascular effect and can be therapeutic for anxiety. Doses for anxiety are generally given at 10–20 mg bid.
4. Trazodone. Mildly sedating antidepressants in low doses can be helpful for anxiety. Relatively quick acting. May be a good bridge medication when waiting for SSRI or SNRI therapeutic effect.

Avoid

1. Benzodiazepines. Helpful in the short-term in younger patients but should be avoided in older adults.
2. Anticholinergics. Drugs like hydroxyzine are helpful in younger adults but should be avoided in older adults.
3. Antipsychotics. Although these drugs can have a calming effect, they should be avoided in the absence of psychosis due to unfavorable side effect profiles and black box warnings regarding use in older adults.

Box 29.3   Psychosocial–spiritual interventions that may be helpful with GAD in older adults

1. Increased pleasant patient-centered activities to combat boredom and loneliness that can exacerbate anxiety.
2. Consider psychotherapy, especially cognitive behavioral therapy (CBT) if available. Psychotherapy can help patients identify dysfunctional thought patterns that may lead to maladaptive reactions to day-to-day minor irritations.
3. Increased physical activity and exercise. Regular exercise can be a good way to combat anxiety.

Box 29.3 (cont.)

4. Increased socialization. More frequent visits with family can be helpful. The family should try to keep visits focused on pleasurable activities and less focused on discussion of various physical complaints or topics of worry.
5. Relaxing techniques such as medication or prayer.
6. Avoid excessive caffeine and consider tapering off caffeine altogether.
7. Music therapy. Consider playing familiar and calming music regularly as an anxiety-relieving technique.

Box 29.4 Considerations for those that do not adequately respond to first-line treatment for GAD

1. Consider the dose of the first-line agent. Often the target dose for anxiety disorders is higher than that needed for response in depression and related disorders. Some providers are overly cautious about titrating the dose of first-line agents to a truly therapeutic dose.
2. Consider adding an augmenting agent to the SSRI or SNRI. For example, add buspirone or trazodone to sertraline or fluoxetine.
3. Switch from an SSRI to an SNRI. Some patients respond better to the mechanism of an SNRI than SSRI.
4. Consider the possibility of psychotic symptoms, especially in those with MNCDs. Soft signs of psychosis in older adults may be an extreme fear response to relatively benign stimuli, talking to oneself (responding to inner stimuli), picking at one's skin as if bugs or irritants were present, or the presence of very disorganized or bizarre behavior.
It may be that SSRIs or SNRIs are not adequate for these patients. A trial of a low dose of atypical antipsychotic may be helpful.

Follow up for those initiating treatment for GAD should be relatively frequent until symptoms are stabilized. Resist the urge to change first-line treatments before an adequately long trial (eight weeks) at an adequate dose has been accomplished. Attempts should be made to taper antipsychotics at least quarterly in those patients that may have benefited from their use for anxiety contributed to by psychosis in MNCD.

Take-Home Points

– It is not uncommon for a resident to try multiple medications to manage an anxiety disorder before finding a tolerated and effective psychotropic. An SSRI or SNRI is usually the first-line agent for pharmacotherapy and GAD.
– Second-line agents or supporting agents may include buspirone, mirtazapine, propranolol, and trazodone. Avoid benzodiazepines and anticholinergics.
– Concern for anxiety is often brought up by caregivers when patients demonstrate disruptive behaviors related to anxiety such as yelling out, resisting care, becoming frightened with personal care, and repetitive behaviors such as pushing a call light many times a day, pacing, or restlessness.
– Strategies to address difficult-to-manage anxiety include reconsidering the first-line agent for appropriate dose and duration, adding an augmenting agent, switching from an SSRI to an SNRI, and considering the possibility of low-grade psychosis as a potential contributing factor to anxiety.

Further Reading

Chen, J. T., Wuthrich, V. M., Rapee, R. M., Draper, B., Brodaty, H., Cutler, H., Low, L. F., Georgiou, A., Johnco, C., Jones, M., Meuldijk, D., & Partington, A. (2022). Improving mental health and social participation outcomes in older adults with depression and anxiety: Study protocol for a randomized controlled trial. *PLoS ONE*, 17 (6), e0269981. https://doi.org/10.1371/journal.pone.0269981

Choi, N. G., Zhou, Y., Marti, C. N., & Kunik, M. E. (2022). Associations between changes in depression/anxiety symptoms and fall worry among community-dwelling older adults. *Journal of Applied Gerontology: the official journal of the Southern Gerontological Society*, 41 (12), 2520–2531. https://doi.org/10.1177/07334648221119464

Hill, N. L., Mogle, J., Bell, T. R., Bhargava, S., Wion, R. K., & Bhang, I. (2019). Predicting current and future anxiety symptoms in cognitively intact older adults with memory complaints. *International Journal of Geriatric Psychiatry*, 34 (12), 1874–1882. doi: 10.1002/gps.5204. Epub 2019 Sep 3. PMID: 31468598; PMCID: PMC6854282.

Lamoureux-Lamarche, C., Berbiche, D., & Vasiliadis, M. (2020). Treatment adequacy and remission of depression and anxiety disorders and quality of life in primary care older adults. *Health and Quality of Life Outcomes*, 19. www.ncbi.nlm.nih.gov/pmc/articles/PMC8444434/

Landreville, P., Gosselin, P., Grenier, S., & Carmichael, P. H. (2021). Self-help guided by trained lay providers for generalized anxiety disorder in older adults: Study protocol for a randomized controlled trial. *BMC Geriatrics*, 21 (1), 324. doi: 10.1186/s12877-021-02221-x. PMID: 34022795; PMCID: PMC8140311.

Nair, P., Walters, K., Aw, S., Gould, R., Kharicha, K., Buszewicz, M. C., & Frost, R. (2021). Self-management of depression and anxiety amongst frail older adults in the United Kingdom: A qualitative study. *PLoS ONE*, 17 (12). https://doi.org/10.1371/journal.pone.0264603

Penninx, B. W., Pine, D. S., Holmes, E. A., & Reif, A. (2021). Anxiety disorders. *Lancet (London, England)*, 397 (10277), 914–927. www.ncbi.nlm.nih.gov/pmc/articles/PMC9248771/

Stavestrand, S. H., Sirevåg, K., Nordhus, I. H., Sjøbø, T., Endal, T. B., Nordahl, H. M., Specht, K., Hammar, Å., Halmøy, A., Martinsen, E. W., Andersson, E., Hjelmervik, H., Mohlman, J., Thayer, J. F., & Hovland, A. (2018). Physical exercise augmented cognitive behavior therapy for older adults with generalized anxiety disorder (PEXACOG): Study protocol for a randomized controlled trial. *Trials*, 20. https://bpsmedicine.biomedcentral.com/articles/10.1186/s13030-023-00280-7

Welzel, F. D., Luppa, M., Pabst, A., Pentzek, M., Fuchs, A., Weeg, D., Bickel, H., Weyerer, S., Werle, J., Wiese, B., Oey, A., Brettschneider, C., König, H., Heser, K., Eisele, M., Maier, W., Scherer, M., Wagner, M., & Riedel-Heller, S. G. (2021). Incidence of anxiety in latest life and risk factors. Results of the AgeCoDe/AgeQualiDe Study. *International Journal of Environmental Research and Public Health*, 18 (23). https://doi.org/10.3390/ijerph182312786

"I Am Not Addicted to Valium"
Panic Disorder

Ms. F was a 70-year-old resident who had a long history of panic disorder with agoraphobia. She had been stable for decades, taking 5 mg of diazepam twice daily for the last 30 years, along with 0.25 mg of alprazolam as needed once a day and imipramine 25 mg daily at bedtime. She was admitted to a nursing facility for rehabilitation after receiving a second kidney transplant. Her PCP, who had prescribed her psychiatric medications for decades, had recently passed away and a young family practitioner took over her care. He felt that Ms. F carried a high risk of falls and confusion due to diazepam, as-needed alprazolam, and imipramine. He also felt that Ms. F had become addicted to diazepam and scheduled a tapering schedule for it. Within a few weeks, Ms. F was severely agitated and required hospitalization in a psychiatric unit. She clearly told the psychiatrist, "I am not addicted to Valium." The psychiatrist discussed treatment options with Ms. F, including switching to an SSRI, mirtazapine, or nortriptyline versus reinstating her original medications. Ms. F chose to restart her original medications, as they had helped her for many years and she was willing to risk the potential adverse effects, including cardiac risks, falls, and cognitive impairment. The psychiatrist reinstated Ms. F's original medication regimen and she was back to her baseline level of functioning within a couple of weeks. The psychiatrist also collaborated with the new PCP and explained the severity of the panic disorder and the plan for frequent outpatient follow-up visits to closely monitor risks for falls and cognitive impairment. The PCP agreed, as long as the psychiatrist would continue to manage Ms. F's panic disorder.

Teaching Points

Panic disorder is a type of anxiety disorder characterized by recurring and unexpected panic attacks. Panic attacks are periods of intense and overwhelming fear that can be accompanied by physical symptoms such as rapid heartbeat, chest pain, dizziness, shortness of breath, tremors, and sweating. The symptoms of these attacks usually escalate very rapidly and may last anywhere from several minutes to an hour or more. People with this condition often live in fear of experiencing another panic attack, which can lead to continuous anxiety and avoidance behaviors. Avoidance behaviors are an attempt to avoid situations or places in which previous panic attacks have occurred. These avoidance behaviors can lead to significant disability in the areas of work, relationships, and general enjoyment of life. Some with panic disorder have comorbid agoraphobia, which is a fear of being in situations where escape might be difficult or embarrassing.

Epidemiologic studies show that an estimated 2% of American adults admit to having had a panic attack in the last 12 months and that around 5% admit to having had a panic attack in their lifetime [1]. The prevalence of panic disorder may actually be higher due to the fact that many patients are likely misdiagnosed as having cardiac or neurologic causes for the panic symptoms. The high prevalence and potential for serious restrictions in normal life activities make panic disorder one of the costliest psychiatric conditions. Thirty years ago a study determined that the cost of anxiety disorders including panic disorder was estimated at $42.3 billion per year in the United States [2]. This was calculated by adding up the direct medical costs (emergency room visits, physician visits, medication), indirect costs (reduced job productivity, absenteeism), and disability and unemployment costs related to anxiety disorders.

Panic disorder is frequently seen with other psychiatric or substance use-related comorbidities, making diagnosis and treatment more difficult [3]. Those with panic disorder are known to have an increased risk of developing substance-use disorders over time, especially alcohol-use disorder and opioid-use disorder.

The causes of panic disorder are likely a complex interplay between genetics, dysfunctional neurophysiology, and psychological and environmental factors. Those with panic disorder can be overly sensitive to physical sensations and may be more likely to interpret benign physical sensations as proof of impending physical catastrophe. Pain is also a well-known potential trigger for panic attacks. Other potential triggers for panic symptoms include relationship conflicts, changes in health status, financial stressors, social outings, and caffeine use.

Biological explanations of panic disorder are explained as imbalances in neurotransmitters in key neural pathways. Involved neurotransmitters include serotonin, norepinephrine, dopamine, and GABA. These mechanisms are supported by the improvement of symptoms with medications that address and modulate the effects of these neurotransmitters in neural pathways [4]. It is also known that gonadal hormones play an influential role in panic disorder. Women are about twice as likely to be diagnosed with the condition as men. Despite the increased biological and psychological stresses of pregnancy, women are less likely to experience panic attacks during pregnancy. The high levels of estrogen, progesterone, and oxytocin during pregnancy are thought to have a protective effect against panic symptoms. Genetic influence is also strong in panic disorder, with 25% of first-degree relatives of those with panic disorder also being diagnosed with panic disorder [5].

The diagnosis of panic disorder is usually via a good medical and psychiatric history. Patients should be encouraged to provide detailed descriptions of their experiences. The detailed description of a panic attack by the patient often clearly points to the diagnosis. Potential diagnoses that can mimic panic disorder include hyperthyroid states, cardiac arrhythmias, and substance use. Once these conditions have been ruled out it is appropriate to proceed toward testing for an anxiety disorder such as panic disorder. The DSM–5–TR criteria for panic disorder are listed in Box 30.1 [6].

There are several options in the treatment of panic disorder. Cognitive behavioral therapy techniques can be quite effective if a patient is motivated and can participate in therapy. It can be limited by the availability of appropriately trained providers, time commitment, and cost. There are several options available for the medical treatment of panic disorder. Selective serotonin reuptake inhibitors are the preferred long-term pharmacologic treatment due to other antidepressant categories producing more adverse

Box 30.1 DSM–5–TR diagnostic criteria for the diagnosis of panic disorder

1. Recurrent unexpected panic attacks. A panic attack is an abrupt surge of intense fear or intense discomfort that reaches a peak within minutes and can occur from a calm or an anxious state. During an attack, four (or more) of the following symptoms occur:

   a. Palpitations, pounding heart, or accelerated heart rate.
   b. Sweating.
   c. Trembling or shaking.
   d. Sensations of shortness of breath or smothering.
   e. Feelings of choking.
   f. Chest pain or discomfort.
   g. Nausea or abdominal distress.
   h. Feeling dizzy, unsteady, lightheaded, or faint.
   i. Chills or heat sensations.
   j. Paresthesias (numbness or tingling sensations).
   k. Derealization (feelings of unreality) or depersonalization (being detached from oneself).
   l. Fear of losing control or "going crazy".
   m. Fear of dying.

   Note: Culture-specific symptoms (e.g., tinnitus, neck soreness, headache, uncontrollable screaming or crying) may be seen. Such symptoms should not count as one of the four required symptoms.

2. At least one of the attacks has been followed by one month (or more) of one or both of the following:

   a. Persistent concern or worry about additional panic attacks or their consequences (e.g. losing control, having a heart attack, "going crazy").
   b. A significant maladaptive change in behavior related to the attacks (e.g. behaviors designed to avoid having panic attacks, such as avoidance of exercise or unfamiliar situations).

3. The disturbance is not attributable to the physiological effects of a substance (e.g. a drug of abuse, a medication) or another medical condition (e.g. hyperthyroidism, cardiopulmonary disorders).

4. The disturbance is not better explained by another mental disorder (e.g. the panic attacks do not occur only in response to feared social situations, as in social anxiety disorder; in response to circumscribed phobic objects or situations, as in specific phobia; in response to obsessions, as in obsessive–compulsive disorder; in response to reminders of traumatic events, as in PTSD; or in response to separation from attachment figures, as in separation anxiety disorder).

effects and the abuse potential of benzodiazepines. Benzodiazepines have been used for many years for the short-term treatment of panic attacks. Prescribing patterns for benzodiazepines have changed over the decades as knowledge has increased regarding the consequences of long-term use. It is not uncommon to encounter older adults who have been on moderate to high doses of benzodiazepines for many years. These patients may be extremely fearful of tapering benzodiazepines due to psychological and physiological dependence that often develops. The treatment options for panic disorder are demonstrated in Box 30.2 [7,8,9].

Box 30.2 Pharmacologic treatment options for those with panic disorder

Acute short-term treatment

Benzodiazepines are recommended for short-term acute treatment of panic disorder. The effects of benzodiazepines on decreasing the severity and frequency of panic symptoms can be seen in as little as days to weeks. They are especially helpful as long-term therapies may take weeks or months for full benefits to be realized. A scheduled dosing is preferred over as-needed dosing.

Long-term therapies

1. SSRIs: First-line agents. Approved medications safe for use in older adults include sertraline and fluoxetine. Avoid paroxetine due to anticholinergic effects in older adults. Doses of citalopram and escitalopram are limited by potential cardiac effects. It may take weeks for clinical response. May require higher doses than typically seen for response in depression.
2. SNRIs: Venlafaxine, duloxetine. Effective, but withdrawal syndromes can be problematic if medications need to be tapered or stopped.
3. Benzodiazepines such as lorazepam, clonazepam. May be required for short-term relief of panic symptoms and for those with inadequate response to SSRIs and SNRIs. Generally avoided in older adults but may be hard to stop in those who have had good responses for years. Use the lowest effective dose [7].

Follow-up for panic disorder should include clinicians asking about the frequency and severity of panic symptoms, the effectiveness of abortive treatments, and continued tolerance of long-term medications. It is important to speak with caregivers in older adults with cognitive impairments.

There are several challenges regarding the treatment of panic disorder that are more specific to older adults. Benzodiazepine use is a well-accepted abortive treatment for panic symptoms in younger adults without a history of substance use disorder. They are fast-acting and generally considered quite safe when used as prescribed. Their use in older adults is more likely to have unwanted side effects such as increased fall risk, worsening cognition, and behavioral disinhibition. For these reasons, every effort should be made to gradually taper older adults off as-needed or scheduled benzodiazepines if possible. Small reductions in dose are likely to be well tolerated but the final discontinuation of even a tiny dose of benzodiazepine may lead to an acute decompensation in panic or anxiety symptoms. For this reason, it may be more prudent to taper the dose of benzodiazepine to the lowest dose possible that does not exacerbate the underlying anxiety/panic. Older adults may by necessity remain on very low doses of benzodiazepines almost indefinitely. Clinicians should not be so averse to benzodiazepine use in older adults as to risk psychiatric decompensation and potential hospitalization. Patients tapering down on benzodiazepines may need up-titration of non-benzodiazepine therapeutics like SSRIs, SNRIs, buspirone, trazodone, gabapentin, and so on.

Those with advanced MNCDs are at higher risk of psychotic symptoms that may trigger anxiety and panic. These patients may benefit from antipsychotic therapy to address this. The lowest dose possible to control psychotic symptoms should be prescribed and periodic trials of tapering the antipsychotic are important due to increased mortality risk when used in older adults with MNCDs.

Take-Home Points

- Panic disorder is a type of anxiety disorder characterized by recurring and unexpected panic attacks. Panic attacks are periods of intense and overwhelming fear that can be accompanied by physical symptoms such as rapid heartbeat, chest pain, dizziness, shortness of breath, tremors, and sweating.
- Benzodiazepines are recommended for short-term acute treatment of panic disorder. The effects of benzodiazepines on decreasing the severity and frequency of panic symptoms can be seen in as little as days or weeks. They are especially helpful as long-term therapies may take weeks or months for full benefits to be realized. A scheduled dosing is preferred over as-needed dosing.
- Pharmacologic treatment options for those with panic disorder can include a short course of benzodiazepines and long-term SSRIs or SNRIs. Cognitive behavioral therapy has proven to be a particularly effective nonpharmacologic approach to the treatment of anxiety and panic.
- Those with advanced MNCDs are at higher risk of psychotic symptoms that may trigger anxiety and panic. These patients may benefit from antipsychotic therapy to address this.

References

1. Hasin, D. S., & Grant, B. F. (2015). The national epidemiologic survey on alcohol and related conditions (NESARC) Waves 1 and 2: Review and summary of findings. *Social Psychiatry and Psychiatric Epidemiology*, 50, 1609–1640.

2. Manjunatha, N., & Ram, D. (2022). Panic disorder in general medical practice: A narrative review. *Journal of Family Medicine and Primary Care*, 11 (3), 861–869. https://doi.org/10.4103/jfmpc.jfmpc_888_21

3. Grant, B. F., Saha, T. D., Ruan, W. J., Goldstein, R. B., Chou, S. P., Jung, J., & Hasin, D. S. (2016). Epidemiology of DSM-5 drug use disorder: Results from the national epidemiologic survey on alcohol and related conditions–III. *JAMA Psychiatry*, 73 (1), 39–47.

4. Kyriakoulis, P., & Kyrios, M. (2022). Biological and cognitive theories explaining panic disorder: A narrative review. *Frontiers in Psychiatry*, 14. https://doi.org/10.3389/fpsyt.2023.957515

5. Nocon, A., Wittchen, H. U., Beesdo, K., Brückl, T., Hofler, M., Pfister, H., & Lieb, R. (2008). Differential familial liability of panic disorder and agoraphobia. *Depression and Anxiety*, 25 (5), 422–434.

6. American Psychiatric Association, DSM–5 Task Force. (2013). *Diagnostic and Statistical Manual of Mental Disorders: DSM–5^{TM}*. 5th ed. (American Psychiatric Publishing, Inc.) https://doi.org/10.1176/appi.books.9780890425596

7. Zulfarina, M. S., Syarifah-Noratiqah, B., Nazrun, S. A., Sharif, R., & Naina-Mohamed, I. (2019). Pharmacological therapy in panic disorder: Current guidelines and novel drugs discovery for treatment-resistant patient. *Clinical Psychopharmacology and Neuroscience*, 17 (2), 145–154. https://doi.org/10.9758/cpn.2019.17.2.145

8. DeMartini, J., Patel, G., & Fancher, T. L. (2019). Generalized anxiety disorder. *Annals of Internal Medicine*, 170 (7), ITC49–ITC64.

9. American Psychiatric Association. (2009). *Practice Guideline for the Treatment of Patients with Panic Disorder*, 2nd ed. (American Psychiatric Association, Ltd.)

Further Reading

Chawla, N., Anothaisintawee, T., Charoenrungrueangchai, K., Thaipisuttikul, P., McKay, G. J., Attia, J., & Thakkinstian, A. (2021). Drug treatment for panic disorder with or without agoraphobia: Systematic review and network meta-analysis of randomised controlled trials.

The BMJ, 376. https://doi.org/10.1136/bmj-2021-066084

Kim, E. J., & Kim, Y. K. (2018). Panic disorders: The role of genetics and epigenetics. *AIMS Genetics*, 5 (3), 177–190. https://doi.org/10.3934/genet.2018.3.177

Melaragno, A. J. (2021). Pharmacotherapy for anxiety disorders: From first-line options to treatment resistance. *Focus: Journal of Life-Long Learning in Psychiatry*, 19 (2), 145–160. https://doi.org/10.1176/appi.focus.20200048

31

"Of Course, I Worry about Him"
Generalized Anxiety Disorder in the
Setting of MNCD

Mrs. B was a 91-year-old woman admitted to an AL home six months ago because of increasing agitation and anxiety. Mr. B, who was 93 years old, could no longer take care of her. Mrs. B had been diagnosed with MNCD due to Alzheimer's disease three years previously. She could not tolerate ChEis due to nausea and diarrhea and had been taking memantine 10 mg twice daily for two years.

Over the last year, Mrs. B had become increasingly anxious and agitated and would start yelling for her husband if she was left alone for even a few minutes. Mrs. B would worry that something terrible had happened to Mr. B and she would not allow him to go anywhere, even if one of their three daughters agreed to stay with her. Mrs. B would try to leave the house to look for her husband and would become aggressive if someone tried to stop her. She showed the same behavior in the AL home, and although lorazepam 0.5 mg three times a day prescribed by her PCP had helped, she became more anxious when started on sertraline 50 mg daily.

The family was growing increasingly frustrated because they would often spend hours with Mrs. B without improvement in her anxiety. Mr. B would become very angry with her, and her daughters could not understand why she was "so stubborn." A geriatric psychiatrist was consulted at this point. The psychiatrist learned from Mrs. B's sister that they had lost their younger brother through accidental drowning when Mrs. B was ten years old. Mrs. B was the oldest of six children and did not have any role in the drowning. Her mother was overwhelmed with working on the farm and raising six children and had put a lot of responsibility on Mrs. B for housework and looking after her younger siblings.

Mrs. B had expressed guilt off and on for years over the death and was described by her family as having been an anxious and shy person who liked to be in her home and take care of her husband and three daughters. There was no history of her anxiety and shyness having caused significant impairment in daily functioning in her younger years.

Mrs. B was otherwise in good health and denied any depressive symptoms during the interview. She reported that she had a difficult life, that her worries about her husband were "normal," and added, "Of course, I worry about him." Mrs. B denied her husband's report that she would become "belligerent." She could not give a detailed history because of her MNCD, her SLUMS score was 16, and her GDS–15 score was seven. A score over five is suggestive of depression. The psychiatrist diagnosed severe anxiety disorder and mild depression in the setting of MNCD. Mrs. B was started on 12.5 mg of sertraline, which was increased every two weeks to a total of 50 mg daily. The psychiatrist informed the care staff at the AL home about Mrs. B's childhood trauma, and both the staff and family were also counseled that MNCD made Mrs. B more susceptible to emotional disorders because of past trauma. The staff became more sympathetic, allowed the medication more time to work, and tried harder to distract Mrs. B during her times of heightened anxiety. The family and staff were educated that SSRIs such as sertraline may cause an initial increase in anxiety before improvements are noted, especially in a patient who is already anxious.

After eight weeks, the staff and family reported a mild improvement in Ms. B's agitation and anxiety, especially her episodes of yelling and disrupting the environment. The psychiatrist further increased sertraline to 62.5 mg daily for two weeks and then to 75 mg daily. After eight more weeks, the anxiety and agitation were substantially less, and yelling episodes were occasional and easily managed. The lorazepam was gradually decreased and changed to as-needed. Mrs. B used it on average once or twice a week.

Teaching Points

Uncontrolled anxiety can adversely affect the ability of an older adult with MNCD to remain successful in a home setting. Anxiety can be very fatiguing to family members and other caregivers as well. Older adults with anxiety and MNCD often have a difficult time with verbal expression, which can make it even more difficult for caregivers to know how to help with anxiety symptoms. Chronic anxiety is highly associated with depression and improvements in anxiety often correlate with improvements in depressive symptoms.

The prevalence of mood and anxiety symptoms in those with MNCD is quite high. A study in 2016 by Zhao et al. showed a prevalence of anxiety in 39% of those with Alzheimer's disease [1]. Another study by Chi et al. in 2015 demonstrated a prevalence of depression of 6–42% depending on the criteria used. It is suggested that depression may be underestimated in those with severe MNCDs as the underlying disease process can lead to a declining ability to both have and express depressive or anxious thoughts [2]. A large meta-analysis examining the prevalence of depression, anxiety, and PTSD in the four most common dementias (Alzheimer's disease, VaD, DLB, and FTD) showed that 25% of these patients were found to have clinically significant levels of depressive symptoms and 14% showed clinically significant anxiety [3].

The prevalence of anxiety likely declines as MNCDs progress in the late stages. It is thought that this may be due to the decline, insight, and awareness that accompanies these later stages of the disease [4].

The pathophysiology of anxiety involves the dysregulation of several neurotransmitter pathways in the CNS. Neurotransmitters implicated include norepinephrine, serotonin, dopamine, and GABA. This dysregulation leads to dysfunction of the sympathetic autonomic nervous system as well, which can lead to physical symptoms such as tachycardia, tachypnea, tremulousness, and elevated blood pressure, for example [5]. The amygdala and limbic system play a pivotal role in controlling anxiety. These structures are connected to the prefrontal cortex. These neural pathways are targets of pharmacologic interventions.

Psychosocial factors influence the experience of anxiety in older adults with or without MNCD. Some factors shown to increase anxiety include very high levels of social contact, dysfunctional patient–caregiver relationships, and high physical dependency [6]. Other factors that can negatively impact anxiety in older adults include boredom, social isolation, and unmet physical needs for proper nutrition, warmth, and cleanliness, for example.

The diagnosis of anxiety in older adults in long-term care should include a physical exam and basic laboratory testing to detect or rule out physical disorders that can cause, exacerbate, or mimic anxiety. See Box 31.1 for medical mimickers of anxiety.

A thorough review of medications is important as some medications are known to influence anxiety. Stimulants are not often used in older adults but are well known to cause or increase anxiety. Corticosteroids are more often seen in older adults and can negatively influence anxiety even at relatively low doses. Some antidepressants are known to cause anxiety, particularly in the initial weeks of treatment. Inhaled and oral medications for asthma such as albuterol and theophylline are also well known to cause anxiety. Some patients can become more sensitive to the effects of caffeine as they get older, and patterns of caffeine use should be explored (Box 31.2).

The treatment of anxiety disorders in older adults in long-term care settings should consider both environmental and pharmacologic interventions. Those who work regularly with older adults with MNCDs will know that an environment that is familiar and consistent, calm and quiet, safe, with protected personal space can go a long way to lessen the symptoms of anxiety. Environmental interventions that may help reduce symptoms of anxiety are listed in Box 31.3.

The pharmacologic treatment of anxiety in older adults in long-term care shares similarities with the treatment of anxiety in younger patients. Both SSRIs and SNRIs are good first-line agents and are generally well tolerated. Selective serotonin reuptake

---

Box 31.1 Medical conditions that can mimic anxiety in older adults

1. Infections. Urinary tract infections are well known to cause an increase in agitation and anxiety in older adults.
2. Chronic pain. Undertreated pain can lead to an increase in depression and anxiety symptoms.
3. Endocrinologic disorders. Hyper or hypoglycemia and hyperthyroid conditions can mimic anxiety. Pheochromocytoma is a rare cause of anxiety.
4. Cardiovascular conditions such as tachyarrhythmias.
5. Pulmonary conditions associated with dyspnea can trigger anxiety symptoms.
6. Neurological conditions associated with anxiety include but are not limited to seizure disorder, multiple sclerosis, and TBI.
7. Substance use or withdrawal. The use or tapering of benzodiazepines, opioids, and alcohol is associated with anxiety.

Box 31.2 Medications known to cause anxiety

1. Corticosteroids. Some patients are intolerant to steroids due to neuropsychiatric side effects.
2. Stimulants. May be used for TRD, excessive fatigue secondary to neurodegenerative diseases, and fatigue in obstructive sleep apnea.
3. Antidepressants. Both SSRIs and SNRIs are well known to potentially increase anxiety in the initial days and weeks of use. Increased anxiety can also be seen with the tapering of these medications.
4. Medications for asthma. Such as inhaled beta-agonists and theophylline.
5. Thyroid supplements prescribed at supratherapeutic doses.

> **Box 31.3** Environmental interventions that may help reduce symptoms of anxiety in older adults in long-term care
>
> 1. Familiar and consistent environment. Avoid changes to the environment. Have familiar objects/furniture in private spaces.
> 2. Adequate lighting. Well-lit private and public spaces with natural light.
> 3. Noise control. A calm and quiet living space.
> 4. Safety. Ensure that the environment has appropriate safety features like handrails and nonslip flooring, for example.
> 5. Structured and predictable daily routine.
> 6. Personalized spaces. Familiar objects and personal items can trigger positive memories and reduce anxiety.
> 7. Supportive social environment that includes visits from loved ones, group activities, and other opportunities for social interaction.

inhibitors commonly prescribed in older adults include sertraline, fluoxetine, citalopram, and escitalopram and are often preferred as there are not as many issues with potentially uncomfortable withdrawal as seen with SNRIs, which include duloxetine and venlafaxine. It should also be noted that starting doses for SSRIs and SNRIs should be roughly only half of the starting dose commonly used in younger adults. This may aid in avoiding the exacerbation of anxiety when initiating treatment. Medication doses should regularly be up-titrated to a dose within the therapeutic range for the medication. Buspirone has long been used and is considered safe for the treatment of anxiety in older adults as well. It can be used as monotherapy or add-on therapy to SSRIs or SNRIs and is generally started at a dose of 5 mg twice daily, increasing to a goal dose of 30 to 60 mg daily (div).

As-needed medications for anxiety can be helpful in the initial weeks of treatment as the therapeutic effect of SSRIs and SNRIs is approached. Useful medications for this include low-dose trazodone (25 or 50 mg every four to six hours as needed), as well as gabapentin, mirtazapine, or low-dose propranolol. Benzodiazepines should generally be avoided due to the increased risk of falls and worsening cognition.

Follow-up monitoring for those treated for anxiety disorders in long-term care includes regular assessments for the control of symptoms. Medication adjustments may be necessary and being alert to the potential side effects of SSRIs and SNRIs is important as well. Some of the more common side effects of these agents are listed in Box 31.4.

There are occasional situations that may make the treatment of anxiety more challenging in long-term care patients. There is a relatively high comorbidity of psychosis in those with MNCDs, especially in later stages. Psychosis may be more difficult to detect in those in the later stages of neurodegenerative disease as the ability to verbalize experiences becomes more difficult. Be aware of potential subtle signs of psychoses such as picking at the air, talking to oneself as if responding to inner stimuli, new onset of bizarre behavior, or paranoia. Anxiety will be difficult to manage if psychotic symptoms are not brought under control with the proper pharmacologic interventions.

Another relatively common presentation is that of situation-specific anxiety such as anxiety that might occur only with bathing. It is not surprising that bath time can be commonly problematic as this is a time of physical vulnerability, often in front of caregivers who might be unfamiliar. Some suggestions to make bath time less threatening are shown in Box 31.5.

Box 31.4 Potential side effects of SSRIs/SNRIs

1. Gastrointestinal side effects. Increases in serotonin activity within the GI tract can potentially trigger diarrhea, nausea, and vomiting.
2. Sleep disturbances. These medications can lead to alterations in sleep. If excessive fatigue is noted, it can be helpful to dose at bedtime. If sleeplessness is noted, it may be best to dose in the morning.
3. Agitation. A transient increase in agitation or anxiety may be noted during the early stages of treatment.
4. Serotonin syndrome (rare). Symptoms may include agitation, confusion, rapid heartbeat, high blood pressure, and tremors. In severe cases, it can be life-threatening.
5. Hyponatremia. Consider evaluating for this if there is a noted change in mental status or alertness. Older adults may be more at risk and risk can be increased with concomitant diuretic use.

Box 31.5 Suggestions for lessening anxiety during bathing

1. Bathe parts of the body one at a time, leaving other parts draped with a towel.
2. Keep the shower area warm.
3. Use hand-over-hand techniques for bathing which may be less threatening.
4. Have a calm and unrushed demeanor during bath times.
5. Keep bathing times consistent.
6. Maintain a safe environment with nonslip mats, grab bars, or shower chairs, and minimize clutter.

Take-Home Points

– Some factors shown to increase anxiety include very high levels of social contact, dysfunctional patient–caregiver relationships, and high physical dependency. Other factors that can negatively impact anxiety in older adults include boredom, social isolation, and unmet physical needs for proper nutrition, warmth, and cleanliness, for example.
– As-needed medications for anxiety can be helpful in the initial weeks of treatment as the therapeutic effect of SSRIs and SNRIs is approached. Useful medications for as-needed treatment of anxiety include low-dose trazodone (25 or 50 mg every four to six hours as needed), as well as gabapentin, mirtazapine, or low-dose propranolol.
– Pharmacologic treatment options for those with panic disorder can include a short course of benzodiazepines and long-term SSRIs or SNRIs. Cognitive behavioral therapy has proven to be a particularly effective nonpharmacologic approach to the treatment of anxiety and panic.
– There is a relatively high comorbidity of psychosis in those with MNCDs, especially in later stages. Psychosis may be more difficult to detect in those with psychosis in the later stages of neurodegenerative disease as the ability to verbalize experiences becomes more difficult. Anxiety can be difficult to control in the setting of untreated psychosis.

References

1. Zhao, Q.-F., Tan, L., Wang, H.-F., Jiang, T., Tan, M.-S., Tan, L., & Yu, J.-T. (2016). The prevalence of neuropsychiatric symptoms in Alzheimer's disease: Systematic review and meta-analysis. *Journal of Affective Disorders*, 190, 264–271. https://doi.org/10.1016/j.jad.2015.09.069

2. Chi, S., Wang, C., Jiang, T., Zhu, X.-C., Yu, J.-T., & Tan, L. (2015). The prevalence of depression in Alzheimer's

disease: A systematic review and meta-analysis. *Current Alzheimer Research*, 12, 189–198. https://doi.org/10.2174/1567205012666150204124310

3. Kuring, J. K., Mathias, J. L., & Ward, L. (2018). Prevalence of depression, anxiety and PTSD in people with dementia: A systematic review and meta-analysis. *Neuropsychology Review*, 28, 393–416.

4. Chen, J. C., Borson, S., & Scanlan, J. M. (2000). Stage-specific prevalence of behavioral symptoms in Alzheimer's disease in a multi-ethnic community sample. *The American Journal of Geriatric Psychiatry*, 8 (2), 123–133.

5. Lahousen, T., & Kapfhammer, H. P. (2018). Anxiety disorders: Clinical and neurobiological aspects. *Psychiatria Danubina*, 30 (4), 479–490. German. doi: 10.24869/psyd.2018.479. PMID: 30439809.

6. Orrell, M., & Bebbington, P. (1996). Psychosocial stress and anxiety in senile dementia. *Journal of Affective Disorders*, 39 (3), 165–173.

Case

32

"Bombs Are Falling! Run, Run!"
PTSD

Mr. M was a 92-year-old resident living in a long-term care facility. He had been experiencing nightmares, verbal and physical aggression, anxiety, and hypervigilance. He would also shout, "Bombs are falling! Run, run!", thereby agitating other residents, and had been isolating himself for several weeks. These symptoms started after Mr. M watched images of recent terrorist attacks on TV. The staff at the nursing home felt that he should be hospitalized in a psychiatric unit, as he was "psychotic." The consulting psychiatrist was asked to help facilitate the hospitalization.

The psychiatrist made an emergency psychiatric evaluation of Mr. M, whose wife reported that he was an army infantryman from 1942 to 1945. He had been in prolonged, intense combat in Sicily and Normandy and experienced mild PTSD symptoms and severe depression from 1946 to 1949. Symptoms gradually decreased after he started meeting regularly with a group of friends who were also in World War II. Married for 57 years, Mr. M had four children and 11 grandchildren. He had a successful career as a banker and never abused drugs or alcohol. His wife reported that Mr. M was an easygoing person who seemed to enjoy life until he entered the nursing home due to multiple medical problems.

He developed severe peripheral vascular disease, resulting in bilateral above-knee amputation of his legs for the treatment of gangrene. He subsequently developed severe CHF and was admitted to the nursing home as his wife could no longer take care of his increasing physical needs at home.

The psychiatrist counseled the family and staff that Mr. M's behaviors could be managed in the long-term care facility if everyone collaborated in helping him. Family and staff were informed that hospitalization carried its own risks of increased confusion, delirium, functional decline, falls, and other iatrogenic problems.

The psychiatrist recommended starting sertraline 12.5 mg daily, increasing it every seven days to a total of 50 mg daily. The psychiatrist also started Mr. M on clonazepam 0.25 mg in the morning and at bedtime but, due to daytime sedation, discontinued the morning dose. The family was encouraged and successful in finding a World War II veteran to visit Mr. M several times a week. Only comedy and game shows were kept on the TV in his room, as well as in other places by astute staff. The psychiatrist also recommended to the family and staff to avoid discussion of the terrorist attacks with Mr. M and to have him avoid watching the news on TV. A list of topics for conversation that did not involve war, politics, religion, or terrorist attacks was devised in consultation with the staff and family.

After two weeks, Mr. M was less agitated but continued to have nightmares, aggression, and nighttime agitation. The psychiatrist discussed the use of prazosin for nightmares but, because of the significant risk of orthostatic hypotension, it was not started. The psychiatrist increased the dosage of clonazepam to 0.5 mg at bedtime, but Mr. M had two falls (no injuries) and the dose was decreased to 0.25 mg. The psychiatrist added mirtazapine 7.5 mg at bedtime and Mr. M started sleeping better over the next two weeks. Over the next three months, Mr. M gradually became significantly less anxious, started sleeping better regularly, and his verbal and physical aggression resolved.

Teaching Points

Post-traumatic stress disorder is a mental health condition that is seen in patients who have experienced or observed a traumatic event. Traumatic events are usually those events that threaten death, serious injury, or sexual assault. Common traumatic experiences that are known to sometimes lead to PTSD include war-related events, serious accidents, natural disasters, physical or emotional abuse, serious illness, or the loss of loved ones. Symptoms may include intrusive memories of the traumatic event, flashbacks, nightmares, anxiety, and avoidance of reminders of the traumatic event. These patients are also at increased risk of psychiatric comorbidities including depression and anxiety. Pharmacologic treatments are often very helpful in lessening the symptoms of PTSD. Nonpharmacologic interventions and support from family and caregivers are also key to optimizing the quality of life in patients with PTSD.

Large epidemiologic studies have found that the lifetime prevalence of PTSD as defined by DSM–5–TR criteria is 6%. Rates are generally higher in women (8%) than in men (4%) [1], and veterans have a much higher prevalence. Lifetime prevalence was 3%, 10%, 21%, and 29% for those veterans that served in World War II/Korean War, the Vietnam War, Persian Gulf War, and Operations Enduring Freedom and Iraqi Freedom, respectively [2]. The declining prevalence with age may reflect that the symptoms of PTSD often improve with time. Improved coping strategies with age may help older adults manage the consequences of experiencing traumatic events more effectively.

The pathophysiology of PTSD is complex and exact mechanisms are still not fully understood but are known to involve neurotransmitter imbalances, hyperactivity of the amygdala, hippocampal changes, prefrontal cortex dysfunction, HPA axis dysregulation, and neuroinflammation. See Box 32.1 for a more detailed description of these factors [3].

The development and maintenance of PTSD symptoms after a traumatic event are influenced by key psychosocial factors. Understanding these factors can help to better understand those with PTSD and design effective psychosocial interventions to help them. Box 32.2 lists some psychosocial factors that are important in the development and maintenance of PTSD [4, 5].

The diagnosis of PTSD is usually through a comprehensive evaluation by a mental health professional, usually a psychiatrist, psychologist, or licensed therapist. The process starts with a detailed assessment of the patient's symptoms, medical history, and any potential traumatic events that the patient has experienced. The DSM–5–TR criteria for PTSD are listed in Box 32.3 [6].

There are some issues particular to the diagnosis of PTSD in older adults [7]. Older adults may be less likely to discuss traumatic experiences due to the perceived stigma of mental health disorders. Cognitive impairment may render older adults less able to describe their symptoms or traumatic events. Older adults are more likely to have medical or neurologic comorbidities with symptoms that can overlap with PTSD

Box 32.1 Mechanisms involved in the pathophysiology of PTSD

1. Neurotransmitter imbalances. Dysregulation of key neural pathways involving serotonin, norepinephrine, and dopamine contributes to the emotional dysregulation and hyperarousal seen in PTSD.
2. Hyperactivity of the amygdala. The amygdala is responsible for processing emotions and fear responses. It is known to be hyperactive in patients with PTSD.
3. Hippocampal changes. The hippocampus is involved in memory consolidation and contextual processing.
4. Prefrontal cortex dysfunction. This can lead to difficulties in controlling emotional responses and inhibiting fear-related memories.
5. Hypothalamic–pituitary–adrenal axis dysregulation. This can result in abnormal cortisol levels that can prolong the symptoms of the stress response.
6. Neuroinflammation due to dysregulation of the immune response, which is reflected by an increase in proinflammatory cytokines and a decrease in anti-inflammatory cytokines.

Box 32.2 Psychosocial factors that are important in the development and maintenance of PTSD

1. Severity, nature, and duration of the traumatic event. Events involving physical harm, sexual violence, or life-threatening situations are more likely to lead to PTSD. Prolonged traumas are also more likely to lead to PTSD.
2. Perceived level of threat. A higher level of perceived threat can increase the likelihood of developing and the severity of PTSD symptoms.
3. Social support. Those with adequate or good social support are less likely to develop PTSD after a traumatic experience.
4. Coping mechanisms. Those individuals with good coping mechanisms, such as the likelihood of seeking professional help, talking about experiences, and engaging in relaxing behaviors, have improved outcomes. Avoiding emotions and relying on maladaptive coping mechanisms such as substance abuse negatively affect outcomes.
5. Pre-existing mental health conditions. Those with pre-existing depression or anxiety disorders are likely more vulnerable to developing PTSD after a traumatic event.
6. Personality traits. Certain personality traits, such as neuroticism or a history of emotional instability, may increase the likelihood of developing and the severity of PTSD symptoms.
7. Childhood factors. Those who have experienced childhood abuse or neglect may have more trouble dealing with trauma later in life.
8. Post-trauma stress. Continued stress after a traumatic event can increase the likelihood of severe or prolonged PTSD symptoms.
9. Avoidance behaviors. Avoidance of thoughts or discussions involving the traumatic event can prevent emotional processing and hinder recovery.

symptoms. They may also have experienced multiple traumatic events during their lifetime which can make identifying a specific event and how that event contributes to the development of PTSD difficult. Grief and loss are common in later life and the symptoms of complex grief can make it challenging to distinguish from PTSD symptoms. Diminished social support in older adults can impact their ability to seek help and access mental health services.

Box 32.3 DSM–5–TR criteria for diagnosing PTSD

1. Exposure to actual or threatened death, serious injury, or sexual violence in one (or more) of the following ways:

   a. Directly experiencing the traumatic event(s).
   b. Witnessing, in person, the event(s) as it occurred to others.
   c. Learning that the traumatic event(s) occurred to a close family member or close friend. In cases of actual or threatened death of a family member or friend, the event(s) must have been violent or accidental.
   d. Experiencing repeated or extreme exposure to aversive details of the traumatic event(s) (e.g. first responders collecting human remains; police officers repeatedly exposed to details of child abuse).

   Note: Criterion 1d does not apply to exposure through electronic media, television, movies, or pictures, unless this exposure is work related.

2. Presence of one (or more) of the following intrusion symptoms associated with the traumatic event(s), beginning after the traumatic event(s) occurred:

   a. Recurrent, involuntary, and intrusive distressing memories of the traumatic event(s).

   Note: In children older than six years, repetitive play may occur in which themes or aspects of the traumatic event(s) are expressed.

   b. Recurrent distressing dreams in which the content and/or effect of the dream are related to the traumatic event(s).

   Note: In children, there may be frightening dreams without recognizable content.

   c. Dissociative reactions (e.g. flashbacks) in which the individual feels or acts as if the traumatic event(s) were recurring. (Such reactions may occur on a continuum, with the most extreme expression being a complete loss of awareness of present surroundings.)

   Note: In children, trauma-specific reenactment may occur in play.

   d. Intense or prolonged psychological distress at exposure to internal or external cues that symbolize or resemble an aspect of the traumatic event(s).
   e. Marked physiological reactions to internal or external cues that symbolize or resemble an aspect of the traumatic event(s).

3. Persistent avoidance of stimuli associated with the traumatic event(s), beginning after the traumatic event(s) occurred, as evidenced by one or both of the following:

   a. Avoidance of or efforts to avoid distressing memories, thoughts, or feelings about or closely associated with the traumatic event(s).
   b. Avoidance of or efforts to avoid external reminders (people, places, conversations, activities, objects, situations) that arouse distressing memories, thoughts, or feelings about or closely associated with the traumatic event(s).

4. Negative alterations in cognitions and mood associated with the traumatic event(s), beginning or worsening after the traumatic event(s) occurred, as evidenced by two (or more) of the following:

   a. Inability to remember an important aspect of the traumatic event(s) (typically due to dissociative amnesia and not to other factors such as head injury, alcohol, or drugs).

Box 32.3 *(cont.)*

    b. Persistent and exaggerated negative beliefs or expectations about oneself, others, or the world (e.g. "I am bad," "No one can be trusted," "The world is completely dangerous," "My whole nervous system is permanently ruined").

    c. Persistent, distorted cognitions about the cause or consequences of the traumatic event(s) that lead the individual to blame themself or others.

    d. Persistent negative emotional state (e.g. fear, horror, anger, guilt, or shame).

    e. Markedly diminished interest or participation in significant activities.

    f. Feelings of detachment or estrangement from others.

    g. Persistent inability to experience positive emotions (e.g. inability to experience happiness, satisfaction, or loving feelings).

5. Marked alterations in arousal and reactivity associated with the traumatic event(s), beginning or worsening after the traumatic event(s) occurred, as evidenced by two (or more) of the following:

    a. Irritable behavior and angry outbursts (with little or no provocation) typically expressed as verbal or physical aggression toward people or objects.

    b. Reckless or self-destructive behavior.

    c. Hypervigilance.

    d. Exaggerated startle response.

    e. Problems with concentration.

    f. Sleep disturbance (e.g. difficulty falling or staying asleep or restless sleep).

6. Duration of the disturbance (Criteria 2, 3, 4, and 5) is more than one month.

7. The disturbance causes clinically significant distress or impairment in social, occupational, or other important areas of functioning.

8. The disturbance is not attributable to the physiological effects of a substance (e.g. medication, alcohol) or another medical condition.

Specify whether:

With dissociative symptoms: The individual's symptoms meet the criteria for PTSD, and in addition, in response to the stressor, the individual experiences persistent or recurrent symptoms of either of the following:

1. **Depersonalization:** Persistent or recurrent experiences of feeling detached from, and as if one were an outside observer of, one's mental processes or body (e.g. feeling as though one were in a dream; feeling a sense of unreality of self or body or of time moving slowly).

2. **Derealization:** Persistent or recurrent experiences of unreality of surroundings (e.g. the world around the individual is experienced as unreal, dreamlike, distant, or distorted).

Note: To use this subtype, the dissociative symptoms must not be attributable to the physiological effects of a substance (e.g. blackouts, behavior during alcohol intoxication) or another medical condition (e.g. complex partial seizures).

Specify if:

With delayed expression: If the full diagnostic criteria are not met by at least six months after the event (although the onset and expression of some symptoms may be immediate).

The pharmacologic treatment of PTSD attempts to alleviate the symptoms associated with the condition including anxiety, depression, and sleep disturbances. Selective serotonin reuptake inhibitors are first-line medications for PTSD and SNRIs such as venlafaxine are also effective, especially in instances where there has been a suboptimal response to SSRIs. Prazosin is particularly helpful with PTSD-related nightmares by blocking the effects of adrenaline on the brain during sleep. Atypical antipsychotics may be required to manage symptoms such as severe agitation, aggression, and dissociation related to PTSD. Benzodiazepines are generally avoided in the treatment of PTSD due to their potential for dependence and the risk of worsening symptoms over time [4].

There are quite a few options for nonpharmacologic therapy in older adults. Outcomes are best in those who participate in both pharmacologic and nonpharmacologic treatments. Some of the best outcomes are seen with CBT combined with pharmacotherapy. Other types of psychotherapy that have shown promise include cognitive processing therapy, group therapy, psychodynamic psychotherapy, and mindfulness-based therapies [8]. Older adults with significant cognitive impairment will likely be poor candidates for psychotherapy-related treatments.

Follow-up for those with PTSD should involve regular visits with a provider to assess response to treatment. Rating scales such as the PTSD Checklist 5 can be quite helpful in objectively assessing the severity and nature of PTSD symptoms over time [9]. Rating scales can also help to guide treatment planning and may allow patients and their families to have a better understanding of the symptoms and treatment-related improvements.

The prognosis of PTSD varies widely among individuals. Some patients may experience significant improvement or even full remission of symptoms over time. Box 32.4 shows some of the variables that can influence outcomes in PTSD [10].

The identification and treatment of PTSD in older adults is an important skill for those who regularly provide psychiatric or primary care in the long-term care setting. Efforts to better understand the condition and assist those with the disorder are often rewarding. Pharmacologic and nonpharmacologic interventions can alleviate suffering, enhance social functioning, reduce healthcare utilization, and improve overall quality of life.

Box 32.4 Variables affecting outcomes in patients with PTSD

1. Early intervention. Those who receive therapeutic interventions early after the traumatic event are likely to have better outcomes.
2. Severity of the trauma. Those patients who experienced physical harm, sexual violence, or life-threatening situations are more likely to have PTSD symptoms that are more difficult to control.
3. Co-occurring conditions. Comorbid psychiatric conditions such as depression or anxiety disorders can influence outcomes.
4. Social support. Those patients with strong support systems including family, friends, and community support are more likely to do better prognostically.
5. Coping skills. Those patients with personality traits including strong resilience tend to do better in the long term.
6. Adherence to treatment. Those patients with better adherence to recommended treatments are likely to have significantly better outcomes.
7. Personal factors such as coping skills, personality traits, spirituality, healthy lifestyle behaviors, and attitudes toward help-seeking can all influence outcomes in the treatment of PTSD.

Take-Home Points

- The pharmacologic treatment of PTSD attempts to alleviate the symptoms associated with the condition including anxiety, depression, and sleep disturbances. SSRIs are first-line medications for PTSD. SNRIs such as venlafaxine are also effective, especially in instances where there has been a suboptimal response to SSRIs.
- Follow-up for those with PTSD should involve regular visits with a provider to assess response to treatment. Rating scales such as the PTSD Checklist 5 can be quite helpful in objectively assessing the severity and nature of PTSD symptoms over time.
- There are quite a few options for nonpharmacologic therapy in older adults. Outcomes are best in those who participate in both pharmacologic and nonpharmacologic treatments. Some of the best outcomes are seen with CBT combined with pharmacotherapy.
- The prognosis of PTSD varies widely among individuals. Some patients may experience significant improvement or even full remission of symptoms over time.

References

1. Goldstein, R. B., Smith, S. M., Chou, S. P., Saha, T. D., Jung, J., Zhang, H., Pickering, R. P., Ruan, W. J., Huang, B. & Grant, B. F. (2016). The epidemiology of DSM–5 posttraumatic stress disorder in the United States: Results from the National Epidemiologic Survey on Alcohol and Related Conditions-III. *Social Psychiatry and Psychiatric Epidemiology*, 51 (8), 1137–1148.

2. Na, P. J., Schnurr, P. P., & Pietrzak, R. H. (2023). Mental health of U.S. combat veterans by war era: Results from the National Health and Resilience in Veterans Study. *Journal of Psychiatric Research*, 158, 36–40. https://doi.org/10.1016/j.jpsychires.2022.12.019

3. Sherin, J. E., & Nemeroff, C. B. (2011). Post-traumatic stress disorder: The neurobiological impact of psychological trauma. *Dialogues in Clinical Neuroscience*, 13 (3), 263–278. DOI: 10.31887/DCNS.2011.13.2/jsherin

4. Albucher, R. C., & Liberzon, I. (2002). Psychopharmacological treatment in PTSD: A critical review. *Journal of Psychiatric Research*, 36 (6), 355–367.

5. Brooks, M., Graham-Kevan, N., Robinson, S., & Lowe, M. (2019). Trauma characteristics and post-traumatic growth: The mediating role of avoidance coping, intrusive thoughts, and social support. *Psychological Trauma: Theory, Research, Practice, and Policy*, 11 (2), 232.

6. American Psychiatric Association. (2022). *Diagnostic and Statistical Manual of Mental Disorders*. 5th ed. text rev. (American Psychiatric Publishing.)

7. Pless Kaiser, A., Cook, J. M., Glick, D. M., & Moye, J. (2019). Post-traumatic stress disorder in older adults: A conceptual review. *Clinical Gerontologist*, 42 (4), 359–376.

8. Schnyder, U., Ehlers, A., Elbert, T., Foa, E. B., Gersons, B. P., Resick, P. A., & Cloitre, M. (2015). Psychotherapies for PTSD: What do they have in common? *European Journal of Psychotraumatology*, 6 (1), 28186.

9. Weathers, F. W., Litz, B. T., Keane, T. M., Palmieri, P. A., Marx, B. P., & Schnurr, P. P. (2013). PTSD Checklist for DSM-5 (PCL-5). Scale available from the National Center for PTSD at www.ptsd.va.gov/professional/assessment/adult-sr/ptsd-checklist.asp

10. Simon, R. I. (1999). Chronic post-traumatic stress disorder: A review and checklist of factors influencing prognosis. *Harvard Review of Psychiatry*, 6 (6), 304–312.

Further Reading

Lee, H., Lee, Y., Hong, Y., Lee, C., Park, W., Lee, R., & Oh, S. (2022). Neuroinflammation in post-traumatic stress disorder. *Biomedicines*, 10 (5). https://doi.org/10.3390/biomedicines10050953

Roberts, N. P., Kitchiner, N. J., Kenardy, J., Robertson, L., Lewis, C., & Bisson, J. I. (2018). Multiple session early psychological interventions for the prevention of post-traumatic stress disorder. *The Cochrane Database of Systematic Reviews*, 2019 (8). https://doi.org/10.1002/14651858 .CD006869.pub3

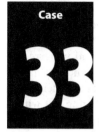

Case

33

"I Used to Do a Bit of Everything"
Substance Use Disorders

Ms. A was a 66-year-old female who was brought to her physician in the geriatric psychiatry clinic by her caseworker to initiate care and for evaluation of "episodes". Ms. A was living on her own in a federally subsidized low-income senior apartment building. Her caseworker provided support to her and others in her building. She had Medicaid-funded chore worker support in the home for two hours per day, five days a week. Ms. A had not driven in some years.

Ms. A was not very forthcoming with any psychiatric history. She said she was doing "fine" and just wanted to be left alone. Her caseworker informed the psychiatrist that Ms. A had not been doing very well in recent months and there was talk of her moving into a long-term care facility due to concerns about appropriateness of her being by herself. Ms. A had three emergency room visits in the previous four months, each after falls and altered mental status/dehydration. A typical scenario would be the chore worker finding Ms. A on the floor in her apartment, groggy and confused. Emergency medical services would be called and the patient taken to the emergency room to be treated as an inpatient for a day or two for dehydration or UTI.

Ms. A did not have much to add to her caseworker's concerns other than to say that she dreaded moving out of her apartment and did not see any reason to go to a nursing home. When asked about her mood she stated that it was generally good but did admit to some anxiety at times. Her PHQ-9 score was nine, indicating mild depression symptoms, and her GAD–7 score was ten, indicating fairly mild anxiety. Her SLUMS exam score was 24/30, indicating mild cognitive impairment. When Ms. A was asked what the psychiatrist could do for her that might help her Ms. A replied, "Tell her [caseworker] I can stay in my apartment."

Ms. A's only known psychiatric diagnosis was mild anxiety and depression for which she took sertraline 100 mg as prescribed by her PCP. Her medical comorbidities included hypothyroidism and hypertension. She did smoke cigarettes and had a history of drug use. "I used to do a bit of everything," she said and admitted to a history of abusing alcohol, prescription pills, and methamphetamine mostly.

Her only living relative was a daughter who was serving time in prison for drug-related charges and she had never been married. She lived on disability from the age of 46 and stated her disability was related to "a bad neck that really doesn't bother me anymore". She had not graduated from high school. Before her approval for disability, she had worked for some years in jobs such as patient care technician, waitress, and convenience store attendant.

The psychiatrist probed Ms. A about her tendency to be hospitalized after being found on the floor of her apartment, as well as being found on the floor in the stairwell of her apartment building. The clinician told Ms. A that his goal was to help her stay as independent as possible and try to assess the appropriateness of her staying in an independent apartment.

When asked about her social life, Ms. A said she had few friends and preferred to keep to herself. She had liked one or two of her chore workers in the past and considered them to be the closest thing to friends that she had in the last several years. When asked about hobbies she admitted to enjoying television and occasionally hanging out with a new friend she had met in the neighborhood. As the interview progressed Ms. A admitted she was smoking crack cocaine in the parking lot of her apartment. Her caseworker appeared shocked and said, "You told me you didn't do that anymore!" to which Ms. A replied, "I don't . . . only when I can afford it."

As the history fleshed out it seemed that Ms. A was smoking crack cocaine in the parking lot with a local dealer who would then help her back into the building. This was happening once or twice per month as Ms. A informed the clinician that it cost her thirty dollars and she was only able to afford that kind of expense once or twice a month at most. If it were not for the cost, Ms. A stated she would use crack every day as it gave her a rush of euphoria and "makes me forget about things".

The psychiatrist and Ms. A's caseworker emphasized to Ms. A that her crack cocaine use was likely the cause of her "episodes" that required hospitalization and that her continued use would likely jeopardize her ability to stay in the senior living apartment. Ms. A refused to admit the crack use was a problem but did agree that she would try not to use it so that she could stay in her apartment and avoid having to live in a nursing home.

On her follow-up visit two months later, Ms. A was relatively unchanged. She had another hospital admission where she presented with dehydration, at which time the emergency room confirmed her urine was positive for cocaine. The caseworker worked to find Ms. A a bed in a skilled nursing facility and, at a subsequent three-month follow-up visit, Ms. A was brought to see her psychiatrist from such a facility where she had been admitted for long-term care. She was doing well medically and had not had any hospital visits. She was quite bitter about being in the long-term care facility but admitted that some of the people were nice. She missed the freedom of being in her apartment.

Teaching Points

As with younger adults, substance abuse among older adults is an increasing burden on the healthcare system. Despite studies showing the increasing prevalence of substance use disorders (SUD) in older adults, they remain underestimated, underdiagnosed, and undertreated in this population. Identification of substance use problems is thought to be more difficult as secondary signs of drug use such as job loss, relationship problems, or legal issues may be lacking. Physical and cognitive declines thought secondary to drug use can be easily misattributed to age-related cognitive or medical conditions. Primary care providers and specialists alike may be less likely to probe into the possibilities of drug use due to a lack of time or a misperception that illicit substance use is more of an issue for younger patients [1]. Other misconceptions now questioned are that most illicit drug use initiation occurs before the age of 30 and rarely occurs after. This may lead to physicians screening less for these conditions in older adults.

Recent studies have indicated that a growing proportion of hospitalizations due to cocaine use are in older adults. In one study in 2006, 21.2% of admissions due to cocaine use were in those over 50 years of age. In contrast, in 2018 43.27% of admissions due to cocaine use were in those over 50 [2].

The health consequences of cocaine use are well documented in the general population, and it is speculated that these effects are likely exacerbated in older adults. Some of the consequences of cocaine use include cardiovascular complications such as left ventricular hypertrophy, ischemic heart disease, aortic or cerebrovascular atherosclerosis, and coronary vasospasm. Other well-known complications of cocaine use include stroke, intracerebral hemorrhage, aneurysm rupture, and psychiatric complications [3].

Treatment of cocaine use disorder in older adults depends on the treatment setting. Those in long-term care may do better in this controlled setting as they will likely have more limited access to controlled substances. Those who are cognitively able may benefit from group or individual psychotherapy to address both triggers and the psychological consequences of substance abuse. Pharmacologic treatment options for cocaine use disorder are limited to treatments that focus on the frequent psychiatric comorbidities that may accompany long-term drug use.

Alcohol use disorder is the most frequent substance use disorder in older adults. A large survey by the Substance Abuse and Mental Health Services Administration in 2019 estimated that 10.7% of adults over the age of 65 engaged in binge alcohol use (defined as more than five drinks on an occasion) and 2.8% had engaged in past-month heavy alcohol use (defined as binge drinking five or more times in the past month) [4]. Older adults are more susceptible to the toxic effects of alcohol due to factors such as increased permeability of the blood–brain barrier, decreased liver metabolism, and increased adiposity/decreased total body water which results in a higher blood alcohol level for a given alcohol intake [5]. Excessive alcohol use in older adults is known to be associated with an increased risk of cognitive dysfunction and MNCDs [6]. Treatment strategies for alcohol use disorder, including psychotherapy and pharmacotherapy, are safe and effective in older adults.

Cannabis use has increased in younger and older adults alike in recent years. This is likely due to the increased availability, decriminalization, and destigmatization of cannabis use. The Substance Abuse and Mental Health Services Administration found that past-year cannabis use increased from 3.3% to 6.0% from 2016 to 2020 [4]. The use of cannabis is thought to be relatively benign by many patients and practitioners but there are some unique risks of cannabis use in older adults that are worth mentioning. Cannabis use has been shown to pose a greater fall risk in older adults compared to younger adults [7]. Older adult cannabis users have also been shown to have a higher risk of past-year MDDs. Those with cannabis use disorder as defined in the DSM–5–TR may experience symptoms familiar to other SUDs such as increased tolerance over time, potential for withdrawal symptoms, and social, professional, or relationship impairment.

The opioid epidemic has impacted both younger and older people. The number of adults over the age of 55 who have entered opioid treatment has tripled from 2007 to 2017 [8]. Opioid use disorder may be influenced by several factors more common in older adults. Older adults are more likely to suffer from chronic pain requiring long-term opiate medication use and are more likely to suffer the effects of loneliness with associated depression and anxiety. Older adults are also more likely to experience major stressful life changes such as retirement, the loss of a spouse, or social isolation that can contribute to increased substance use. Interventions for opioid use disorders in older adults can be similar to treatment in younger adults and can include medication-assisted treatment (buprenorphine), psychotherapy, support groups, alternative pain management plans, and increased social support to help with loneliness and social isolation.

The use of methamphetamines has increased alongside that of the use of other illicit substances in recent years. Some parts of the country have experienced epidemic levels of methamphetamine abuse, with contributing factors including wide availability due to low cost and ease of manufacture. Methamphetamines are often used along with other illicit substances to enhance the euphoric effects or mitigate the side effects of other substances. They are highly addictive and medication treatment options are limited. Rates of use are particularly high in lower socioeconomic groups who may have more limited access to medical treatment. Besides addiction, chronic methamphetamine use can lead to multiple health consequences including cognitive impairment, increased risk of mood disorders, dental decay, malnutrition, and social and legal problems. The epidemic of methamphetamine use in some areas of the country has not spared older adults and a high index of suspicion should be maintained when evaluating older adults with neuropsychiatric symptoms [9].

Take-Home Points

- The potential of SUDs in older adults is often overlooked in a general health assessment. Substance use disorders have a high comorbidity with other psychiatric disorders.
- Cannabis use is increasing in all age groups, including older adults. Be aware that older adults may be using cannabis to self-medicate psychiatric conditions such as anxiety and depression or to treat chronic pain despite limited evidence for long-term improvement.
- Psychological changes in older adults make them more susceptible to the negative effects of alcohol use. With the proper support and resources, older adults with alcohol use disorder can live a healthier, happier life free from alcohol.
- Older adults may be at risk of opiate use disorder due to chronic pain issues, multiple medical comorbidities, and psychiatric comorbidities. Treatment options for opioid use disorder, such as medications, outpatient treatment programs, and psychosocial supports are often as effective in older adults as in younger patients.

References

1. Yarnell, S. C. (2015). Cocaine abuse in later life: A case series and review of the literature. *The Primary Care Companion for CNS Disorders*, 17 (2). https://doi.org/10.4088/PCC.14r01727

2. Gangu, K., Bobba, A., Basida, S. D., Avula, S., Chela, H., & Singh, S. (2022). Trends of cocaine use and manifestations in hospitalized patients: A cross-sectional study. *Cureus*. 14 (2), e22090. doi: 10.7759/cureus.22090. PMID: 35165645; PMCID: PMC8830384.

3. Yarnell, S., Li, L., MacGrory, B., Trevisan, L., & Kirwin, P. (2020). Substance use disorders in later life: A review and synthesis of the literature of an emerging public health concern. *The American Journal of Geriatric Psychiatry*, 28 (2), 226–236.

4. Substance Abuse and Mental Health Services Administration. National Survey on Drug Use and Health. 2017–2020. www.samhsa.gov/data/data-we-collect/nsduh-national-survey-drug-use-and-health. Access June 2022.

5. Lin, J., Arnovitz, M., Kotbi, N., & Francois, D. (2023). Substance use disorders in the geriatric population: A review and synthesis of the literature of

a growing problem in a growing population. *Current Treatment Options in Psychiatry*, 1–20. www.ncbi.nlm.nih.gov/pmc/articles/PMC10241125/

6. Koch, M., Fitzpatrick, A. L., Rapp, S. R., Nahin, R. L., Williamson, J. D., Lopez, O. L., DeKosky, S. T., Kuller, L. H., Mackey, R. H., Mukamal, K. L., Jensen, M. K., & Sink, K. M. (2019). Alcohol consumption and risk of dementia and cognitive decline among older adults with or without mild cognitive impairment. *JAMA Network Open*, 2, e1910319. doi: 10.1001/jamanetworkopen.2019.10319.

7. Workman, C. D., Fietsam, A. C., Sosnoff, J., & Rudroff, T. (2021). Increased likelihood of falling in older cannabis users vs. non-users. *Brain Sciences*, 11 (2), 134.

8. Lynch, A., Arndt, S., & Acion, L. (2021). Late- and typical-onset heroin use among older adults seeking treatment for opioid use disorder. *The American Journal of Geriatric Psychiatry*, 29, 417–425.

9. Han, B., Compton, W. M., Jones, C. M., Einstein, E. B., & Volkow, N. D. (2021). Methamphetamine use, methamphetamine use disorder, and associated overdose deaths among US adults. *JAMA Psychiatry*, 78 (12), 1329–1342. doi: 10.1001/jamapsychiatry.2021.2588. PMID: 34550301; PMCID: PMC8459304.

Case

34

"No One Here Is on My Level"
Narcissistic Personality Disorder

Ms. G was an 82-year-old female. She had recently moved into long-term care after a stay in rehab following a fall at home and a left hip fracture. She was now confined to a wheelchair and needed assistance with many ADLs such as showering, dressing, toileting, and incontinence care. She was cognitively intact and could direct her care but had a difficult time adjusting to her new home in long-term care. In the short time she had been a resident at the facility she had shown a tendency toward not getting along with others, including care staff. Some staff had gone as far as to refuse to work an assigned shift if they knew it would involve caring for Ms. G. She was described as demanding, hypercritical, demeaning to others, and snobbish. Staff asked her provider to evaluate her for a potential untreated psychiatric condition that could be making it difficult for Ms. G to fit in at the facility.

On the initial visit with Ms. G, she was found in her room dressed in a fluffy bathrobe, a large string of pearls, large earrings, and rings on every finger of a costume jewelry style. The walls of her room were covered with photos of herself, and several of were of the "glamour shot" style that was popular in the mid-1990s. Ms. G's greeting was warm and almost before introductions were finished, she delved into a 30-minute monologue describing the accomplishments of her life and her associations with many important people in the community. Attempts to interrupt Ms. G by the provider were greeted with acidic irritation. The provider listened quietly for some time, largely out of fascination for the outlandishness of the narrative that unfolded. Ms. G described a life that was full of meaningful and close relationships with many successful people in all areas including politics, the arts, and business. She described her talents in business, the arts, and later-life philanthropic ventures in great detail.

When asked about her family, Ms. G admitted to having three children who she described as "wildly successful". She had married three times and divorced three times. When asked if the provider could speak with one of her children, Ms. G stated that they were all "terribly busy" and would likely not have time to speak with a doctor. When asked about the facility and her adjustment to it she had little good to say. She described the perceived incompetencies of the staff, the inedible nature of the food, and the drab decor. She mentioned she was at the facility only long enough for her to find accommodations she was more accustomed to. When asked about activities she enjoyed she mentioned that she found none of the activities enjoyable as none of the other residents were "on my level".

Ms. G was on no psychiatric medications. She stated she had no history of mental health issues and had never been hospitalized for mental health reasons. She had no history of drug or alcohol abuse but admitted that she needed a good martini every evening to "stay sane" and was furious that there was not a bartender in the facility who could accommodate her.

Ms. G's SLUMS score was 26. She showed no outward signs of clear cognitive impairment although she was at times hard to keep on topic.

The clinician called Ms. G's youngest daughter who was listed as her power of attorney. The daughter was quite willing to discuss her mother's psychiatric history and stated that Ms. G had been a "difficult woman" her entire life. Her life was dotted with troubled relationships; she had been married three times and each divorce was non-amicable. She tended to alienate any new friends she would make after only a short time. During recent years she began needing more and more help at home and her daughter had personally arranged for a total of eight different caregivers in a year who each quit – usually after a matter of days or weeks due to her mother's demanding nature and queen-like attitude. Ms. G's daughter encouraged the provider to believe less than half of what Ms. G said as she greatly exaggerated her achievements and the perceived incompetencies of others. Ms. G was moved into the nursing home as her family could find no others to care for her at home.

After a long conversation with the daughter and conversations with care staff at the facility the long-term care provider felt that Ms. G met no criteria for any clinical mood or anxiety disorders. She did not appear to have more than mild cognitive dysfunction and had no signs of any psychosis. The pattern of current and past relationship dysfunction suggested a diagnosis of narcissistic personality disorder. Staff were informed of the provider's opinion on the patient's mental health diagnosis and gave them strategies to better deal with the challenging behaviors of Ms. G. The provider also recommended regular psychotherapy to focus on potential ways that she could improve her interactions with others and make for a more pleasurable living situation for her and a better work environment for those who helped care for her.

Teaching Points

Personality traits are patterns of thoughts, feelings, and behaviors that remain relatively stable over a person's life and strongly influence how they interact with and perceive the world. These traits can be adaptive and lead to improved psychosocial function or be maladaptive and lead to impairment in psychosocial function. When personality traits come together in particular maladaptive patterns and lead to dysfunction and significant impairment in personal, family, social, educational, occupational, or other important areas of functioning they can be classified as a personality disorder. Personality disorders are relatively common. Estimates are that about 12% of the general population, 25% of primary care patients, and at least 50% of psychiatric outpatients meet the criteria for a personality disorder [1].

Those with personality disorders usually show signs of personality traits and behavioral patterns in adolescence that can later solidify into a recognized personality disorder in late adolescence or early adulthood.

The DSM–5 lists ten distinct personality disorders, which can be classified into three subgroups. Cluster A personality disorders are characterized by traits and behaviors that are often seen as odd or eccentric and these patients may have difficulty with social relationships due to their unusual behaviors and thought patterns. Cluster A personality disorders include paranoid personality disorder, schizoid personality disorder, and

Personality Disorder Clusters

Cluster A disorders

Odd, eccentric behaviors.

Paranoid, Schizoid, Schizotypal.

Cluster B disorders

Dramatic, emotional, impulsive behaviors.

Antisocial, Borderline, Histrionic, and
Narcissistic

Cluster C disorders

Anxious, worried behaviors.

Avoidant, Dependent, Obsessive-
compulsive.

Figure 34.1 The three clusters of personality disorders.

schizotypal personality disorder. Cluster B personality disorders are marked by behaviors that are theatrical, impulsive, self-destructive, and emotionally intense. These behaviors can lead to interactions with others that are often perplexing or difficult to understand. Cluster C personality disorders are characterized by anxious and fearful behaviors. Individuals with these disorders tend to experience high levels of worry, anxiety, and apprehension. The three personality disorders in Cluster C are avoidant personality disorder, dependent personality disorder, and obsessive–compulsive personality disorder (Figure 34.1). A brief description of the ten recognized personality disorders is shown in Table 34.1 [2].

The causes of personality disorders are complex and involve an interplay between genetic factors, environmental factors, and psychological factors. Personality disorders develop over time and are likely influenced by a variety of environmental factors. Genetic heritability of personality disorders is estimated to be anywhere from 0.2 to 0.4 (1.0 being 100% heritable) depending on the disorder [3], but some of these studies are older and findings have been difficult to repeat. These same studies have suggested environmental contribution to be from 0.62 to 0.79, depending on the disorder.

Early childhood experiences are thought to play a significant role in the potential to develop personality disorders later in life. Issues including abuse, neglect, inconsistent parenting, and disruptions in attachment can all negatively impact personality development. Chronic stress in childhood can also lead to maladaptive personality traits.

Personality disorders can vary in their outcomes. Several personality disorders are more likely to create pervasive life problems than others. Cluster B personality disorders are more likely to be the most disruptive to an individual's success in life and relationships.

A better knowledge of personality disorders can help the clinician in several ways. Identification may help a provider refer a patient to the appropriate mental health professional promptly. Psychotherapy can assist patients in better self-awareness of their thoughts, feelings, and behaviors that may be contributing to personal and interpersonal difficulties. Therapy can help patients develop coping skills to manage emotions, stress, and interpersonal conflicts that may trigger maladaptive behaviors. Therapists can assist

Table 34.1 Brief descriptions of the ten personality disorders.

Antisocial	Characterized by a widespread disregard for and violation of the rights of others
Avoidant	Individuals show inhibited behaviors and feelings of inadequacy in interpersonal interactions; there is hypersensitivity to negative evaluation
Borderline	Patients show instability in interpersonal interactions, sense of self, and affect; there is marked impulsivity
Dependent	Demonstrate a pervasive need to be cared for; often depend on and submit to the control of others
Histrionic	Individuals show excessive emotionality and a tendency toward attention-seeking
Narcissistic	Characterized by grandiosity, need for admiration, and lack of empathy
Obsessive–Compulsive	There is a preoccupation with orderliness, perfection, morality, and control
Paranoid	Characterized by distrust and suspiciousness of others
Schizoid	Patients demonstrate detachment from social relationships; there is a restricted range of emotional expression in interpersonal interactions
Schizotypal	Individuals have patterns of odd, eccentric behavior or thinking; perceptual distortions; there is discomfort with interpersonal interactions

patients in developing better relationship skills such as communication and boundary setting.

A provider's understanding of personality disorders can assist in communication issues that may arise with these patients and can improve treatment planning. Understanding can also enhance the therapeutic alliance that can be challenging to establish and maintain with these patients. Providers will also often be asked to provide support and advice to caregivers and families of these patients. Personality disorders can sometimes be mistaken for other psychiatric conditions. Familiarity with personality disorders can avoid misdiagnosis and help a provider be aware of the high likelihood of psychiatric comorbidity.

Take-Home Points

- Personality traits are patterns of thoughts, feelings, and behaviors that remain relatively stable over a person's life and strongly influence how people interact with and perceive the world.
- Personality disorders are personality traits that cluster in recognizable patterns and produce dysfunction in multiple areas of life.
- Personality disorders do not respond well to pharmacologic interventions but are often accompanied by other psychiatric comorbidities that can be treated medically.
- Recognizing personality disorders can help a provider avoid misdiagnosing psychiatric conditions, anticipate future care challenges, and better counsel family and caregivers.

References

1. Bach, B., & First, M. B. (2018). Application of the ICD-11 classification of personality disorders. *BMC Psychiatry*, 18.

2. American Psychiatric Association. (2022). *Diagnostic and Statistical Manual of Mental Disorders*. 5th ed. text rev. (American Psychiatric Association.)

3. Kendler, K. S., Aggen, S. H., Czajkowski, N., Røysamb, E., Tambs, K., Torgersen, S., Neale, M. C., & Reichborn-Kjennerud, T. (2008). The structure of genetic and environmental risk factors for DSM-IV personality disorders: A multivariate twin study. *Archives of General Psychiatry*, 65 (12), 1438. https://doi.org/10.1001/archpsyc.65.12.1438

Further Reading

Brudey, C. (2021). Personality disorders in older age. *Focus: Journal of Life Long Learning in Psychiatry*, 19 (3), 303–307. https://doi.org/10.1176/appi.focus .20210007

Ekselius, L. (2018). Personality disorder: A disease in disguise. *Upsala Journal of Medical Sciences*, 123 (4), 194–204. https://doi.org/10.1080/03009734.2018 .1526235

Green, A., MacLean, R., & Charles, K. (2022). Female narcissism: Assessment, aetiology, and behavioural manifestations. *Psychological Reports*, 125 (6), 2833–2864. https://doi.org/10.1177/ 00332941211027322

Hutsebaut, J., Willemsen, E., Bachrach, N., & Van, R. (2020). Improving access to and effectiveness of mental health care for personality disorders: The guideline-informed treatment for personality disorders (GIT-PD) initiative in the Netherlands. *Borderline Personality Disorder and Emotion Dysregulation*, 7 (16).

Veenstra, M. S., Bouman, R., & Oude Voshaar, R. C. (2022). Impact of personality functioning and pathological traits on mental wellbeing of older patients with personality disorders. *BMC Psychiatry*, 22 (214).

Case

35

"I Cannot Wait to Get out of This Miserable Place"

Borderline Personality Disorder

Ms. L was a 64-year-old woman admitted to a nursing home for rehabilitation after a prolonged hospital stay (three months) for nephrectomy and post-nephrectomy complications (infection, bleeding, and delirium with agitation). The long-term care provider was asked to help manage the resident's hostile and aggressive behavior toward staff. The staff expressed anger and resentment at having to provide personal care for Ms. L because of her persistent name-calling, yelling at the staff, and demeaning them almost daily. Some staff members had started to call in sick if they found out that they had to care for Ms. L, and some refused to care for her.

The provider found Ms. L to be an intelligent person who had relatively intact cognitive function (SLUMS score 26) and was quick to take offense but also willing to accept help from "competent" professionals. She repeatedly expressed, "I cannot wait to get out of this miserable place."

Ms. L was taking sertraline, 100 mg daily, for MDD. After interviewing Ms. L, the provider met with the staff to explain that, in his opinion, Ms. L had been experiencing moderate to severe depression (MDD) (PHQ–9 score was 20) with an underlying long-standing personality disorder. Ms. L had confided in the provider that she had been severely physically and emotionally abused as a child and had experienced three "horrible" marriages. She had expressed to the provider that she "hated everyone," liked animals more than people, had lots of pets that she took care of, and helped the Humane Society in caring for sick pets.

The provider provided emotional support to the staff, validated their feelings related to dealing with Ms. L's negative behaviors, discussed specific therapeutic ways the staff could respond to these negative behaviors, and explained the treatment plan (increase in antidepressants and individual psychotherapy). The provider (with Ms. L's permission) shared minor details about her abusive childhood and spousal relationships and the good volunteer work she was doing with the Humane Society. This helped the staff feel supported, improved their compassion for Ms. L, and enabled them to be more patient with her so that treatment could be given time to help.

The long-term care provider increased the dosage of sertraline from 100 to 150 mg and encouraged the staff to tell Ms. L that she was being disrespectful when she used foul language or yelled at them. Staff was also encouraged to respond calmly (without resentment) and appreciatively when Ms. L talked respectfully. The provider gently helped Ms. L understand that her hostile behavior put her at a much higher risk of prolonged stay in the nursing home because the staff would be less likely to meet her needs diligently or promptly. Ms. L agreed to go to an outpatient clinic once a week for counseling with a social worker. Over the next few weeks, the frequency and intensity of hostile comments by Ms. L decreased modestly, the staff was able to meet more of her needs, and Ms. L made significant progress in physical therapy.

Teaching Points

Depressive disorders are common among residents who have personality disorders and are often underrecognized and undertreated. A resident who has a personality disorder also generates strong negative feelings in others that may result in staff being less likely to meet the resident's needs. Interventions should be designed with the intention of making at least modest changes in behavior possible to achieve a desired result. Interventions may include pharmacotherapy for comorbid mood or anxiety disorder, staff education, or counseling for the patient. Behavior goals may include less name-calling by the resident toward staff, resulting in an increased likelihood that staff will be able to meet the resident's needs.

Psychotherapy is useful for residents who have personality disorders and relatively intact cognitive function. Optimization of treatment of comorbid mental disorder (MDD in this situation) and specific guidance for staff of therapeutic ways to respond to negative behaviors are also crucial for a successful outcome.

Borderline personality disorder (BPD) is a complex mental health condition. Those with the condition have unstable moods, a history of difficulty functioning in relationships, and a dysfunctional self-image. Patients with BPD have emotional dysregulation that can lead to impulsive behaviors, self-harm, and fear of abandonment. They also struggle with chronic feelings of emptiness and loneliness. Caring for those with BPD can be particularly challenging. Knowledge of the condition by healthcare professionals can provide insight into patients suffering from BPD and help providers have more compassionate and therapeutic interactions with them.

The prevalence of BPD is estimated to be between 1 and 6% [1]. Those with diagnosed BPD are more likely to be female (75%) than male (25%) [2]. The symptoms are usually recognized first in late adolescence or early adulthood, but it is also possible to be diagnosed in late adulthood. Those with BPD use a disproportionately high amount of psychiatric services and are more likely to have a history of multiple psychiatric hospital admissions [3]. Studies also show that those with BPD are more likely to have comorbid mood disorders.

The causes of BPD are complex. As with many mental health conditions, there is an interplay between genetics and environmental factors. Although no specific gene or genes have been identified, it is known that BPD tends to run in families. Individuals with BPD have been shown to have a higher incidence of structural and functional abnormalities of regions of the brain involved in emotional regulation and impulse control. Those who have had childhood trauma, abuse, or neglect are more likely to develop BPD.

Those with BPD have significant challenges in life that can lead to poor psychosocial outcomes. Interpersonal relationships can often be intense and dysfunctional and demonstrate frequent conflicts. Those with BPD may have a hard time maintaining long-term relationships. Emotional dysregulation can lead to rapid and intense mood swings, which often makes functioning in work environments very difficult. Impulsivity can lead to issues such as reckless spending, risky sexual behaviors, and substance abuse. Those with BPD are less likely to achieve educational goals, more likely to have legal issues, and

Box 35.1 DSM–5–TR criteria for the diagnosis of BPD

A pervasive pattern of instability of interpersonal relationships, self-image, and affects, and marked impulsivity, beginning in early adulthood and present in a variety of contexts, as indicated by five (or more) of the following:

1. Frantic efforts to avoid real or imagined abandonment. (Note: Do not include suicidal or self-mutilating behavior covered in Criterion 5.)
2. A pattern of unstable and intense interpersonal relationships characterized by alternating between extremes of idealization and devaluation.
3. Identity disturbance: Markedly and persistently unstable self-image or sense of self.
4. Impulsivity in at least two areas that are potentially self-damaging (e.g. spending, sex, substance abuse, reckless driving, binge eating). (Note: Do not include suicidal or self-mutilating behavior covered in Criterion 5.)
5. Recurrent suicidal behavior, gestures or threats, or self-mutilating behavior.
6. Affective instability due to a marked reactivity of mood (e.g. intense episodic dysphoria, irritability, or anxiety usually lasting a few hours and only rarely more than a few days).
7. Chronic feelings of emptiness.
8. Inappropriate, intense anger or difficulty controlling anger (e.g. frequent displays of temper, constant anger, recurrent physical fights).
9. Transient, stress-related paranoid ideation or severe dissociative symptoms.

have less access to consistent treatment. Those with BPD are also at much higher risk of suicide than the general population [4].

The diagnosis of BPD is usually made by a psychiatrist, psychologist, or other mental health professional. The DSM–5–R criteria for the diagnosis of BPD are listed in Box 35.1 [2].

The treatment of BPD is largely through long-term psychological therapy and the gold standard approach is dialectical behavior therapy (DBT). This therapy focuses on optimizing emotional regulation, distress tolerance, interpersonal effectiveness, and mindfulness skills. Other therapies that have been used with success are CBT, schema-focused therapy, and supportive psychotherapy, among others. There is no specific medication approved for the treatment of BPD but those who have it often have comorbid anxiety or depression that require pharmacologic interventions. Research has suggested that approximately half of people who receive psychotherapy do not respond to the treatment independent of psychotherapy modality or length of treatment [5]. Issues with access to appropriately trained therapists are also widespread.

There are currently no FDA-approved medications for the treatment of BPD. Off-label use of medications is common. A list of medication classes sometimes used to treat BPD-associated symptoms is shown in Box 35.2 [6].

Interactions between healthcare providers and those with BPD can be challenging and patients in the long-term care setting are at risk of poor outcomes as they are often perceived as unpleasant and demanding. Setting boundaries is important when dealing with these patients. Regular empathetic validation of feelings by the provider can strengthen the therapeutic relationship between those with BPD and their providers.

The prognosis for borderline personality is generally mixed. Thankfully, a majority of patients with BPD have a decline in symptoms during adulthood. It is estimated that up

Box 35.2 Pharmacologic treatments for BPD-associated symptoms

1. Anticonvulsants. These can target affective dysregulation such as mood lability, angry outbursts, suicidal thoughts and behavior, and impulse behavioral dyscontrol.
2. Antidepressants. These agents can be used to target affective dysregulation associated with BPD such as depression, anxiety, mood lability, suicidal thoughts and behaviors.
3. Antipsychotics. Have been used for severe affective dysregulation in the setting of BPD.
4. Benzodiazepines. Can be helpful in the treatment of acute anxiety, agitation, and impulsiveness.
5. Sedative–hypnotic medications. These can help address comorbid sleep disorders associated with BPD.
6. Melatonin. Used with BPD-related sleep disturbances.

to 85% of patients with BPD reach a diagnostic remission within ten years of diagnosis. Some residual symptoms may persist, leading to lifelong challenges. These may include fear of abandonment, impulsivity, intense anger issues, and an unstable self-image that can lead to lifelong social and occupational challenges [7]. Those with persistent BPD do have a higher risk of death from suicide and medical comorbidities. The clinical course is often marked by multiple suicidal attempts and up to 10% of those with BPD will die by suicide. Common practice is still to admit those patients who make suicidal threats despite the lack of evidence that hospitalization reduces the risk of actual suicide. There is also no evidence that pharmacologic interventions reduce the risk of suicide in BPD patients although they are effective in reducing the symptoms of comorbid mood or anxiety symptoms [8].

The nature of BPD is generally chronic and persistent dysfunction, but the level of dysfunction may actually decline with age. It is thought that age and maturity may mellow the symptoms of the condition over the course of a lifetime. Cumulative treatment and support can have a slow, steady, and positive effect in helping those with BPD to manage their symptoms more effectively. The stable environment that a supportive long-term care setting can provide may also have a positive impact on the outcomes of older adults with BPD.

Therapeutic relationships between providers and those with BPD can be challenging. A better understanding of the etiologic factors, treatment interventions, and comorbidities can foster more empathy and understanding of these patients and allow the provider to guide the treatment team in the long-term care setting more effectively.

Take-Home Points

- Borderline personality disorder is a complex mental health condition. Those with the condition have unstable moods, a history of difficulty functioning in relationships, and a dysfunctional self-image. Patients with BPD have emotional dysregulation that can lead to impulsive behaviors, self-harm, and fear of abandonment.
- The treatment of BPD is largely through long-term psychological therapy and the gold standard approach is DBT. This therapy focuses on optimizing emotional regulation, distress tolerance, interpersonal effectiveness, and mindfulness skills.
- Those with BPD have significant challenges in life that can lead to poor psychosocial outcomes. Interpersonal relationships can often be intense and dysfunctional and demonstrate frequent

conflicts. Emotional dysregulation can lead to rapid and intense mood swings. Impulsivity can lead to issues such as reckless spending, risky sexual behaviors, and substance abuse.

— The nature of BPD is generally chronic and persistent dysfunction, but the level of dysfunction may decline with age. It is thought that age and maturity may mellow the symptoms of the condition over the course of a lifetime. Cumulative treatment and support can have a slow, steady, and positive effect in helping those with BPD to manage their symptoms more effectively.

References

1. Skodol, A., Stein, M., & Hermann, R. (2019). *Borderline Personality Disorder: Epidemiology, Pathogenesis, Clinical Features, Course, Assessment, and Diagnosis.* (Waltham, MA: UpToDate.)

2. American Psychiatric Association, D. S. M. T. F., & American Psychiatric Association. (2013). *Diagnostic and Statistical Manual of Mental Disorders: DSM-5* (Vol. 5, No. 5). (Washington, DC: American Psychiatric Association.) p. 663.

3. Evans, L. J., Harris, V., Newman, L., & Beck, A. (2017). Rapid and frequent psychiatric readmissions: Associated factors. *International Journal of Psychiatry in Clinical Practice*, 21 (4), 271–276.

4. Broadbear, J. H., Dwyer, J., Bugeja, L., & Rao, S. (2020). Coroners' investigations of suicide in Australia: The hidden toll of borderline personality disorder. *Journal of Psychiatric Research*, 129, 241–249.

5. Woodbridge, J., Townsend, M., Reis, S., Singh, S., & Grenyer, B. F. (2022). Non-response to psychotherapy for borderline personality disorder: A systematic review. *The Australian and New Zealand Journal of Psychiatry*, 56 (7), 771–787. https://doi.org/10.1177/00048674211046893

6. Gartlehner, G., Crotty, K., Kennedy, S., Edlund, M. J., Ali, R., Siddiqui, M., & Viswanathan, M. (2021). Pharmacological treatments for borderline personality disorder: A systematic review and meta-analysis. *CNS drugs*, 35 (10), 1053–1067.

7. Niesten, I. J., Karan, E., Franjenburg, F. R., Fitzmaurice, G. M., & Zanarini, M. C. (2016). Description and prediction of the income status of borderline patients over 10 years of prospective follow-up. *Personal Mental Health*, 10 (4), 285–292.

8. Paris, J. (2019). Suicidality in borderline personality disorder. *Medicina (Kaunas)*, 55 (6), 223.

Further Reading

Bozzatello, P., Garbarini, C., Rocca, P., & Bellino, S. (2021). Borderline personality disorder: Risk factors and early detection. *Diagnostics*, 11 (11). https://doi.org/10.3390/diagnostics11112142

Gunderson, J. G., Stout, R. L., McGlashan, T. H., Shea, M. T., Morey, L. C., Grilo, C. M., & Skodol, A. E. (2011). Ten-year course of borderline personality disorder: psychopathology and function from the collaborative longitudinal personality disorders study. *Archives of General Psychiatry*, 68 (8), 827–837.

Soloff, P. H., & Chiappetta, L. (2019). 10-year outcome of suicidal behavior in borderline personality disorder. *Journal of Personality Disorders*, 33 (1), 82–100.

Veenstra, M. S., Bouman, R., & Oude Voshaar, R. C. (2022). Impact of personality functioning and pathological traits on mental wellbeing of older patients with personality disorders. *BMC Psychiatry*, 22.

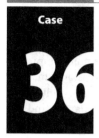

Case

36

"Can I Have a Hug?"
Sexually Inappropriate Behavior

Mrs. M was a 91-year-old female who was a resident of a skilled nursing facility in a rural area served via virtual visits from her geriatric psychiatrist. She had a history of Alzheimer's disease with behavioral disturbances, anxiety, insomnia, peripheral vascular disease, adrenal insufficiency, and osteoporosis. Her cognitive impairment was moderate to severe and she needed assistance with most ADLs. Mrs. M. was described as very sociable and had been nicknamed "The Hostess" by staff as she liked to attend to other residents in the unit and make sure they were comfortable. Sometimes she was confused and perturbed as she felt that she was at home and that the other residents were guests who would not leave, and she expressed fears that she would not be able to cover the cost of the food and entertainment.

She was also described by staff as "a very sexual lady". Her sexual behaviors had become increasingly problematic over the course of weeks to months. Staff noted that Mrs. M had lost her modesty, as demonstrated by often leaving her room without any underwear or pants on. She was also noted to often be masturbating in common areas. When attempts were made to redirect her to a more appropriate and private place she would become angry and also verbally and physically aggressive to staff or other residents. She had been noted to be more frequently touching male staff and residents and had also been found trying to crawl into bed with other male residents. Staff brought up these behaviors with the patient's family but they found it hard to accept that their mother could be doing these things as she had always been very proper and modest as a younger adult.

The patient's mood was described as mostly pleasant and content much of the time, but she had been having increasing episodes of acting sad, anxious, or restless. During the virtual interview with the patient, she was calm, pleasant, and was appropriately and modestly dressed. She was unable to give any history due to her confusion and was oriented to person only.

Her medication list was relatively short and included a multivitamin daily, hydrocortisone tab 10 mg daily, acetaminophen 650 mg twice daily, quetiapine 25 mg daily, melatonin 20 mg qhs, and hydroxyzine 25 mg twice daily as needed for anxiety.

A medical workup including blood work and urine tests was unrevealing. Her psychiatrist decided to discontinue hydroxyzine due to anticholinergic effects in older adults, her nightly melatonin dose was decreased from 20 to 5 mg, and her quetiapine dose was increased from 25 g daily to 25 mg twice daily in an attempt to help her anxiety and restlessness in the setting of advanced cognitive impairment. She was also started on duloxetine 30 mg daily as her psychiatrist felt that she was showing signs of depression and anxiety with an increase in agitation and restlessness.

At a follow-up appointment four weeks later, nursing staff reported that she was possibly engaging in less sexually inappropriate behaviors than a month prior but the behaviors were still thought to be problematic. Her duloxetine was then increased to 60 mg daily and nursing staff reported that the patient's behaviors were much improved at the subsequent four-week follow-up visit. She was still engaging in occasional masturbation in common areas but was easily redirected to her room. She was generally much less irritable and anxious. It was decided to continue the low-dose quetiapine and the 60 mg daily dose of duloxetine.

Teaching Points

This is an interesting case on several fronts. It brings into focus issues involving sexuality and sexual expression in older adults with cognitive impairment.

Disinhibited behavior is commonly demonstrated in seniors with MNCD. This can be demonstrated by such things as pilfering, swearing, physical aggression, diminished social graces, and unwanted sexual expression. Prevalence of sexually inappropriate behavior (SIB) varies depending on the type of MNCD, but reports have shown rates of 2–25% depending on the setting. Behavioral variant FTD patients likely have the highest prevalence of SIB with estimates ranging from 8% to 18% [1]. Some examples of SIB that can be demonstrated by those with MNCD are listed in Box 36.1.

It is a misconception that all those with MNCD lose the desire for sexual touch and sexual expression as their disease progresses from the mild to more moderate or severe stages of the disease. As with those younger patients unaffected by MNCD, the spectrum of "normal" sexual behavior is wide and undoubtedly influenced by a patient's underlying personality or past sexual experiences. Those with advanced MNCD may even confuse those they encounter in day-to-day life with a spouse or significant other that has passed away.

Sexual expression in those with MNCD therefore should not be universally discouraged, shamed, or medically treated as an aberrant behavior. Sexual expression such as consensual physical touch, holding hands, and kissing can be essential to mental health for those with MNCD who have the desire.

The workup of SIB in long-term care residents starts with a good history, often obtained from caregivers. It is important to assess the context of SIB by answering questions such as (1) what exactly is the behavior being demonstrated? (2) what is the context of the behavior? (3) how often is the behavior occurring? (4) who is being impacted by the behavior? (5) is the sexual behavior greatly out of proportion to other disinhibited behaviors? (Figure 36.1).

Box 36.1 Examples of SIB in older adults with MNCD

1. Inappropriate sexual comments.
2. Inappropriate exposure.
3. Being overly flirtatious, making others uncomfortable.
4. Using sexual language that is different from a person's premorbid personality.
5. Requesting genital care in the absence of need.
6. Reading pornographic material in public areas.
7. Overt sexual acts including groping, grabbing, or public masturbation.

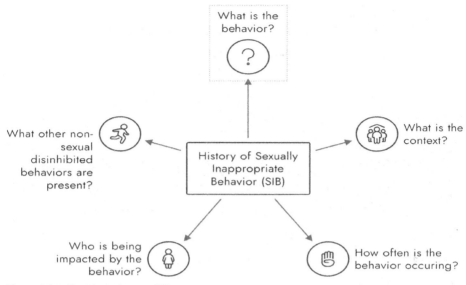

Figure 36.1 Obtaining a history of SIB.

Box 36.2 Medications well known to potentially contribute to SIB.

1. Dopamine agonist agents such as carbidopa/levodopa, pramipexole, and ropinorole.
2. Anticholinergic agents can lead to increased confusion and disinhibited behavior.
3. Bupropion may increase inappropriate sexual behavior through dopaminergic pathways.
4. Benzodiazepines may lead to increased confusion and disinhibited sexual behavior.

Box 36.3 Nonpharmacologic interventions to address SIB

1. Attempt to identify and remove patient-specific triggers of SIB.
2. Give patients more meaningful social activities to address issues of boredom and lack of human interaction that may contribute to SIB.
3. Provide patients with easily accessible private areas to engage in solo sexual expression.
4. Encourage social interactions with family members, friends, and other residents in a supervised and appropriate setting.

Medications should be examined as there are medications well known to have an impact on disinhibited sexual behaviors. Carbidopa/levodopa is commonly used in those with Parkinson's disease and has been well-known to increase hypersexuality. Bupropion is also known to increase hypersexual behavior in some patients and benzodiazepines are well known to lead to disinhibited behavior. Box 36.2 provides some additional details regarding meds that can be implicated in SIB.

Management strategies for SIB should focus on nonpharmacologic and pharmacologic interventions. Nonpharmacologic management strategies for SIB are listed in Box 36.3.

EVALUATION AND TREATMENT OF SEXUALLY INAPPROPRIATE BEHAVIOR

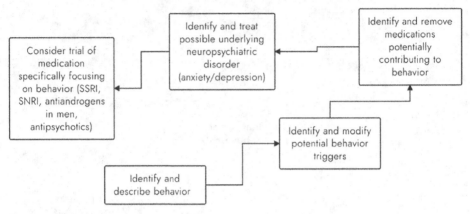

Figure 36.2 Evaluation and treatment of SIB.

Pharmacologic management strategies of SIB in those with MNCD are not predictable as there are no randomized controlled trials to establish the efficacy or safety of various medication interventions. A good general approach to management involves first addressing modifiable environmental factors that could be leading to SIB. Secondly, medications known to possibly increase changes in SIB should be identified and removed if possible (benzodiazepines, dopamine agonists). Finally, pharmacologic treatments specific to the SIB can be trialed. Antidepressants such as SSRIs, trazodone, and mirtazapine have been used with some success and are generally well tolerated. Antiandrogens such as medroxyprogesterone, estrogen, and finasteride can be used in men and have shown benefit. Anticonvulsants such as gabapentin and tegretol have been used for SIB (Figure 36.2).

In the case presented here, the patient's behavior was considered problematic as her sexual behavior was in common areas among other staff and residents. Other residents were uncomfortable. The dignity of the patient could not be ensured with sexual behaviors occurring in public places.

Of interest to the psychiatrist was the fact that these behaviors seemed to escalate in the setting of Mrs. M's increasing outward signs of depression and anxiety. Although studies specific to older adult patients are lacking, it is known that anxiety and depression have been linked to hypersexual behavior. Also, anxiety and depression are the most common mental health diagnoses in those who could be considered to have dysfunctional sexual behaviors. It was reasoned that the patient's dysfunctional sexual expression could be one of her manifestations of depression or anxiety. This was the impetus to initiate more aggressive treatment with an SNRI/atypical antipsychotic combination. Staff were encouraged to continue attempts to redirect Mrs. M to private areas of the facility where she could express herself without offending others and while maintaining her dignity. It was hoped that as the treatment of her potential underlying mood disorder took effect, she would be less angry and upset with attempts at redirection.

> **Take-Home Points**
>
> − Sexually inappropriate behavior can be a manifestation of disinhibited behavior seen in older adults with MNCD.
> − The evaluation of SIB should include a detailed history of what the behavior is, who is involved, what the context of the behavior is, who is being impacted, and if the behavior is out of proportion with other disinhibited behaviors.
> − Sexual expression in older adults with MNCD is normal and should not be universally discouraged when in the appropriate setting and when the rights of others are not violated.
> − Look for and potentially remove medications that could be contributing to SIB including dopamine agonists, anticholinergic agents, and benzodiazepines.

References

1. Mendez, M. F., Chen, A. K., Shapira, J. S., & Miller, B. L. (2005). Acquired sociopathy and frontotemporal dementia. *Dementia and Geriatric Cognitive Disorders*, 20 (2–3), 99–104.

Further Reading

Alkhalil, C., Tanvir, F., Alkhalil, B., & Lowenthal, D. T. (2004). Treatment of sexual disinhibition in dementia: Case reports and review of the literature. *American Journal of Therapeutics*, 11 (3), 231–235.

Joller, P., Gupta, N., Sitz, D. P., Frank, C., Gibson, M., & Gill, S. S. (2013). Approach to inappropriate sexual behavior in people with dementia. *Canadian Family Physician*, 59, 255–260.

Lesser, J. M., Hughes, S. V., Jemelka, J. R., & Griffith, J. (2005). Sexually inappropriate behaviors. Assessment necessitates careful medical and psychological evaluation and sensitivity. *Geriatrics (Basel, Switzerland)*, 60 (1), 34–36.

Mendez, M. F., & Shapira, J. S. (2013). Hypersexual behavior in frontotemporal dementia: A comparison with early-onset Alzheimer's disease. *Archives of Sexual Behavior*, 42 (3), 501–509. doi: 10.1007/s10508-012-0042-4. Epub 2013 Jan 8. PMID: 23297146; PMCID: PMC3596488.

Raymond, N. C., Coleman, E., & Miner, M. H. (2003). Psychiatric comorbidity and compulsive/impulsive traits in compulsive sexual behavior. *Comprehensive Psychiatry*, 44, 370–380.

Sarangi, A., Jones, H., Bangash, F., & Gude, J. (2021). Treatment and management of sexual disinhibition in elderly patients with neurocognitive disorders. *Cureus*, 13 (10), e18463. doi: 10.7759/cureus.18463. PMID: 34745786; PMCID: PMC8563511.

Series, H., & Dégano, P. (2005). Hypersexuality in dementia. *Advances in Psychiatric Treatment*, 11 (6), 424–431. doi:10.1192/apt.11.6.424

Torrisi, M., Cacciola, A., Marra, A., De Luca, R., Bramanti, P., & Calabrò, R. S. (2017). Inappropriate behaviors and hypersexuality in individuals with dementia: An overview of a neglected issue. *Geriatrics and Gerontology International*, 17 (6), 865–874. doi: 10.1111/ggi.12854. Epub 2016 Aug 4.

37

"Everyone Is Just So Good to Me!"
Pseudobulbar Affect

Mr. P was a 78-year-old who had been a resident of a local long-term care facility since the death of his wife several years earlier. He had a history of coronary artery disease, hypertension, mild obesity, diet-controlled diabetes, benign prostatic hyperplasia, and a stroke. Before his stroke, Mr. P was quite functional and independent. The stroke left Mr. P with left-sided weakness but after extensive rehab he was able to ambulate with the assistance of a walker. He was also left with some mild cognitive impairment. He could generally complete his own ADLs with reminders from his wife or other caregivers. Sadly, after the death of his wife from breast cancer the patient was forced to enter a long-term care facility as his children did not live close and were very active in their own careers and with their own families. Mr. P did surprisingly well with the transition to long-term care. He made friends at the facility, enjoyed participating in social activities, and got along well with others. He adapted well to the day-to-day routine of his facility.

The geriatric psychiatry team was consulted for the evaluation of potential depression. Mr. P was noted to become very emotional and have episodes of crying at times, which were usually short-lived but disturbing to the patient and those around him. His primary physician had placed Mr. P on escitalopram 5 mg daily and this was subsequently increased to 10 mg daily. He had been on the 10 mg daily dose for approximately six weeks prior to psychiatry being consulted but there was little improvement noted in his emotional lability.

Mr. P was on an additional medication regimen of low-dose aspirin, atorvastatin, metformin, lisinopril, multivitamin, and tamsulosin. He did not have any prior significant psychiatric history.

When interviewed Mr. P was friendly and pleasant. He scored 22/30 on the SLUMS exam and scored 3 on the PHQ–9. He had left-sided weakness and some mild dysarthria consistent with his history of stroke. His mood was described as euthymic and his thought processes were thought to be logical. He had no evidence of any hallucinations or delusions. He was noted to become suddenly tearful when the conversation came around to discussing one or two of the caregivers at the facility when he mentioned how grateful he was for the day-to-day help and care they provided him with. He was also quite tearful when offering thanks to the consulting psychiatrist for the attention provided to him. "Everyone is just so good to me!" he sobbed. When asked, he felt that the escitalopram started six weeks before had maybe been a little helpful with his episodes of crying.

After reviewing the patient's medical records and speaking to caregivers a presumptive diagnosis of MNCD–vascular type–mild with secondary pseudobulbar affect (PBA) was made. The patient scored 14 on the Center for Neurologic Study – Lability Scale (CNS–LS scale). This score was suggestive of pseudobulbar affect.

Mr. P was prescribed dextromethorphan/quinidine 10/20 mg once daily for seven days. This was then increased to twice daily. A follow-up visit four weeks later showed Mr. P in good spirits. He was thrilled that his new treatment had improved his episodes of pathologic crying a good deal and he had no negative side effects from the medication. The escitalopram dose was decreased to 5 mg daily and then discontinued. At a follow-up four weeks later Mr. P continued to have what could be described as a good response to the dextromethorphan/quinidine and plans were made to see the patient every three months or so.

Teaching Points

Pseudobulbar affect is described as episodes of involuntary, unprovoked, and sudden episodes of crying or laughing that happen as a result of CNS pathology. Pseudobulbar affect can be easily overlooked or misdiagnosed as a primary mood disorder. Over the years it has been called a number of different names including emotional incontinence, pathological laughter and crying, and excessive emotionalism, among others. Pseudobulbar affect is seen in a wide variety of neuropsychiatric disorders including Parkinson's disease, ALS, Alzheimer's disease, multiple sclerosis, history of stroke, TBI, and CNS malignancies. The burden of this disorder can be high, causing embarrassment and distressing impairment in social situations. The displays of emotion cannot be prevented or aborted by the patient, leading to social isolation and contributing to anxiety and depression. Symptoms can include emotionally congruent reactions that are pathologically intense. Patients can also demonstrate emotionally incongruent affect reactions such as crying during a happy occasion or while watching a TV sitcom.

The exact pathophysiology behind the disorder is poorly understood but thought to involve several pathways in the brain that control motor, cognitive, and affective function. Pathological crying seems to be more common than pathological laughter.

There can be a good deal of overlap in the symptomatology of patients with PBA and primary mood disorders. Many of the primary neurological disorders associated with PBA also have a high incidence of comorbid anxiety and depression. When trying to distinguish anxiety and depression from PBA it should be noted that symptoms of depression and anxiety tend to be more persistent throughout the day, whereas PBA symptomatology tends to be more sporadic.

There are four major diagnostic criteria for PBA. These include the presence of an emotional response that is situationally inappropriate, the patient's feelings and the effective response not being closely related, the patient being unable to control the duration and severity of the episodes, and expressions of emotion not leading to a feeling of relief.

Diagnosis is usually made by an appropriate history with congruent symptomatology, but rating scores do exist that are helpful. A common one is the CNS–LS. It is a seven-item questionnaire that can be self-administered or administered by a healthcare professional.

Several classes of medications have been used with varying success [1] (see Box 37.1). Treatments generally focus on the neuromodulation of norepinephrine, serotonin, or glutamate. Most treatments have been used off-label until dextromethorphan/quinidine (Nuedexta) was approved in 2010. Dextromethorphan acts as a noncompetitive NMDA receptor antagonist and is rapidly and extensively converted in the liver to a compound that is unable to cross the blood–brain barrier. Quinidine helps to slow this hepatic

> **Box 37.1 Pharmacologic options for treatment of PBA**
>
> 1. Selective serotonin reuptake inhibitors such as fluoxetine and sertraline. Use is off-label. Studies showing benefits are older and with relatively small sample sizes. Inexpensive and well-tolerated option [2].
> 2. Tricyclic antidepressants. Nortriptyline is preferred in older adults due to a lower anticholinergic burden than some alternatives.
> 3. Dextromethorphan/quinidine (Nuedexta). Brand-only medication FDA approved in 2010. Use often requires insurance prior to authorization. Cost issues may be a factor.

metabolism, allowing more of the dextromethorphan to reach the CNS. Dextromethorphan/quinidine is the newest treatment option and is still under patent protection. For this reason, it can be a less appealing treatment option financially. It is reasonable to start a patient on an SSRI and titrate to a therapeutic dose. Tricyclic antidepressants have also been used but are less desirable in the elderly due to side effects.

> **Take-Home Points**
>
> - Pseudobulbar affect is described as episodes of involuntary, unprovoked, and sudden episodes of crying or laughing that happen as a result of CNS pathology.
> - Several classes of medications have been used to treat PBA with varying success. These include SSRIs, SNRIs, and tricyclic antidepressants.
> - Pseudobulbar affect can be easily overlooked or misdiagnosed as a primary mood disorder.
> - Dextromethorphan/quinidine (Neudexta) was approved in 2010 for the treatment of PBA.

References

1. Hakimi, M., & Maurer, C. W. (2019). Pseudobulbar affect in Parkinsonian disorders: A review. *Journal of Movement Disorders*, 12 (1), 14–21. https://doi.org/10.14802/jmd.18051

2. Ahmed, A., & Simmons, Z. (2013). Pseudobulbar affect: Prevalence and management. *Therapeutics and Clinical Risk Management*, 9, 483–489.

Further Reading

Choi-Kwon, S., Han, S. W., Kwon, S. U., Kang, D. W., Choi, J. M., & Kim, J. S. (2006). Fluoxetine treatment in poststroke depression, emotional incontinence, and anger proneness: A double-blind, placebo-controlled study. *Stroke*, 37 (1), 156–161.

Fitzgerald, K. C., Salter, A., Tyry, T., Fox, R. J., Cutter, G., & Marrie, R. A. (2018). Pseudobulbar affect: Prevalence and association with symptoms in multiple sclerosis. *Neurology: Clinical Practice*, 8 (6), 472–481. https://doi.org/10.1212/CPJ.0000000000000523

Fralick, M., Sacks, C. A., & Kesselheim, A. S. (2019). Assessment of use of combined dextromethorphan and quinidine in patients with dementia or Parkinson disease after US Food and Drug Administration approval for pseudobulbar affect. *JAMA Internal Medicine*, 179 (2). https://doi.org/10.1001/jamainternmed.2018.6112

Miller, A., Pratt, H., & Schiffer, R. B. (2011). Pseudobulbar affect: The spectrum of clinical presentations, etiologies and treatments. *Expert Review of Neurotherapeutics*, 11 (7), 1077–1088. DOI: 10.1586/ern.11.68

Pioro, E. P., Brooks, B. R., Cummings, J., Schiffer, R., Thisted, R. A., Wynn, D., Hepner, A., & Kaye, R. (2010). Dextromethorphan plus ultra-low-dose quinidine reduces pseudobulbar affect. *Annals of Neurology*, 68 (5), 693–702.

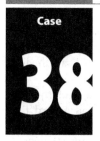
"Why Do They Say I Have Dementia?"

ADD in Older Adults

Mr. A was a boisterous 78-year-old gentleman who resided at a long-term care facility. He was quite popular with other residents and staff alike as he was very sociable and friendly and enjoyed participating in many of the facility's activities. He moved into the long-term care facility two years prior after a fall at home which resulted in a hip fracture. Before this, he was living in a small travel trailer on a piece of land owned by a friend. He had never been married and had no children.

During hospitalization after the fall, a psychiatry consultation was ordered after the care team questioned his ability to live alone due to possible dementia. He was evaluated by a psychiatric nurse practitioner who diagnosed the patient with mild to moderate MNCD, likely Alzheimer's type. Mr. A's SLUMS score was 18/30 at that time. After input from the mental health practitioner, the medical team recommended the patient be transferred to an acute rehab facility and likely to long-term care afterward due to the inability to care for himself secondary to dementia.

Mr. A had several medical problems that contributed to his physical decline, including poorly controlled diabetes, COPD, CHF, and mild renal disease. All of these conditions became well controlled as he was having his medications reliably administered by facility staff and getting regular medical checkups. In the long-term care facility, he was able to perform his basic ADLs without problem. Despite the diagnosis of probable Alzheimer's disease, Mr. A had no apparent declines in either cognition or independence in the two years he had been at the facility.

Over the course of several months, Mr. A's long-term care PCP observed him to be quite cheerful and socially appropriate. He knew the names of nearly all the other residents. He liked to play bingo, loved to eat, and slept well. His only visitor from outside the facility was his friend who owned the land where he used to live. During one of the visits the provider met the patient's friend and he and Mr. A reminisced. Mr. A had lived on the piece of property in his travel trailer for 20 years. He had never worked a "real job" but always seemed able to support himself with the help of food stamps and odd jobs, mostly consisting of small engine repairs for his friend who owned an equipment rental shop. His front yard was well known to be piled high with various machines and small engine parts, most rusted beyond recognition.

Mr. A had never graduated high school. He had made it through the eighth grade but dropped out of his small country school at the age of 13. He mentioned that he had been a terrible student but had always been good at "figuring out how things work". There was a time in his life when Mr. A admitted that he abused alcohol. He lost his driver's license due to several DUIs in his 30s and it had never been reinstated. He quit drinking altogether in his 40s after he had a bad fall at home and hit his head, suffering a bad concussion. He did not smoke or have any history of using recreational drugs.

His parents had both died when he was relatively young and he had no siblings. He had come close to getting married on a couple of occasions but says, "I saw the light before it was too late!"

Mr. A said his hobby had always been fixing things. He did not particularly enjoy television, except for game shows and a few sitcoms, as he says he had a hard time following along during a movie or an hour-long drama-type show.

Mr. A asked, "Why do they say I have dementia?" He saw people around the facility with dementia and did not feel that he had similar issues. Another SLUMS exam was performed and the patient scored 18/30. It was noted that Mr. A had a very difficult time staying focused on the SLUMS as it was being administered, taking about twice as long as it does for most other people.

The provider began to suspect that Mr. A's cognitive difficulties were due to inattention and possible adult attention deficit disorder (ADD). With further questioning, Mr. A revealed that he did quite poorly in school when he was young. He relayed that he had hated school, always felt picked on by the teachers, and his desk was always placed in the front corner of the room away from the other children for speaking out of turn. He was always getting in trouble for daydreaming and never turning in his homework. At one point his parents were told that Mr. A had a learning disability but Mr. A says "they didn't know what to do about it back then".

Mr. A was informed by his provider about the likelihood that he had ADD and how this diagnosis could sometimes cause symptoms that can be confused with dementia in older adults or learning disabilities and behavioral problems in children. Mr. A was not inclined to consider any treatment for the condition as he felt he was doing well and felt well-adjusted to his new life and community. He also stated, "I already take too many pills!"

Teaching Points

Attention deficit hyperactivity disorder (ADHD) was for many years considered to be a condition primarily affecting children and adolescents. We now know that up to 60% of children and adolescents retain symptoms of ADD into adulthood [1]. Symptoms such as difficulty concentrating, forgetfulness, and difficulty with organization or executive function can mimic cognitive issues seen in those with early MNCDs. This distinction can be particularly difficult in those older adults who present with cognitive complaints.

Approximately 5–7% of children and adolescents are thought to have ADHD. The condition also affects an estimated 2.5% of adults across the world [2]. The condition is more commonly diagnosed in males than females with a male-to-female ratio of about 2:1. The effects of ADHD in adults and older adults can involve multiple areas of life including professional activities, social activities, financial health, and relationships. In this age of heightened awareness of ADHD, it has now become less likely for a patient to present to a healthcare provider with a many-year history of undiagnosed or untreated ADD.

The pathophysiology of ADD is complex and not completely understood but, as with many neuropsychiatric conditions, it is believed to involve a combination of genetic, neurobiological, and environmental factors. One leading theory involves the dysregulation of neurotransmitters, particularly dopamine and norepinephrine. Dopamine is the neurotransmitter associated most with reward, motivation, and executive functions such as planning and decision-making. Norepinephrine is involved in arousal and attention. Some studies suggest that individuals with ADD may have lower levels of dopamine and norepinephrine in certain brain regions which play a critical role in executive functioning. The fact that ADD and ADHD tend to run in families shows that the condition also has a strong genetic component. Multiple genes are thought to be involved [3].

Those with ADHD may experience lower self-esteem and self-worth secondary to personal and professional problems attributed to the diagnosis. The condition can have a significant impact on education and career choices. Those with ADHD may struggle with work-related task completion and maintaining attention. It can also affect interpersonal relationships with impulsivity, forgetfulness, and inattentiveness leading to relationship conflicts with partners, friends, and family members. Those with ADHD are at increased risk of developing comorbid psychiatric conditions such as anxiety or depression. They are also more likely to have substance use disorders [4].

Diagnostic criteria for ADHD in adults are laid out in detail in the DSM–5-TR. Symptoms can be classified as either primarily inattentive or hyperactive/impulsive. The diagnostic criteria for ADHD described in DSM–5-TR are listed in Box 38.1 [5].

Diagnosing adult ADHD can be particularly challenging if a patient is also at risk of MNCDs. Many of the symptoms of ADHD can mimic cognitive impairments seen in early MNCDs. Older adults with ADHD may be misdiagnosed with a MNCD as was likely true with the case presented here.

The need for treatment of adult ADHD depends on the degree of dysfunction, psychiatric comorbidities, patient preference, and side effect profiles of medications. Stimulant medication such as methylphenidate or amphetamine-based medications can help improve focus and attention by modifying dopamine and norepinephrine-dependent pathways in the brain. Stimulant medications for ADHD are more effective than non-stimulant medications but also have a higher likelihood of misuse, diversion, and abuse [4]. Non-stimulant medications can also sometimes be effective and include atomoxetine, guanfacine, and clonidine. Bupropion is used mainly as an antidepressant but it is sometimes prescribed off-label for adult ADHD due to its effects on both dopamine and norepinephrine [6]. Counselors and psychologists can also provide many valuable insights to help those with ADHD better adapt to the challenges of living with the condition.

Several treatment challenges are more commonly encountered by older adults with ADHD. They often have medical comorbidities such as cardiovascular conditions that may make the use of stimulant medications more problematic. Those with poorly controlled cardiovascular conditions such as CHF, arrhythmias, or hypertension may best be treated with non-stimulant medications. Those with well-controlled or stable cardiovascular conditions are likely to tolerate lower or moderate doses of stimulant medications without issue but may warrant extra monitoring.

Treating ADHD in the setting of comorbid psychiatric illness can present unique challenges. Those patients with comorbid bipolar disorder are at higher risk of psychiatric instability with the introduction of stimulant medication. These patients may best be treated under the guidance of a psychiatrist. Also, those patients with psychotic disorders may become psychiatrically unstable with the introduction of stimulant medications that may modulate dopamine pathways.

Box 38.1 Inattentive symptoms seen in adult ADHD

1. A persistent pattern of inattention and/or hyperactivity–impulsivity that interferes with functioning or development, as characterized by a. and/or b.:

   a. **Inattention:** Six (or more) of the following symptoms have persisted for at least six months to a degree that is inconsistent with developmental level and that directly impacts negatively on social and academic/occupational activities:

   Note: The symptoms are not solely a manifestation of oppositional behavior, defiance, hostility, or failure to understand tasks or instructions. For older adolescents and adults (age 17 and older), at least five symptoms are required.

   i. Often fails to give close attention to details or makes careless mistakes in schoolwork, at work, or during other activities (e.g. overlooks or misses details, work is inaccurate).
   ii. Often has difficulty sustaining attention in tasks or play activities (e.g. has difficulty remaining focused during lectures, conversations, or lengthy reading).
   iii. Often does not seem to listen when spoken to directly (e.g. mind seems elsewhere, even in the absence of any obvious distraction).
   iv. Often does not follow through on instructions and fails to finish schoolwork, chores, or duties in the workplace (e.g. starts tasks but quickly loses focus and is easily sidetracked).
   v. Often has difficulty organizing tasks and activities (e.g. difficulty managing sequential tasks; difficulty keeping materials and belongings in order; messy, disorganized work; has poor time management; fails to meet deadlines).
   vi. Often avoids, dislikes, or is reluctant to engage in tasks that require sustained mental effort (e.g. schoolwork or homework; for older adolescents and adults, preparing reports, completing forms, reviewing lengthy papers).
   vii. Often loses things necessary for tasks or activities (e.g. school materials, pencils, books, tools, wallets, keys, paperwork, eyeglasses, mobile telephones).
   viii. Is often easily distracted by extraneous stimuli (for older adolescents and adults, may include unrelated thoughts).
   ix. Is often forgetful in daily activities (e.g. doing chores, running errands; for older adolescents and adults, returning calls, paying bills, keeping appointments).

   b. **Hyperactivity and impulsivity:** Six (or more) of the following symptoms have persisted for at least six months to a degree that is inconsistent with developmental level and that directly impacts negatively on social and academic/occupational activities:

   Note: The symptoms are not solely a manifestation of oppositional behavior, defiance, hostility, or a failure to understand tasks or instructions. For older adolescents and adults (age 17 and older), at least five symptoms are required.

   i. Often fidgets with or taps hands or feet or squirms in seat.
   ii. Often leaves seat in situations when remaining seated is expected (e.g. leaves his or her place in the classroom, in the office or other workplace, or in other situations that require remaining in place).
   iii. Often runs about or climbs in situations where it is inappropriate. (Note: In adolescents or adults, may be limited to feeling restless.)
   iv. Often unable to play or engage in leisure activities quietly.
   v. Is often "on the go," acting as if "driven by a motor" (e.g. is unable to be or uncomfortable being still for extended time, as in restaurants, meetings;

Box 38.1 (*cont.*)

      may be experienced by others as being restless or difficult to keep up with).

  vi. Often talks excessively.

  vii. Often blurts out an answer before a question has been completed (e.g. completes people's sentences; cannot wait for turn in conversation).

  viii. Often has difficulty waiting his or her turn (e.g. while waiting in line).

  ix. Often interrupts or intrudes on others (e.g. butts into conversations, games, or activities; may start using other people's things without asking or receiving permission; for adolescents and adults, may intrude into or take over what others are doing).

2. Several inattentive or hyperactive–impulsive symptoms were present prior to age 12 years.

3. Several inattentive or hyperactive–impulsive symptoms are present in two or more settings (e.g. at home, school, or work; with friends or relatives; in other activities).

4. There is clear evidence that the symptoms interfere with, or reduce the quality of, social, academic, or occupational functioning.

5. The symptoms do not occur exclusively during the course of schizophrenia or another psychotic disorder and are not better explained by another mental disorder (e.g. mood disorder, anxiety disorder, dissociative disorder, personality disorder, substance intoxication or withdrawal).

Specify whether:

F90.2 Combined presentation: If both Criterion 1a (inattention) and Criterion 1b (hyperactivity–impulsivity) are met for the past six months.

F90.0 Predominantly inattentive presentation: If Criterion 1a (inattention) is met but Criterion 1b (hyperactivity–impulsivity) is not met for the past six months.

F90.1 Predominantly hyperactive/impulsive presentation: If Criterion 1b (hyperactivity–impulsivity) is met and Criterion 1a (inattention) is not met for the past six months.

Specify if: In partial remission: When full criteria were previously met, fewer than the full criteria have been met for the past six months, and the symptoms still result in impairment in social, academic, or occupational functioning.

Specify current severity:

Mild: Few, if any, symptoms in excess of those required to make the diagnosis are present, and symptoms result in no more than minor impairments in social or occupational functioning.

Moderate: Symptoms or functional impairment between "mild" and "severe" are present.

Severe: Many symptoms in excess of those required to make the diagnosis, or several symptoms that are particularly severe, are present, or the symptoms result in marked impairment in social or occupational functioning.

The prognosis for adult ADHD is generally good with appropriate treatment and follow-up. These patients can function well in professional, social, and relationship arenas. Older adults may potentially have less need for treatment as their symptoms may be less disruptive to day-to-day function.

Take-Home Points

- Symptoms of adult ADHD can mimic early MNCD in older adults.
- Deficits uncovered in standard cognitive tests can be due to impaired attention in older adults with ADHD.
- Treatment of adult ADHD in older adults is similar to that in younger patients and includes stimulant and non-stimulant medications. Extra caution should be used when prescribing stimulant medications to those with medical or psychiatric comorbidities.
- About 60% of children or adolescents with ADHD go on to experience adult ADHD. Symptoms of adult ADHD may lessen or be less problematic in older adults. Some older adults may still benefit from treatment.

References

1. Callahan, B. L., Bierstone, D., Stuss, D. T., & Black, S. E. (2017). Adult ADHD: Risk factor for dementia or phenotypic mimic? *Frontiers in Aging Neuroscience*, 9. https://doi.org/10.3389/fnagi.2017.00260

2. Dobrosavljevic, M., Solares, C., Cortese, S., Andershed, H., & Larsson, H. (2020). Prevalence of attention-deficit/hyperactivity disorder in older adults: A systematic review and meta-analysis. *Neuroscience & Biobehavioral Reviews*, 118, 282–289. https://doi.org/10.1016/j.neubiorev.2020.07.042

3. Kessi, M., Duan, H., Xiong, J., Chen, B., He, F., Yang, L., Ma, Y., Bamgbade, O. A., Peng, J., & Yin, F. (2022). Attention-deficit/hyperactive disorder updates. *Frontiers in Molecular Neuroscience*, 15. https://doi.org/10.3389/fnmol.2022.925049

4, Faraone, S. V., Banaschewski, T., Coghill, D., Zheng, Y., Biederman, J., Bellgrove, M. A., Newcorn, J. H., Gignac, M., Al Saud, N. M., Manor, I., Rohde, L. A., Yang, L., Cortese, S., Almagor, D., Stein, M. A., Albatti, T. H., Aljoudi, H. F., Alqahtani, M. J., Asherson, P., & Wang, Y. (2021). The World Federation of ADHD International Consensus Statement: 208 evidence-based conclusions about the disorder. *Neuroscience and Biobehavioral Reviews*, 128, 789. https://doi.org/10.1016/j.neubiorev.2021.01.022

5, American Psychiatric Association. (2022). *Diagnostic and Statistical Manual of Mental Disorders*. 5th ed. text rev. (American Psychiatric Association.)

6. Elliott, J., Johnston, A., Husereau, D., Kelly, S. E., Eagles, C., Charach, A., Hsieh, C., Bai, Z., Hossain, A., Skidmore, B., Tsakonas, E., Chojecki, D., Mamdani, M., & Wells, G. A. (2020). Pharmacologic treatment of attention deficit hyperactivity disorder in adults: A systematic review and network meta-analysis. *PLoS ONE*, 15 (10). https://doi.org/10.1371/journal.pone.0240584

Further Reading

Anbarasan, D., Kitchin, M., & Adler, L. A. (2020). Screening for adult ADHD. *Current Psychiatry Reports*. 22 (12), 72. doi: 10.1007/s11920-020-01194-9. PMID: 33095375.

Antshel, K. M., & Barkley, R. (2020). Attention deficit hyperactivity disorder. *Handbook of Clinical Neurology*, 174, 37–45. doi: 10.1016/B978-0-444-64148-9.00003-X. PMID: 32977893.

Posner, J., Polanczyk, G. V., & Sonuga-Barke, E. (2020). Attention-deficit hyperactivity disorder. *Lancet (London, England)*, 395 (10222), 450.

Young, J. L., & Goodman, D. W. (2016). Adult attention-deficit/hyperactivity disorder diagnosis, management, and treatment in the DSM–5 era. *Primary Care Companion for CNS Disorders*, 18 (6). doi: 10.4088/PCC.16r02000. PMID: 27907271.

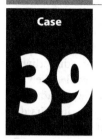

Case

39

"I Hate That Guy ... I Can't Get Any Sleep!"

Sleep–Wake Cycle Disorders

Mr. R was an 82-year-old gentleman who had resided in a long-term care facility for three months. He possessed an outgoing personality and was generally a favorite among the facility care staff and other residents. He had a history of mild MNCD, likely Alzheimer's type, mild COPD, psoriasis, and osteoarthritis involving multiple joints. Before moving to the long-term care facility he had lived with his daughter, who had experienced a decline in her own health necessitating his move to long-term care.

Mr. R was quite content with his move to the long-term care facility, actively participating in activities and enjoying communal dining. He mentioned that living with his daughter had often left him feeling bored and, at times, like a burden. He was considered eccentric in one or two ways, such as his preference to have his evening meal as early as possible and often being found in bed asleep for the night around 6 or 6:30 pm. Despite sleeping soundly, he would frequently wake up around 2 am and could be found sitting at the nurse's station, engaging in conversations with the night shift staff and watching old westerns on the television in the common area.

About a month before a psychiatric consultation was requested, Mr. R acquired a roommate, allowing him to pay a significantly lower monthly fee for his room and board at the facility. Several weeks after getting the new roommate, Mr. R was reportedly irritable and less pleasant to be around. The facility staff began to wonder if Mr. R was becoming depressed because of the dramatic change in his personality, leading to the request for a consultation with the long-term care psychiatrist.

During the initial visit, Mr. R was observed in his room at 2 pm in the afternoon, nodding off to sleep in his wheelchair. While he was cooperative with the interviewer, he was best described as irritated and appeared tired. He was reasonably well-groomed and appeared well-nourished. He was oriented to person and place and able to answer all direct, in-the-moment questions but struggled as a historian and exhibited some forgetfulness. His mood was described as irritable. When asked about his feelings toward the day-to-day routine at the facility and the staff, he reported having no complaints, except for his roommate. Under his breath, he expressed, "I hate that guy ... I can't get any sleep! He's up till one or two in the morning watching Fox News and then sleeps all morning, expecting me to be quiet so he can sleep till noon!"

Mr. R was not taking any psychiatric medications. He denied feelings of sadness or depression but admitted to irritability and fatigue. He also denied experiencing any hallucinations. When questioned about his early bedtime, he explained that during his 35 years working in construction, he had to leave his house at 4 am in the morning, leading him to become accustomed to going to bed early and waking up very early.

Mr. R mentioned to the provider that his new roommate had worked the overnight shift at a large brewery for 30 years.

The psychiatrist found no evidence of mood disorder, anxiety disorder, thought disorder, or rapidly progressing MNCD. Mr. R was informed that his circadian rhythm or "internal clock" was now set for sleep times much earlier than most people, likely due to his years of working early mornings in construction. This pattern, known as advanced sleep phase syndrome, is not inherently problematic unless it significantly impairs day-to-day functioning. Ironically, his new roommate likely had delayed sleep phase syndrome due to years of working nights. The suggested options to address this issue were to either change roommates or, for both Mr. R and his roommate, to gradually adjust their sleep cycles to a more conventional schedule.

Mr. R and his roommate both expressed a desire to make their current living situation work and were open to efforts to bring about change. Mr. R agreed to delay his bedtime by half an hour every week until he reached a more conventional schedule. Simultaneously, his roommate agreed to advance his bedtime by half an hour per week until reaching a more conventional time.

During a follow-up visit six weeks later, both men were doing well. Mr. R was now going to bed at around 9:30 pm at night, spending some time watching Fox News with his roommate before they retired to bed at approximately 10 pm. Both men had gradually adjusted to their new sleep schedules and were developing a friendship in the process.

Teaching Points

Sleep-related complaints are quite common in the long-term care setting. Some may be symptoms of psychiatric disorders, but many can be attributed to primary sleep disorders. It is estimated that 40–70% of older adults experience some form of chronic sleep-related complaints, and up to 50% of these cases go undiagnosed [1].

The physiology of sleep in older adults is well known to exhibit differences when compared to that of younger adults. Box 39.1 lists some age-related changes to sleep physiology [2,3].

Poor sleep quality and fatigue can result from other physiological or psychiatric conditions, but they can also be primary issues related to circadian rhythm disturbances. Circadian rhythms encompass physical, mental, and behavioral patterns that follow a

---

Box 39.1 Some age-related changes to sleep physiology seen in older adults

Increased:

Time awake after sleep onset (wakefulness at night).
Number of sleep arousals.
Sleep latency-time to fall asleep.

Decreased:

Total sleep time.
Slow wave sleep.
REM sleep.
Sleep efficiency.

24-hour cycle. The most evident example of a circadian rhythm is the sleep–wake cycle, which typically involves sleep during the night and wakefulness during the day. Various other bodily systems are closely linked to circadian rhythms as well, including endocrinologic hormone release, eating habits and digestion, urine production, and body temperature, among others.

The neurons of the suprachiasmatic nucleus (SCN) of the anterior hypothalamus are the heart of the circadian rhythm in mammals. They influence other parts of the brain via efferent neurons and the humoral effects of melatonin released from the pineal gland. The activity of the SCN runs autonomously but is regulated by environmental signals. It resets daily and is heavily influenced by light inputs from the retina during the day and melatonin secretion at night [4].

Significant distress and dysfunction can arise when there is a misalignment between the endogenous biological clock and the external light–dark cycle. External factors influencing circadian rhythms can include light exposure, work schedules, eating schedules, and exercise.

Disturbances in the sleep–wake cycle are also referred to as circadian rhythm disorders. Box 39.2 lists some of the more common sleep–wake cycle disturbances.

The treatment of sleep disorders in older adults depends on the primary diagnosis. Long-term care physicians are often the ones tasked with making these diagnoses, as access to a sleep medicine specialist may be challenging for long-term care residents. Some general principles to encourage higher-quality sleep in older adults are listed in Box 39.3.

Box 39.2 Some common sleep–wake cycle disturbances seen in older adults

Insomnia: These patients have trouble initiating sleep, often lying awake for an extended period before falling asleep. Insomnia also includes those who have trouble with maintaining sleep, who may have frequent awakenings during the night and difficulty returning to sleep.

Delayed sleep phase syndrome: These patients tend to go to bed and wake up later than what is considered normal. This can lead to difficulties in day-to-day life and social function.

Advanced sleep phase syndrome: This is considered the opposite of delayed sleep phase syndrome. These patients tend to go to bed and wake up earlier than is conventionally considered normal.

Irregular sleep–wake rhythm: This sleep disorder can lead to multiple short sleep episodes throughout a 24-hour day. There may be no clear pattern of consolidated sleep at night.

Non-24-hour sleep–wake disorder: These patients may have longer than 24-hour circadian rhythms, causing their sleep–wake pattern to be later and later each day, making it difficult to maintain a schedule.

Sleep state misperception (paradoxical insomnia): These patients consistently underestimate the amount of sleep they get. They may complain of insomnia, but objective measurements of sleep duration and quality are normal.

Hypersomnia: Patients with hypersomnia have excessive daytime sleepiness that can be due to poor quality sleep, sleep disorders, or underlying medical or psychiatric conditions.

Narcolepsy: A relatively rare neurological disorder that leads to excessive daytime sleepiness, sudden loss of muscle tone, and other REM sleep-related symptoms.

Box 39.3 Good nonpharmacologic principles beneficial to sleep quality in older adults

Sleep hygiene practices: These may include maintaining a consistent sleep schedule, creating a comfortable and dark sleeping environment, avoiding stimulating activities and bright screens before bedtime, and limiting caffeine intake in the latter part of the day.

Sleep restriction: Limiting time spent in bed to improve the quality of sleep while in bed.

Physical activity: Physical activity during the day can promote better sleep at night. Limit physical activity around bedtime.

Limiting naps: Daytime napping can reduce sleep quality at night.

Light exposure: Bright natural light exposure during the day can help maintain circadian rhythms and better sleep quality at night.

The pharmacologic treatment of primary sleep disorders in older adults is somewhat limited due to the sensitivity of this population to side effects. Several pharmacologic options are considered potentially safe and well-tolerated in many older adults. Trazodone, a sedating antidepressant, is generally regarded as a safer alternative for individuals experiencing difficulty in sleep onset and maintenance. Starting doses of 25 mg or 50 mg at bedtime are typically effective. Melatonin is considered a relatively benign pharmacologic option for older adults with difficulty initiating sleep, although there is limited data supporting its efficacy. Doses of 3–10 mg at bedtime are often used. Mirtazapine can produce a generally safe sedative/hypnotic effect at relatively low doses, but caution is advised in those who are overweight, as it can stimulate hunger [5]. A newer class of medications, orexin antagonists suvorexant and lemborexant, show promise for safety and efficacy in older adults but is still limited by cost and insurance coverage at the time of this publication [6].

The list of potentially inappropriate medications for older adults with sleep disturbances is longer than the list of potentially appropriate meds. Benzodiazepines are best avoided in older adults due to increased rates of falls and delirium associated with these medications. Additionally, these medications quickly lead to tolerance and dependence. Antihistamines, despite being somewhat effective for insomnia in younger adults, are best avoided in older adults due to their strong anticholinergic effects. Non-benzodiazepine hypnotics such as zolpidem and eszopiclone are well known to trigger confusion and delirium in older adults and also carry some risk of tolerance and dependence.

Take-Home Points

- Sleep-related complaints are quite common in the long-term care setting. It is estimated that 40–70% of older adults have some type of chronic sleep-related complaint. Up to 50% of these go undiagnosed.
- Older adults are known to have increased wakefulness at night, increased number of sleep arousals, and increased sleep latency, alongside decreased total sleep time, slow wave sleep, REM sleep, and sleep efficiency.
- Some common sleep–wake cycle disturbances seen in older adults include primary insomnia, delayed sleep phase syndrome, advanced sleep phase syndrome, irregular sleep–wake rhythm, non-24-hour sleep–wake disorder, sleep state misperception, hypersomnia, and narcolepsy.
- Good nonpharmacologic principles beneficial to sleep quality are often safer and more effective than pharmacologic therapies. These include good sleep hygiene practices, sleep restriction, increased physical activity, limiting daytime naps, and daytime bright light exposure.

References

1. Avidan, A. Y. (2014). Normal Sleep in Humans. In H. A. A. Y. Kryger Meir and B. Berry Richard (eds.) *Atlas of Clinical Sleep Medicine*. 2nd ed. (Philadelphia, PA: Saunders). pp. 70–97.

2. Miner, B., & Kryger, M. H. (2017). Sleep in the aging population. *Sleep Medicine Clinics*, 12 (1), 31. https://doi.org/10 .1016/j.jsmc.2016.10.008

3. Tatineny, P., Shafi, F., Gohar, A., & Bhat, A. (2020). Sleep in the elderly. *Missouri Medicine*, 117 (5), 490–495. www.ncbi .nlm.nih.gov/pmc/articles/PMC7723148/

4. Weldemichael, D. A., & Grossberg, G. T. (2010). Circadian rhythm disturbances in patients with Alzheimer's disease: A review. *International Journal of Alzheimer's Disease*, 2010. https://doi.org/ 10.4061/2010/716453

5. Brewster, G., Riegel, B., & Gehrman, P. R. (2018). Insomnia in the older adult. *Sleep Medicine Clinics*, 13 (1), 13–19. https:// doi.org/10.1016/j.jsmc.2017.09.002

6. Mogavero, M. P., Silvani, A., Lanza, G., DelRosso, L. M., Ferini-Strambi, L., & Ferri, R. (2023). Targeting orexin receptors for the treatment of insomnia: From physiological mechanisms to current clinical evidence and recommendations. *Nature and Science of Sleep*, 15, 17–38. https://doi.org/10.2147/ NSS.S201994

Further Reading

Auger, R. R., Burgess, H. J., Emens, J. S., Deriy, L. V., Thomas, S. M., & Sharkey, K. M. (2015). Clinical practice guideline for the treatment of intrinsic circadian rhythm sleep–wake disorders: Advanced sleep-wake phase disorder (ASWPD), delayed sleep–wake phase disorder (DSWPD), non-24-hour sleep–wake rhythm disorder (N24SWD), and irregular sleep–wake rhythm disorder (ISWRD). An update for 2015: An American Academy of Sleep Medicine Clinical Practice Guideline. *Journal of Clinical Sleep Medicine*, 11 (10), 1199–1236. https://doi.org/10.5664/jcsm .5100

Fifel, K., & Videnovic, A. (2020). Circadian and sleep dysfunctions in neurodegenerative disorders: An update. *Frontiers in Neuroscience*, 14. https://doi .org/10.3389/fnins.2020.627330

Jaqua, E. E., Hanna, M., Labib, W., Moore, C., & Matossian, V. (2023). Common sleep disorders affecting older adults. *The Permanente Journal*, 27 (1), 122–132. https://doi.org/10.7812/TPP/22.114

Jha, V. M. (2023). The prevalence of sleep loss and sleep disorders in young and old adults. *Aging Brain*, 3. https://doi.org/10.1016/j .nbas.2022.100057

Kim, J. H., Elkhadem, A. R., & Duffy, J. F. (2022). Circadian rhythm sleep–wake disorders in older adults. *Sleep Medicine Clinics*, 17 (2), 241. https://doi.org/10.1016/ j.jsmc.2022.02.003

Palagini, L., Manni, R., Aguglia, E., Amore, M., Brugnoli, R., Bioulac, S., Bourgin, P., Franchi, A. M., Girardi, P., Grassi, L., Lopez, R., Mencacci, C., Plazzi, G., Maruani, J., Minervino, A., Philip, P., Parola, S. R., Poirot, I., Nobili, L., & Geoffroy, P. A. (2021). International expert opinions and recommendations on the use of melatonin in the treatment of insomnia and circadian sleep disturbances in adult neuropsychiatric disorders. *Frontiers in Psychiatry*, 12. https://doi.org/10.3389/fpsyt .2021.688890

Sun, Y., & Chen, H. (2022). Treatment of circadian rhythm sleep–wake disorders. *Current Neuropharmacology*, 20 (6), 1022–1034. https://doi.org/10.2174/ 1570159X19666210907122933

Case
40

"Just One Kiss"
Sexuality in Long-Term Care

Ms. H was a 78-year-old woman who had been living in a nursing home for two years. Since she was admitted, staff had noticed that Ms. H had tried to invite various male residents to her room and had tried to kiss them or would ask for "just one kiss." A consultant psychiatrist was requested because of the staff's report that Ms. H was "sexually aggressive" toward male residents.

After a detailed interview and input from various staff members, the psychiatrist discovered that the nursing assistants who were involved in caring for Ms. H for the first year and a half had left. The new nursing assistants had just obtained their certifications and were unsure how to deal with Ms. H's SIB. One nursing assistant felt that the behavior was "cute" and "funny" and even giggled when Ms. H exhibited SIB, while another felt the behavior was "abhorrent" and needed to be stopped. In fact, the latter nursing assistant had told Ms. H that she was not behaving like a "lady" and another staff member found Ms. H crying after this exchange.

The "sexually aggressive" behavior that precipitated the consult was that Ms. H had succeeded in getting a male resident into her room and they were found kissing. During the interview, Ms. H was a cheerful woman who asked the psychiatrist to give her "just one kiss." The psychiatrist showed her his wedding ring, but Ms. H responded by stating, "Your wife will not know." The psychiatrist told her that he loved his wife and could not grant Ms. H's wish. The clinician was pleasant and nonjudgmental during the entire interview and shook Ms. H's hand at the end. The psychiatrist spent a lot of time educating the staff caring for Ms. H that her need for sexual gratification was normal, although expressed inappropriately because of her MNCD, and emphasized the importance of being nonjudgmental and the need for a consistent staff approach. The psychiatrist also discussed the role of damage to the frontal lobe or its connections in predisposing the resident to sexually disinhibited behavior.

Over the next eight weeks, Ms. H responded well to a nonjudgmental approach and firm and consistent redirection by all staff. Ms. H was encouraged to hug and hold hands with male residents who liked it (and whose family agreed with such contact) and her SIB became much more manageable. The psychiatrist also met with the director of nursing and administrator and together they decided to have facility-wide in-service training for all staff addressing this topic.

Teaching Points

A significant percentage of older adults remain sexually active [1]. Studies have shown that sexual activity in older adults is associated with better cognitive and mental health and better sleep. Quality of life and general satisfaction may also be adversely affected by the decline in sexual activity with age [2].

The development of MNCDs in patients does not preclude the need for a sexual life but does alter the way love is given and received. The misconception that those with cognitive impairment are asexual is commonly used by caregivers to discourage them from seeking fulfillment of their sexual needs.

Major neurocognitive disorders are a common cause of SIB. Despite the few studies discussing sexual aspects in MNCD, existing reports indicate that up to 25% of patients suffering from Alzheimer's disease have inappropriate sexual behavior, including increased sexual urge and hypersexuality [3,4]. These behaviors can result in increased burden on caregivers and clinicians, increased use of psychotropic medications, increased utilization of healthcare resources, and earlier transition to long-term care facilities [3].

Neurobiological changes in MNCDs may result in a stronger impulse to have sex, decreased sex drive, sexual aggression, anger in response to rejection, or even a complete loss of interest in sexual expression. During the early stages of Alzheimer's disease specifically, the sexual desire frequently increases or, alternatively, there is a complete loss of desire for sexual expression [5].

Dysfunction of various anatomical areas of the brain has been implicated in the neurobiology of inappropriate sexual behavior. Anatomic areas of particular importance in SIB include the frontal lobe, the temporal limbic system, the striatum, and the hypothalamus. Frontal lobe pathology can lead to more disinhibited behaviors such as public exposure or public masturbation. Degeneration of the striatum can be more associated with OCD sexual behaviors. Pathology of the temporal limbic system can lead to increased sexual drive as seen in Kluver–Bucy syndrome. Lesions in the hypothalamus can also be seen in those with hypersexuality [6].

Definitions of SIB in patients with MNCD can vary widely depending on who is asked the question. Definite acts of SIB include making explicit sexual comments, touching someone other than a partner on the breasts or genitals, touching a partner on the breasts or genitals in public, requesting unneeded genital care, and exposing the genitals or breasts in public. More ambiguous demonstrations of SIB can involve being undressed outside of the bedroom or bathroom, seeking out non-genital intimate touch such as kissing or caressing another, or self-touch of genitals through one's clothes [7]. Since there is no widely agreed-upon definition of SIB the distinction is usually based on the judgment of what is normal for a person in a particular situation or on the level of risk or discomfort of others.

Nursing assistants at long-term care facilities are responsible for the brunt of the day-to-day patient care. Despite their importance, they likely receive little instruction on issues relating to mental health in those with MNCD, especially sexuality. Turnover rates are also quite high in many long-term care facilities, which makes education even more challenging. Nursing assistants and other care staff should be made aware via educational opportunities that sexual behavior can increase in those with MNCD due to the following reasons: (1) there is brain dysfunction due to the underlying disease process, (2) there can be disease-related disinhibition of sexual behaviors, (3) normal etiquette can be forgotten in illnesses with cognitive impairment, (4) delusions and hallucinations may impact sexual behavior. Staff should also be informed about social and environmental factors that can play a role in increased SIB. Examples of this include the loss of a

Box 40.1 Questions pertinent in the assessment of a patient's ability to consent to sexual activity in the long-term care setting

1. Is the patient aware of who is initiating sexual contact?
2. Is delusion or misidentification affecting the patient's choice (e.g. is the patient mistaking the other person for their spouse)?
3. Can the patient express what level of sexual intimacy they would be comfortable with?
4. Can the patient avoid exploitation?
5. Is the behavior consistent with previously held beliefs and values?
6. Does the patient have the capacity to say no to uninvited sexual contact?
7. Is the patient aware of potential risks?
8. Does the patient realize that the relationship might be time-limited (e.g. if a placement is temporary)?
9. Can the patient describe how they will react when or if the relationship ends?

usual sexual partner, lack of privacy, an under stimulating environment, and loss of the ability to properly interpret social cues. Staff should also be made aware that certain medications have the potential to increase SIB. Understanding the reasons for SIB can be helpful for those who must deal with these behaviors on a day-to-day basis [7].

There are instances when the sexual expression of long-term care residents should be particularly protected and encouraged. It is not uncommon for a married or partnered couple to room together in an AL or long-term care setting. One or both of the couple can have cognitive challenges. In these situations, it may become important to assess a person's capacity to consent to sexual activity and to possibly reassess capacity should cognition continue to decline [8].

The ability of patients to consent to sexual relations may be underestimated by healthcare staff. Therefore, the issue of capacity to consent to sexual activity is an important point of discussion among staff members and each case should be assessed separately. Some experts recommend assessment of these situations by a geriatrician, an internist experienced in the care of older adults, or a geriatric psychiatrist [9]. The need for expert opinion supports the notion that assessing a patient's capacity to consent to sexual activity can be difficult. Questions pertinent to assessing a patient's ability to consent to sexual activity are shown in Box 40.1.

Take-Home Points

- A significant percentage of older adults remain sexually active. Studies have shown that sexual activity in older adults is associated with better cognitive and mental health and better sleep.
- Major neurocognitive disorders are a common cause of SIB. Despite the few studies discussing the sexual aspects of MNCD, existing reports indicate that up to 25% of patients suffering from Alzheimer's disease have inappropriate sexual behavior, including increased sexual urge and hypersexuality.
- The ability of patients to consent to sexual relations may be underestimated by healthcare staff. Therefore, the issue of consent is an important point of discussion among staff members and each case should be assessed separately.
- Long-term care facilities should have policies in place that address the evaluation of a patient's capacity to consent to sexual activity.

References

1. DeLamater, J. (2012). Sexual expression in later life: A review and synthesis. *Journal of Sex Research*, 49 (2–3), 125–141.

2. Persson, G. (1980). Sexuality in a 70-year-old urban population. *Journal of Psychosomatic Research*, 24 (6), 335–342.

3. Black, B., Muralee, S., & Tampi, R. R. (2005). Inappropriate sexual behaviors in dementia. *Journal of Geriatric Psychiatry and Neurology*, 18 (3), 155–162.

4. Derouesné, C. (2009). The so-called hypersexual behaviors in dementia. *Psychologie & NeuroPsychiatrie du vieillissement*, 7 (2), 101–108.

5. Tabak, N., & Shemesh-Kigli, R. (2006). Sexuality and Alzheimer's disease: Can the two go together? In G. C. Cooper (ed.) *Nursing Forum* (Vol. 41, No. 4) (Malden, USA: Blackwell Publishing Inc.). pp. 158–166.

6. Nordvig, A. S., Goldberg, D. J., Huey, E. D., & Miller, B. L. (2019). The cognitive aspects of sexual intimacy in dementia patients: A neurophysiological review. *Neurocase*, 25 (1–2), 66–74.

7. Series, H., & Dégano, P. (2005). Hypersexuality in dementia. *Advances in Psychiatric Treatment*, 11 (6), 424–431. doi:10.1192/apt.11.6.424

8. Eshmawey, M., Fredouille, J., & Bianchi-Demicheli, F. (2020). Advanced age, cognitive decline and sexuality in healthcare institutions. *Revue Medicale Suisse*, 16 (686), 548–551.

9. Rosen, T., Lachs, M. S., & Pillemer, K. (2010). Sexual aggression between residents in nursing homes: Literature synthesis of an underrecognized problem. *Journal of the American Geriatrics Society*, 58 (10), 1970–1979.

Case

41

"I Don't Feel Well"

Anticholinergic Medications, Incontinence, and Overactive Bladder

Mrs. S was a 72-year-old woman who had multiple chronic medical problems (diabetes for 30 years, hypertension, osteoarthritis, chronic liver disease due to alcoholism, peripheral neuropathy) and recently had right-sided hemiplegia due to stroke. After some initial anxiety and depression upon moving into an AL home, she had been doing well for three months. Mrs. S was a frail, petite woman who had a body mass index of 17. She was taking 12 different medications for her many medical conditions, including 10 mg of amitriptyline for peripheral neuropathic pain and insomnia. For several weeks, Mrs. S had developed urinary frequency and incontinence and was started on oxybutynin 5 mg daily for suspected overactive bladder (OAB). Her urine analysis was negative for infection.

The staff noticed that over five days the resident had become more confused and irritable, had two falls (without injury), and was unable to sleep more than two or three hours at night. The provider recommended discontinuing amitriptyline, but the resident and family refused because she had been taking it for more than 15 years and it had helped her peripheral neuropathy pain and insomnia. A psychiatric consult was obtained.

Mrs. S told the psychiatrist, "I don't feel well," but could not clarify what was bothering her. After the assessment, the psychiatrist recommended discontinuing oxybutynin and following a scheduled toileting program to treat OAB. Over the next 72 hours Mrs. S's delirium resolved, and she was back to her level of functioning before starting oxybutynin.

The psychiatrist then met with the resident and her family, explaining the risk of cognitive impairment with amitriptyline and the potential benefits of alternatives, such as gabapentin or nortriptyline. The family agreed to try switching to gabapentin with the assurance that if it did not help, the resident could restart the amitriptyline. The psychiatrist checked the resident's renal function before she started taking the gabapentin. Her serum creatinine was 1.8, indicating mild chronic kidney disease. Amitriptyline was decreased to 5 mg daily at bedtime for two weeks and then discontinued. Gabapentin was added at 100 mg daily at bedtime and over two weeks increased to 300 mg at bedtime. The resident had mild insomnia for a few days but no increase in peripheral neuropathy pain. To improve sleep, the staff was recommended to encourage Mrs. S to increase physical activity, increase exposure to sunlight, and minimize daytime napping. After two weeks of taking gabapentin, discontinuing amitriptyline, and beginning a regimen of individualized psychosocial–spiritual interventions, Mrs. S felt she was doing "quite well." The staff noticed that her constipation was replaced with mild diarrhea, which resolved once the medications for constipation (docusate sodium and senna) were discontinued.

Teaching Points

Adding an anticholinergic medication such as oxybutynin for a frail resident who is already taking other medications with high anticholinergic activity (amitriptyline in this case) and compromised neurological status (cerebrovascular disease in this case) puts that resident at high risk of drug-induced delirium. Drugs for OAB such as tolterodine and oxybutynin and other anticholinergic drugs (diphenhydramine, hydroxyzine) may precipitate delirium and should be used with great caution in residents who are frail, have pre-existing MNCD, have a history of liver disease, or are taking multiple drugs metabolized through the Cytochrome PCY450 system [1]. A rigorous trial of scheduled toileting should be considered before prescribing drugs for OAB.

Each assessment for change in mental status is also an opportunity to review the resident's medications and reduce the anticholinergic load. Gabapentin has no anticholinergic activity and is a much better choice than amitriptyline for the treatment of peripheral neuropathy in long-term care residents. Because gabapentin is primarily excreted by the kidneys, it is important to start with a low dose in residents who have chronic kidney disease, and a very low dose may be sufficient for a therapeutic response. Additionally, for a resident who has been taking psychiatric medication for a long time, discontinuing such medication is a major decision and may be associated with significant anxiety. Hence, it is important that the healthcare provider discuss the risks of continuing current psychiatric medications and the benefits of safer alternatives before instituting any change. Finally, anticholinergic medications are constipating, and most residents need medication to treat constipation caused by anticholinergic drugs. By reducing the anticholinergic load, the healthcare professional may help residents decrease the need for medication to treat constipation, thus reducing polypharmacy and its harmful consequences.

The commonly encountered issues of urinary incontinence in the older patient population are such that it warrants further discussion here. The prevalence of urinary incontinence in women aged 70 years and older in long-term care settings is estimated to be around 50–80%. The prevalence of urinary incontinence in men over 70 in long-term care settings varies depending on the study and population examined but is thought to be closer to about 45%. Urinary incontinence in older patients can have significant psychiatric implications, including depression, anxiety, social isolation, and decreased quality of life. Incontinence can cause embarrassment, shame, and loss of dignity, leading to feelings of frustration, helplessness, and hopelessness. Nygaard et al. reported that 80% of women with severe urinary incontinence are likely to develop depression compared with 40% of those with mild incontinence [2]. Incontinence can also interfere with daily activities, including work and social engagements, further exacerbating feelings of isolation and depression. Patients with incontinence may become more reliant on caregivers and may experience a loss of autonomy, leading to decreased self-esteem and negative self-image. It is important to address the psychological impact of incontinence in older patients and provide appropriate support and treatment to improve the overall quality of life.

There are six major categories of urinary incontinence. They include stress incontinence, urge incontinence, mixed incontinence, overflow incontinence, functional incontinence, and total incontinence. Stress incontinence occurs when urine leaks due to physical activity such as coughing, sneezing, laughing, or exercising. Urge incontinence

Box 41.1 Causes of urinary incontinence in older adults

1. Weak pelvic floor muscles: Weakening of the muscles that support the bladder and control urine flow is a common cause of urinary incontinence, especially in older adults. This can occur due to factors such as aging, childbirth, hormonal changes (in women), or certain medical conditions.
2. Urinary tract infections: Infections in the urinary tract, such as bladder infections, can irritate the bladder and lead to urinary incontinence.
3. Medications: Certain medications, such as diuretics, sedatives, muscle relaxants, and some antihypertensive medications, can affect bladder control and contribute to urinary incontinence.
4. Neurological conditions: Conditions that affect the nervous system, such as Parkinson's disease, multiple sclerosis, stroke, or spinal cord injuries, can disrupt the nerve signals between the bladder and the brain, leading to urinary incontinence.
5. Benign prostatic hyperplasia (BPH): In men, an enlarged prostate gland, such as occurs in BPH, can obstruct the urinary flow and cause urinary incontinence or urgency.
6. Cognitive impairment: Patients with dementia or cognitive decline may experience difficulties recognizing the need to urinate or finding their way to the bathroom in time, resulting in urinary incontinence.
7. Restricted mobility: Physical limitations, such as mobility impairment or musculoskeletal conditions, can make it challenging for geriatric patients to reach the bathroom quickly, leading to urinary incontinence.
8. Chronic constipation: Chronic constipation can put pressure on the bladder and lead to urinary incontinence or OAB symptoms.
9. Chronic diseases: Certain chronic conditions, such as diabetes, obesity, cardiovascular diseases, or COPD can contribute to urinary incontinence.

involves a sudden and strong urge to urinate, followed by an involuntary loss of urine. It may be caused by OAB or other neurological conditions. Mixed incontinence is a combination of stress and urge incontinence. Overflow incontinence happens when the bladder does not empty completely and leads to constant dribbling of urine. Functional incontinence occurs when physical or cognitive impairment makes it difficult for a person to reach the bathroom in time. Finally, total incontinence refers to the continuous and total loss of urinary control, which may result from a congenital abnormality or injury.

The differential diagnosis of urinary incontinence in older adults is broad. Box 41.1 includes a list of potential causes [3].

The workup of incontinence in older adults can be time-consuming, inconvenient, and costly. The most basic and practical workup includes a complete history, physical exam, medication review, and urinalysis. Those in long-term care often have significant logistic barriers to seeing a urologist in an outpatient setting for a more complete workup that might include urodynamics and cystoscopy. For this reason, it is not uncommon to see patients affected with incontinence trialed on one of the medications that are approved for OAB in lieu of a full urologic workup to evaluate for other types of incontinence.

Overactive bladder and its treatment are often encountered by those treating older adults in long-term care. The definition of OAB by the International Continence Society describes it as the presence of urinary urgency, with or without urgency urinary incontinence, often accompanied by frequency and nocturia, without any apparent underlying UTI or other visible abnormalities. There are two general classes of medications used to treat OAB. These include antimuscarinic (anticholinergic) agents such as oxybutynin and tolterodine and beta-3 adrenergic agonists such as mirabegron and vibegron. Antimuscarinic agents block muscarinic receptor stimulation by acetylcholine and reduce smooth muscle contraction of the bladder. The beta-3 adrenergic agonists work by stimulating the receptors in the bladder responsible for smooth muscle relaxation [4]. Antimuscarinic agents are often prescribed first as they are inexpensive, and physicians tend to be well-versed in their use. However, their use comes at a different cost. As with most anticholinergic medications, side effects of antimuscarinics include dry mouth, constipation, blurred vision, sedation, and confusion. For this reason, they are included on the Beers list (a list of medications known to be potentially harmful for use in older adults). The beta-3 adrenergic agents are preferred as they are not anticholinergic and are not included on the Beers list [1].

It is recommended to attempt a trial of bladder training before initiating medication in patients with suspected OAB, the purpose of which is to help individuals regain control over their bladder function by improving the bladder's ability to store urine and reducing the urge to urinate frequently. This is accomplished through various techniques, including timed voiding, delaying urination when the urge to urinate arises, and increasing the time between bathroom breaks. The goal of bladder training is to increase the amount of urine the bladder can hold, reduce the frequency of urination, and improve the individual's quality of life [5].

Take-Home Points

— Drugs for OAB such as tolterodine and oxybutynin and other anticholinergic drugs (diphenhydramine, hydroxyzine) may precipitate delirium and should be used with great caution in frail residents, those with pre-existing MNCD, those with a history of liver disease, or those who are taking multiple drugs metabolized through the Cytochrome PCY450 system.
— Urinary incontinence in older patients can have significant psychiatric implications, including depression, anxiety, social isolation, and decreased quality of life.
— There are six major categories of urinary incontinence. They include stress incontinence, urge incontinence, mixed incontinence, overflow incontinence, functional incontinence, and total incontinence.
— There are two general classes of medications used to treat OAB. These include antimuscarinic (anticholinergic) agents such as oxybutynin and tolterodine and beta-3 adrenergic agonists such as mirabegron and vibegron. The beta-3 adrenergic agents are preferred as they are not anticholinergic and are not included on the Beers list.

References

1. American Geriatrics Society. (2023). Updated AGS Beers Criteria® for potentially inappropriate medication use in older adults. *Journal of the American Geriatrics Society*, 71 (7), 2052–2081. https://doi.org/10.1111/jgs.18372

2. Nygaard, I., Turvey, C., Burns, T. L., Crischilles, E., & Wallace, R. (2003). Urinary incontinence and depression in middle-aged United States women. *Obstetrics & Gynecology*, 101 (1), 149–156.

3. Batmani, S., Jalali, R., Mohammadi, M., & Bokaee, S. (2021). Prevalence and factors

related to urinary incontinence in older adult women worldwide: A comprehensive systematic review and meta-analysis of observational studies. *BMC Geriatrics*, 21 (1), 212. doi: 10.1186/s12877-021-02135-8. Erratum in: BMC Geriatr. 2022 May 25;22(1):454. PMID: 33781236; PMCID: PMC8008630.

4. Andersson, K. E. (2017). On the site and mechanism of action of β3-adrenoceptor agonists in the bladder. *International Neurourology Journal*, 21 (1), 6–11. doi: 10.5213/inj.1734850.425. PMID: 28361520; PMCID: PMC5380826.

5. InformedHealth.org [Internet]. Cologne, Germany: Institute for Quality and Efficiency in Health Care (IQWiG); 2006-. Bladder training. 2013 Nov 12 [Updated 2016 Dec 30]. Available from: www.ncbi.nlm.nih.gov/books/NBK279430/

Further Reading

Corcos, J., Przydacz, M., Campeau, L., Witten, J., Hickling, D., Honeine, C., Radomski, S. B., Stothers, L., & Wagg, A. (2017). CUA guideline on adult overactive bladder. *Canadian Urological Association Journal*, 11 (5), E142. https://doi.org/10.5489/cuaj.4586

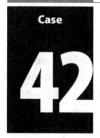

"I Like Food"

Binge Eating Disorder

Mr. W was an 81-year-old resident living in an AL home for two years. He was doing well, taking 10 mg daily escitalopram for the treatment of MDD-like symptoms and anxiety symptoms secondary to MNCD due to Alzheimer's disease. Over two years he gained 50 pounds, and in the last three months he gained 14 pounds (for a final BMI of 42), primarily due to a sedentary lifestyle and excessive eating during and between meals.

Mr. W had struggled with obesity for most of his life and intermittently went to Weight Watchers to reduce weight and eat healthier. However, due to Alzheimer's disease, he had stopped going to Weight Watchers. A psychiatrist was consulted, as Mr. W had become irritable, had expressed feeling "upset" about gaining weight, and his wife felt his depression was coming back and antidepressants should be adjusted. The psychiatrist found Mr. W to be sociable but upset about his weight gain.

Mr. W told the psychiatrist, "I like food." Certain other pertinent facts came out while taking a thorough history from the patient, his family, and staff. Mr. W was often found to have rather large collections of candy, packaged baked goods, sodas, and salty snacks under his bed. He was found by staff several times per week in bed, surrounded by crumbs, empty soda cans, and wrappers. This would usually happen several times per week. On a couple of occasions, Mr. W had eaten so much that he became ill and vomited. He became defensive and irritable when staff attempted to discuss these behaviors with him. Mr. W's wife admitted that she would regularly bring in goodies for her husband but she felt the amounts were fairly modest (one or two boxes of snack cakes or bags of chips per week). The staff mentioned that the patient would also regularly visit the snack area of the facility and use food found there to add to his under-the-bed collection.

Mrs. W revealed that Mr. W had experienced a complex relationship with food for most of his adult life and said he had always been "a big man". When he was younger, he was well known to consume large quantities of food and to frequent buffet restaurants alone, eating to the point of being quite uncomfortable. He would later feel guilty for this and become depressed, irritable, and socially withdrawn. He started his career as an attorney with great promise, but the stress involved with success and advancing responsibilities would often trigger more dysfunctional eating behavior. Eventually, the patient's weight became such that it interfered with his ability to go to work, and he worked more at home. This hindered his career advancement.

The psychiatrist shared with Mr. W, his wife, and staff that he did not think antidepressants needed to be adjusted. They recommended a program of exercise (five minutes of strength training and 15 minutes of assisted ambulation daily) and nutritional strategies. Nutritional strategies involved a portion-controlled diet (smaller portions given during the three meals), replacing consumption of unhealthy snacks (crackers, candy, ice cream) with fruits and vegetables Mr. W liked (blueberries, mangoes, carrots, celery with a vegetable dip), and replacing intake of soda with diet soda and water.

Mr. W's wife was encouraged to bring in healthier snack options for her husband. Interventions to help add patient-specific enjoyable activities were helpful as well since boredom was thought to be a trigger for his dysfunctional eating. Weekly supportive psychotherapy was initiated to further explore Mr. M's emotional triggers for eating and to help him with more productive strategies to deal with them.

Mr. W initially resisted this change in diet but, with the staff's support and his wife's encouragement, he acquiesced. Over the next eight weeks, not only did Mr. W lose four pounds, he also seemed to have more energy, started getting out of the chair on his own (previously he needed one-person assistance to do this), and began walking around the facility. Staff also noticed that Mr. W seemed to carry on longer conversations and showed less irritability.

Teaching Points

For some residents who are obese, simple nutritional changes with a modest increase in physical activity and lots of support and encouragement can lead not only to modest but significant weight loss and also improvement in mood and function.

Eating disorders are complex chronic medical conditions that have both psychological and medical consequences. They are characterized by abnormal eating behaviors that can lead to significant morbidity and even mortality. Well-characterized eating disorders that are described in the DSM–5–TR include anorexia nervosa, binge eating disorder, and restrictive/avoidant food intake disorder, among others. Eating disorders are more commonly thought of as affecting younger adults but they can also occur or continue in older adults [1].

The case here depicts a patient with binge eating disorder. The DSM–5–TR diagnostic criteria for binge eating disorder are presented in Box 42.1[2].

There is relatively little research focusing on eating disorders in older adults and they may be easily overlooked. Stigmas associated with eating disorders and age-related misconceptions might contribute to underreporting and underdiagnosis of eating disorders in older adults. Studies have estimated that between 1.8 and 3.8% of women over the age of 60 have indications of an eating disorder [1]. It is known that the most common eating disorder in older adults is anorexia nervosa. Binge eating disorder is less common, being reported by 0.6–1.8% of women and 0.3–0.7% of men [3].

The pathophysiology of binge eating disorder involves both biological and psychological factors. Just as in substance use disorders, dysregulation in neurocircuitry related to reward and emotional processing might contribute to the development and maintenance of binge eating behavior. Neurotransmitters such as dopamine, which are involved in pleasure and reward, might be implicated in the compulsive nature of binge eating. Neuroimaging studies have shown hyperactivity of the medial orbitofrontal cortex and hypoactivity in the prefrontal network in individuals with binge eating disorder. One theory suggests that people exhibiting elevated impulsiveness and heightened responsiveness to rewards can develop addictive-like reactions to specific foods, such as those rich in sugar and fats. This can contribute to and maintain binge eating behaviors [4].

Diagnosing binge eating disorder is largely through a comprehensive history. Clinicians should ask about the age of onset of binge eating episodes, frequency of

---

Box 42.1 DSM–5–TR criteria for the diagnosis of binge eating disorder

1. Recurrent episodes of binge eating. An episode of binge eating is characterized by both of the following:

   a. Eating, in a discrete period of time (e.g. within any two-hour period), an amount of food that is definitely larger than what most people would eat in a similar period of time under similar circumstances.

   b. A lack of control when eating during the episode (e.g. a feeling that one cannot stop eating or control what or how much one is eating).

2. The binge eating episodes are associated with three (or more) of the following:

   a. Eating much more rapidly than normal.
   b. Eating until feeling uncomfortably full.
   c. Eating large amounts of food when not feeling physically hungry.
   d. Eating alone because of feeling embarrassed by how much one is eating.
   e. Feeling disgusted with oneself, depressed, or very guilty afterward.

3. Marked distress regarding binge eating is present.
4. Binge eating occurs, on average, at least once a week for three months.
5. Binge eating is not associated with the recurrent use of inappropriate compensatory behavior as in bulimia nervosa and does not occur exclusively during the course of bulimia nervosa or anorexia nervosa.

Specify if:

In partial remission: After full criteria for binge eating disorder were previously met, binge eating occurs at an average frequency of less than one episode per week for a sustained period of time.

In full remission: After full criteria for binge eating disorder were previously met, none of the criteria have been met for a sustained period of time.

Specify current severity: The minimum level of severity is based on the frequency of episodes of binge eating. The level of severity may be increased to reflect other symptoms and the degree of functional disability.

Mild: 1–3 binge eating episodes per week.
Moderate: 4–7 binge eating episodes per week.
Severe: 8–13 binge eating episodes per week.
Extreme: 14 or more binge eating episodes per week.

---

episodes, amounts of food consumed, emotions associated with the behavior, comorbid medical problems, potential triggers for the behavior, history of substance abuse, and family history of binge eating.

Pharmacologic treatment options for binge eating disorder have provided disappointing results. Comorbid mood and anxiety disorders are more common in this population and treatment of these conditions may produce related improvements in comorbid eating disorders. Cognitive behavioral therapy and interventions focused on behavioral weight loss have been shown to be effective in reducing the frequency and severity of binge eating episodes [5].

In the case here, Mr. W responded well to behavioral-focused techniques and emotional support, with the family encouraged to provide healthier options for snacks. Boredom was thought to be a significant trigger for Mr. W's binge eating so individualized interventions were focused on finding frequent and engaging activities for him to participate in.

The long-term outlook for older adults with binge eating disorder will usually include periodic setbacks or relapses. Individualized efforts to prevent relapses should focus on identifying and mitigating triggers of emotional eating. Areas of future research may involve medications with newer indications for the treatment of obesity such as injectable GLP-1 agonists that increase the feeling of satiety, delay gastric emptying, and may inhibit the pleasurable feedback mechanisms that contribute to dysfunctional behaviors in those with binge eating disorder [6].

Ethical challenges can present themselves in dealing with those with eating disorders in the long-term care setting. Patients have as much right to engage in legal, albeit self-destructive, behaviors as those outside of long-term care. An overly paternalistic approach to the treatment of those in long-term care can undermine a resident's right to autonomy, dignity, and self-determination. A patient such as Mr. W should not be disallowed access to foods that are central to his dysfunctional eating. A better approach is to give Mr. W and his family/caregivers the best biopsychosocial support to encourage him to make better choices for himself.

In past decades it was commonplace for patients to be placed on restrictive diets by their healthcare providers in the long-term care setting. Very restrictive diets are generally contraindicated in older adults. These include salt-free diets for those with hypertension or CHF, no-sugar diets for diabetics, low-fat diets for hyperlipidemia, and very low-protein diets for those with chronic kidney disease. These restrictive diets are often so unpalatable as to risk malnutrition. Nutritional goals in long-term care patients should be a well-balanced diet with a good balance of macro and micronutrients. Also, patients should generally not be disallowed their favorite foods when in the final stage of life.

Take-Home Points

- Eating disorders are complex chronic medical conditions that have both psychological and medical consequences. They are characterized by abnormal eating behaviors that can lead to significant morbidity and even mortality.
- The pathophysiology of binge eating disorder involves both biological and psychological factors. Just as in substance use disorders, dysregulation in neurocircuitry related to reward and emotional processing might contribute to the development and maintenance of binge eating behavior.
- Pharmacologic treatment options for binge eating disorder have provided disappointing results. Comorbid mood and anxiety disorders are more common in this population and treatment of these conditions may produce related improvements in comorbid eating disorders.
- Ethical challenges can present themselves in dealing with those with eating disorders in the long-term care setting. Patients have as much right to engage in legal, albeit self-destructive, behaviors as those outside of long-term care.

References

1. Mulchandani, M., Shetty, N., Conrad, A., Muir, P., & Mah, B. (2021). Treatment of eating disorders in older people: A systematic review. *Systematic Reviews*, 10 (1), 1–20.

2. American Psychiatric Association. (2022). *Diagnostic and Statistical Manual of Mental Disorders*. 5th ed. text rev. (American Psychiatric Association.)

3. Keski-Rahkonen, A. (2021). Epidemiology of binge eating disorder: Prevalence, course, comorbidity, and risk factors. *Current Opinion in Psychiatry*, 34 (6), 525–531.

4. Schulte, E. M., Grilo, C. M., & Gearhardt, A. N. (2016). Shared and unique mechanisms underlying binge eating disorder and addictive disorders. *Clinical Psychology Review*, 44, 125–139.

5. Grilo, C. M., Reas, D. L. & Mitchell, J. E. (2016). Combining pharmacological and psychological treatments for binge eating disorder: Current status, limitations, and future directions. *Current Psychiatry Reports*, 18, 55.

6. McElroy, S. L., Mori, N., Guerdjikova, A. I., & Keck, P. E. (2018). Would glucagon-like peptide-1 receptor agonists have efficacy in binge eating disorder and bulimia nervosa? A review of the current literature. *Medical Hypotheses*, 111, 90–93. https://doi.org/10.1016/j.mehy.2017.12.029

Further Reading

Atwood, M. E., & Friedman, A. (2020). A systematic review of enhanced cognitive behavioral therapy (CBT-E) for eating disorders. *International Journal of Eating Disorders*, 53 (3), 311–330.

Dingemans, A., Danner, U., & Parks, M. (2017). Emotion regulation in binge eating disorder: A review. *Nutrients*, 9 (11).

Hay, P. (2020). Current approach to eating disorders: A clinical update. *Internal Medicine Journal*, 50 (1), 24–29.

Samuels, K. L., Maine, M. M., & Tantillo, M. (2019). Disordered eating, eating disorders, and body image in midlife and older women. *Current Psychiatry Reports*, 21, 1–9.

"I Like the Way She Laughs"

43 Sexuality in Long-Term Care

Mr. T, a resident of a long-term care facility for 12 months, was increasingly depressed because his wife had reduced the frequency of her visits to once a week and would visit for only a few minutes. His wife reported that visiting him was too depressing, as he was not the active and intelligent person she married. Over time, Mr. T lost weight and stopped going to group activity programs he previously attended.

He was about to be put on an antidepressant when his mood started to improve. He began eating better, started taking part in activities, and seemed to be genuinely happy. This was because Mr. T had developed a friendship with a female resident and they would spend several hours per day together, watching TV or sharing stories. When asked what he liked about this new friend, Mr. T replied, "I like the way she laughs."

Mr. T had documented moderately advanced MNCD, mixed type – Alzheimer's and vascular. His last SLUMS exam score was 19/30 and was performed three months prior. His medical comorbidities included mild CHF, well-controlled Type 2 diabetes, and hypertension. His history of falls and nighttime wandering triggered his admission to long-term care one year before.

Mrs. T and the patient's daughter attended a monthly care plan meeting virtually. The long-term care facility staff at the meeting also included the director of nursing, administrator, and social worker. Mr. T's improved mental health was discussed. Both Mrs. T and the patient's daughter were clearly shocked and upset when they found out that Mr. T had taken up a presumed romantic relationship with another resident at the facility. They were also angered by the fact that this situation was allowed to happen. The social worker pointed out that, even though Mr. T had dementia and needed support with several ADLs, he still had the same emotional needs for closeness and intimacy that he had prior to his admission to the long-term care environment. It was also pointed out that the relationship between Mr. T and his new romantic interest was mutual and consensual and that they both had the ability to voice and act on their wishes to continue in the relationship. The relationship was not clearly intimate physically beyond sitting closely together and hand-holding but should they express the desire for this the facility was required to honor their right to privacy and dignity.

At the next care plan meeting Mrs. T and her daughter were present again and inquired about the relationship between Mr. T and his new companion. The facility staff told his family that the two appeared to be continuing to enjoy each other's company and they could nearly always be found together. The family of Mr. T's girlfriend was very happy that she had found companionship and love when she previously seemed sad and lonely.

Mrs. T and her daughter expressed that, after many conversations and time, they felt more comfortable with the fact that Mr. T had a romantic relationship outside of his marriage that added comfort and meaning where there was loneliness and boredom before.

Teaching Points

This case illustrates the power of friendship, attachment, and intimacy in healing emotional pain. It also illustrates the resiliency of Mr. T (and many other residents) in the face of overwhelming adversity.

The topic of sexuality and sexual expression within the context of long-term care is complex. Medical providers, administrators, nursing staff, and social workers should all be familiar with the basics when it comes to matters of sexuality in the long-term care facility.

It is a misconception that the need for physical intimacy and sexual expression declines with age. Although normal biological changes that occur with age can lead to declining libido, the inner drive for physical and emotional connection will often remain in older adults indefinitely.

The prevalence of loneliness in long-term care is high despite the large number of interpersonal interactions possible on a given day between patients, their co-residents, and care staff. Loneliness is a function of both the number and depth of human relationships. The depth and quality of connection of an older adult with a romantic partner in the long-term care setting can lead to a huge boost in quality of life.

The rights of residents of long-term care facilities are clearly stated in the Code of Federal Regulations (CFR) section 483.10. The CFR is a set of regulations that govern various aspects of healthcare, including nursing homes and long-term care facilities, in the United States. Some of these rights guaranteed to residents of long-term care facilities include the right to dignity and respect, the right to make one's own choices including the right to refuse medical treatment, the right to privacy and confidentiality, the right to freedom from abuse and restraints, the right to have visitors of their choice, and the right to participate in care planning, among others.

Although the CFR is updated every year it does not specifically address matters of rights to sexual expression in the long-term care setting. However, Appendix PP in the CFR does and is also updated regularly. This document states, "Residents have the right to engage in consensual sexual activity. However, any time the facility has reason to suspect that a resident may not have the capacity to consent to sexual activity, the facility must take steps to ensure that the resident is protected from abuse. These steps should include evaluating whether the resident has the capacity to consent to sexual activity."

The concept of capacity is key to the discussion of sexual activity in older adults in the long-term care setting. Evaluating a person's capacity to consent to sexual activity is key to ensuring the safety of residents from sexual abuse or exploitation. Capacity is not a blanket determination but is situational. For instance, the capacity to understand and evaluate the complexities of estate planning necessary to guide one's financial affairs may be lacking when the capacity for entering a romantic or sexual relationship remains. Also, there can be no surrogate decision-maker when it comes to consent for sexual activity. Universally accepted criteria for the capacity to consent to sexual activity are lacking and legal criteria vary state by state.

Individual long-term care facilities should have clearly stated policies involving sexuality that address a resident's capacity to consent to consensual physical contact of a sexual nature. Some important questions to be addressed are shown in Box 43.1 [1].

Box 43.1 Important questions to be asked when assessing a patient's capacity to consent to sexual activity in the long-term care setting

1. Recognition. Can both parties in the relationship consistently recognize their potential sexual partner? Or, is the person in question mistaking the potential sexual partner for another individual (as can sometimes happen in MNCD)?
2. Is there a sign of interest in sexual activity from both parties of the relationship? Do both parties have the ability to communicate said interest?
3. Is there the ability to communicate needs or emotions by both parties either verbally or nonverbally?
4. Does each party in the relationship have the ability to express the level of relationship desired (friendship, companionship, romantic intimacy)?
5. Does each person in the relationship retain the ability to communicate unwanted physical or sexual contact?
6. Does each person in the relationship retain the ability to recall recent prior sexual encounters to the degree necessary to proceed with potential future encounters free of fear of abuse?
7. Effect on quality of life. Does the relationship appear to improve the quality of life of both parties involved?
8. Is the potential relationship free of concern for exploitation of either person by the other?

The challenges of family involvement in situations concerning intimate relationships among residents in long-term care are real. Family members may need time to adjust to their loved one forming a new romantic relationship, especially if they were in a long-term marriage or partnership before entering the nursing home. This adjustment can involve mixed emotions, including happiness for the resident's newfound companionship and concern about the potential impact on the existing family dynamic. It can also be difficult for families to understand and respect the privacy and other boundaries of the resident in the new relationship. Families may need guidance when communicating their concerns about a new relationship to their loved one. They may have concerns over the perceived undue influence of the new partner in matters of family dynamics, finances, or health decisions. Cultural and religious beliefs can influence the family dynamics of a developing new relationship. The depth and breadth of complicating an established family dynamic with a new relationship may be such that the help of a professional counselor or psychologist may be of significant benefit.

Education of staff is important for providing appropriate and patient-centered responses to new relationships in the long-term care setting. Providers are often engaged to educate staff in formal and informal ways. Long-term care communities should include education on the rights of residents including rights specific to romantic relationships and awareness of potential abuse situations as part of their comprehensive new staff training. Staff need to be regularly reminded of the rights of privacy and dignity of each resident. Management personnel with a higher knowledge of concepts and policies involving sexual expression in the long-term care setting should be readily available for questions or concerns.

Rarely, situations may arise involving sexual contact between residents that are unplanned or unknown to providers and staff at long-term care facilities. Facilities must adequately investigate and report these occurrences when there is any suspicion of non-consensual sexual activity. A resident's consent to engage in sexual activity is invalid if it is obtained from a resident lacking the capacity to consent, or if consent is obtained through intimidation, coercion, or fear. Any forced, coerced, or extorted sexual activity with a resident, regardless of the existence of a pre-existing or current sexual relationship, is considered to be sexual abuse. A facility is required to investigate and protect a resident from non-consensual sexual relations any time the facility has reason to suspect that the resident does not wish to engage in sexual activity or may not have the capacity to consent. If voluntary sexual activity has occurred between two individuals in the long-term care setting with the capacity to consent to that sexual activity, no abuse has occurred and efforts should be made to ensure privacy and dignity for the residents going forward.

The presence of companionship, emotional connection, and potential physical intimacy that comes with a romantic partnership in later life can inject joy and meaning into the lives of older adults. These relationships should be respected and protected in those patients who are cognitively able to safely participate.

Take-Home Points

— Older adults retain the need for physical and emotional intimacy far into their later years despite the presence of cognitive impairment.
— The capacity to consent to sexual activity is possible for residents who are able to correctly recognize a potential partner, express interest in sexual activity, communicate needs and wants either verbally or nonverbally, and communicate a lack of desire for sexual contact.
— The involvement of families in discussions of romantic relationships in the long-term care setting can be challenging but is improved by education and experience on behalf of providers and staff.
— Federal regulations regarding long-term care facilities indicate that residents have the right to engage in consensual sexual activity if they have the capacity to consent.

References

1. American Bar Association Commission on Law and Aging/American Psychological Association. (2008). *Assessment of Older Adults with Diminished Capacity: A Handbook for Psychologists.* www.apa.org/pi/aging/programs/assessment/capacity-psychologist-handbook.pdf

Further Reading

Esmail, S., & Concannon, B. (2022). Approaches to determine and manage sexual consent abilities for people with cognitive disabilities: Systematic review. *Interactive Journal of Medical Research,* 11 (1). https://doi.org/10.2196/28137

Jackson, S. E., Firth, J., Veronese, N., Stubbs, B., Koyanagi, A., Yang, L., & Smith, L. (2019). Decline in sexuality and wellbeing in older adults: A population-based study. *Journal of Affective Disorders,* 245, 912–917.

Lichtenberg, P. A. (2014). Sexuality and physical intimacy in long-term care: Sexuality, long-term care, capacity assessment. *Occupational Therapy in Health Care,* 28 (1), 42. https://doi.org/10.3109/07380577.2013.865858

Smith, L., Yang, L., Veronese, N., Soysal, P., Stubbs, B., & Jackson, S. E. (2019). Sexual activity is associated with greater enjoyment of life in older adults. *Sexual Medicine,* 7 (1), 11–18.

Srinivasan, S., Glover, J., Tampi, R. R., Tampi, D. J., & Sewell, D. D. (2019). Sexuality and the older adult. *Current Psychiatry Reports,* 21, 1–9.

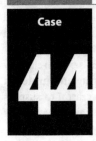

Case

44

"This Is So Hard"
Caring for the Caregiver

Mr. L, the 90-year-old husband of Mrs. L, an 85-year-old woman who had advanced MNCD, commented during an interview with Mrs. L's physician, "My wife is there, but she is not there. She needs a wheelchair now and her speech is almost gone. She recognizes me by face at times but calls me 'Dad' when she says a few words that I can make sense of. She is starting to be combative. This is so hard. I find myself getting angry even though I know that it is her disease that makes her behave this way. Then I get depressed. This is so unlike her."

The psychiatrist treating Mrs. L provided emotional support to Mr. L, suggesting that he see a social worker or therapist who specializes in helping spouses adjust to MNCD in their loved one. Mr. L was reluctant but agreed after his daughter promised to accompany him on the first visit to the social worker. After several weekly meetings with the social worker, Mr. L gradually felt less guilty, was able to express his grief and loss, and learned ways to make his visits with his wife meaningful and even fun at times. He also started attending spousal support groups run by the local chapter of the Alzheimer's Association. Mr. L resumed his regular exercise program at a local health club after the psychiatrist indicated that, if he keeps himself physically healthy, he would better be able to support his wife emotionally through her journey with MNCD. Mr. L also became more mindful of "little" gifts from his wife, such as her breaking into a big smile when she saw him approach.

Teaching Points

The devastating effects of MNCDs on those afflicted with them are the focus of a major portion of this book. They experience loss of physical health, loss of mental health, and sadly a gradual loss of personality and self. We who care for those with MNCDs understand that care must be provided, not only to the patients suffering from MNCD but also to those who care for them. Primary caregivers play a pivotal role in the lives of those with MNCD by providing essential support and assistance. The demands of the role can lead to significant stress, adversely affecting the caregiver's physical, psychological, and financial well-being. Addressing the grief and stress of a family caregiver can have the added benefit of improving the emotional well-being of a resident in long-term care.

Caregivers of those with MNCDs may have a multitude of responsibilities. These can include, but may not be limited to, assisting with ADLs, providing emotional support, overseeing medication and medical care, and looking after a loved one's financial interests, all while balancing their own needs. Caregiving often becomes increasingly demanding as the disease process progresses and caregivers may experience physical demands related to their role. Earlier in the course of the disease caregivers will often gradually assume full responsibility for the major activities of the household, including cooking, shopping and meal planning, financial planning, and managing medical care and appointments. This can leave a caregiver with less and less time for self-care. Later in the course of the disease, caregivers may be responsible for providing or overseeing care involving even basic ADLs such as bathing, feeding, and mobility.

The source of caregiver stress can include the physical and practical demands of caregiving. The physical demands often lead primary caregivers to seek outside help in the home or may necessitate a move to a long-term care facility. The emotional and behavioral manifestations of advancing neurocognitive disorders can be distressing to caregivers. Those who provide care or care oversight can experience social isolation as much of their time is spent in the care of their loved ones. This can lead to loneliness, anxiety, and depression. Caregivers may experience financial stressors related to the care of their loved one in the form of lost wages due to caregiving responsibilities or paying for expensive in-home or out-of-home care. Some caregivers may lack sufficient support from family and friends and the strain of an uncertain future can also weigh heavily on their minds.

Providing excellent direct medical care and mental healthcare to seniors with MNCDs is invaluable. However, those who provide medical care to those with MNCDs should become familiar enough with outside resources to offer guidance to caregivers. A list of terms applicable to the resources available for advancing care needs of those with MNCD is presented here.

- **Senior apartments.** Communities generally for those 55 and over or with disabilities that may have very limited on-site services such as group transportation or a senior social worker to help with some ADLs. Rent is often subsidized or income-based. Senior apartments are appropriate for those with no cognitive impairment to mild cognitive impairment. Cost=$
- **Independent living.** Communities for seniors that provide additional services such as meals and transportation. Often comes with the option of privately paid ADL assistance from home health aides. Appropriate for those with no cognitive impairment to mild or moderate MNCD. Cost=$$
- **Residential care homes.** Facilities that provide care to those with MNCD are more home-like and tend to have a higher caregiver-to-resident ratio. Usually for those with moderate to severe MNCD. Cost=$$$
- **Assisted living.** Communities for seniors that provide meals, some transportation, activities, medication oversight and administration, and usually some licensed practical nurse or registered nurse care oversight. May provide specialized memory care units for those with MNCDs. Appropriate for those with no cognitive impairment to advanced MNCD. Cost: $$$
- **Continuing care retirement communities.** Ascribe to the concept of "age in place". The facilities provide care to seniors of all levels of disability from independent to long-term care. Seniors can move up or down the levels of care as necessary depending on care needs. Cost=$$$$
- **Long-term care.** Communities for those who need assistance with multiple basic ADLs. Full medication management is provided. On-site physician and nursing care.

Registered nurse or licensed practical nurse care oversight is provided 24/7. Appropriate for those with no cognitive impairment to those with advanced MNCD. Cost=$-$$$$ (depending on Medicaid eligibility)

- **Respite care.** Short-term care is provided in a long-term care or AL facility for those who usually live at home. Useful for providing care needs when a caregiver needs a break or temporary assistance. Appropriate for those with no cognitive impairment to those with advanced MNCD depending on facility. Cost $$$
- **Home care.** Services are usually provided in the home setting and paid for at an hourly rate. Services can be for as little as several hours per week to 24/7 in-home care. Appropriate for those with mild to late stage MNCD. Cost=$-$$$$
- **Hospice care.** Provided in private homes, independent living, AL, and long-term care settings. Provides additional care and supplies/services tailored to those with terminal illness, including those with end-stage MNCDs. Cost=n/a. Medicare-funded service.

The options for care settings and levels of support are many and differences between them can be nuanced. For this reason, it may be helpful to involve a professional to guide caregivers in these decisions. Agencies exist that are able to provide advice and guidance to caregivers from licensed clinical social workers who specialize in geriatric care.

There are several other ways that providers can assist caregivers in optimizing their quality of life. Many cities and towns have support groups for caregivers of those with dementia. The Alzheimer's Association has multiple chapters and a very helpful website offering links to resources for caregivers. Providers can also provide referrals to local therapists or counselors who may be experienced in assisting caregivers through the challenges inherent in having a loved one with MNCD. Caregivers may also ask providers for referrals to legal counsel to assist with legal issues related to the care of seniors with MNCD.

Providers are in a position to care for partners by providing advice on how best to optimize time spent with a loved one in long-term care. Some suggestions to offer loved ones are listed here.

1. Be aware of your body language. Interactions with your partner in long-term care should be calm and pleasant. Those with dementia can sense and may mirror your emotional state.
2. Limit distractions. Visits with your partner are best in areas of the facility that are quiet, peaceful, and relatively free from distractions.
3. Discuss pleasant, shared memories with your partner. Patients with MNCD may be able to remember their younger years well into the moderate stages of their disease.
4. Speak slowly and clearly. Try not to raise your voice if frustrated with a lack of understanding on the part of your partner. Try to calmly rephrase statements or move on.
5. When asking questions of your partner with MNCD, try to stick to questions that are easily answered such as yes/no type questions. Open-ended questions or questions with multiple potential answers can seem overwhelming to those with dementia.
6. It may be best to distract your partner with a new topic or a new environment if your partner becomes agitated.

Take-Home Points

- Health providers of those with MNCD are in a unique position to provide support to primary caregivers who may be struggling with the many responsibilities of being a primary caregiver.
- Be sensitive to the presence of potential caregiver stress. Offer suggestions to caregivers that may assist in better interactions with their loved one with MNCD.
- Become familiar with the various support resources and supported living environments available to those with MNCD. Having a connection with a social worker or geriatric case manager can be helpful as a referral source for those families that may need more extensive assistance in planning for care needs.
- Be familiar with and ready to refer family members of those with MNCD to local support groups such as the Alzheimer's Association for ongoing caregiver support.
- Have a couple of book recommendations on hand that may offer assistance to caregivers such as *The 36-Hour Day: A Family Guide to Caring for People Who Have Alzheimer's Disease and other Dementias* or *What to Do Between the Tears: A Practical Gide to Dealing with a Dementia or Alzheimer's Diagnosis in the Family.*

Further Reading

Baharudin, A. D., Din, N. C., Subramaniam, P., & Razali, R. (2019). The associations between behavioral-psychological symptoms of dementia (BPSD) and coping strategy, burden of care and personality style among low-income caregivers of patients with dementia. *BMC Public Health*, 19 (Suppl 4).

Boucher, A., Haesebaert, J., Freitas, A., Adekpedjou, R., Landry, M., Bourassa, H., Stacey, D., Croteau, J., Geneviève, G., & Légaré, F. (2019). Time to move? Factors associated with burden of care among informal caregivers of cognitively impaired older people facing housing decisions: Secondary analysis of a cluster randomized trial. *BMC Geriatrics*, 19.

Gérain, P., & Zech, E. (2019). Informal caregiver burnout? Development of a theoretical framework to understand the impact of caregiving. *Frontiers in Psychology*, 10. https://doi.org/10.3389/fpsyg.2019.01748

Koca, E., Taşkapilioğlu, Ö., & Bakar, M. (2017). Caregiver burden in different stages of Alzheimer's disease. *Archives of Neuropsychiatry*, 54 (1), 82–86.

Martin-Cook, K., Trimmer, C., Svetlik, D., & Weiner, M. (2000). Caregiver burden in Alzheimer's disease: Case studies. *American Journal of Alzheimer's Disease*, 15 (1), 47–52.

Vu, M., Mangal, R., Stead, T., Lopez-Ortiz, C., & Ganti, L. (2022). Impact of Alzheimer's disease on caregivers in the United States. *Health Psychology Research*, 10 (3). https://doi.org/10.52965/001c.37454

Index

Printed in the United States
by Baker & Taylor Publisher Services